Archives of Family Practice

*Selected Papers and Abstracts Representing
Original Work Advancing the Specialty of
Family Practice*

Volume III
1982

Edited by

John P. Geyman, M.D.

Professor and Chairman
Department of Family Medicine
School of Medicine
University of Washington
Seattle, Washington

 APPLETON-CENTURY-CROFTS / *Norwalk, Connecticut*

Prentice-Hall International, Inc., London
Prentice-Hall of Australia, Pty. Ltd., Sydney
Prentice-Hall of India Private Limited, New Delhi
Prentice-Hall of Japan, Inc., Tokyo
Prentice-Hall of Southeast Asia (Pte.) Ltd., Singapore
Whitehall Books Ltd., Wellington, New Zealand

ISBN 0-8385-0326-8
ISSN 0270-9074
LC 80-648565

PRINTED IN THE UNITED STATES OF AMERICA

This series is dedicated to family physicians around the world and to the continued refinement of their specialized roles in providing continuing personal and comprehensive health care to their patients and families.

Contents

SECTION TWO: QUALITY OF CARE ASSESSMENT IN FAMILY PRACTICE

Abstracts

Preface

The process of specialization in family practice is by no means limited to national boundaries. Whether known as *family practice* or *general practice*, the field is actively involved in the development of educational programs at undergraduate, graduate, and postgraduate levels, improvement of clinical standards, and strengthening of the research base in general/ family practice in many countries. Tremendous progress has been made in these areas in the last 10 years in the United States, Canada, United Kingdom, Israel, Australia, and New Zealand. More recently, progress is being made toward these goals in Western Europe, Scandinavia, South Africa, Japan, and elsewhere. Although the education and health care systems may vary considerably from one country to another, there is much that can be learned from the experience of other countries concerning the many common interests in this effort.

The literature of record presenting original work in general/family practice not only involves parallel efforts in different countries but is also published in a variety of journals and related publications, many of which are not customarily read by family physicians and others involved in the field. The need, therefore, exists to bring together in a collated form the important works advancing the field.

Archives of Family Practice is unique among existing books in the field as the first to focus *exclusively* on the clinical, educational, and research development of the specialty in its own right and in its own settings. This approach was not possible in the past due to the specialty's relative immaturity as a teachable clinical discipline with an active area of research. The overall goal of *Archives of Family Practice* is therefore to reflect the advancing state of the art in the clinical, educational, and research elements of this growing specialty.

As a series of annual volumes, *Archives of Family Practice* includes a collection of papers in both full and abstract form in three general content areas related to (1) the specialty and its clinical applications, (2) education for family practice, and (3) research in family practice. Papers and abstracts are drawn from the literature of record in numerous journals, reports, and related documents and are selected for their value in best reflecting the advancing field within each content area. Where appropriate, authors have been asked to add current comments to update their papers to the year of publication.

This volume, the third in the series, will focus on: (1) *Clinical Research in Family Practice,* (2) *Quality of Care Assessment,* and (3) *Continuing Educa-*

tion in Family Practice. In contrast to the first two volumes, this book is much more heavily weighted toward *clinical* advances within the field. This emphasis will be continued in future volumes, so that this series can be expected to be increasingly useful for clinical reference purposes as research activity matures and expands within the field.

This series is directed primarily to medical students, family practice residents, family physicians, and educators involved in family practice teaching programs. *Archives of Family Practice* will also be of interest to others in medicine desiring to better appreciate, in a single volume, the emerging roles of family practice in medical practice and in medical education.

John P. Geyman, M.D.
Seattle, Washington

Acknowledgments

The papers and abstracts appearing in *Archives of Family Practice 1982* have been selected from the following journals:

American Journal of Medicine
Annals of Internal Medicine
Archives of Internal Medicine
Australian Family Physician
Canadian Family Physician
Continuing Education for the Family Physician
Diabetes Care
Journal of American Medical Association
Journal of Chronic Disease
Journal of Family Practice
Journal of Medical Education
Journal of Royal College of General Practitioners
Lancet
New England Journal of Medicine
Postgraduate Medicine
Stroke

I am grateful to my son Sabin for his excellent editorial assistance in preparing the abstracts and other materials for this volume, and to Rowena de Saram for her help in assembling the final manuscript. I am further indebted to Richard Lampert, and Anne Friedman of Appleton-Century-Crofts for their diligent efforts in publishing this volume. Special thanks are extended to Mr. David Stires, president of Appleton-Century-Crofts, for his continued encouragement and early recognition of the vital role of the generalist physician in the health care of families.

John P. Geyman, M.D.

Clinical Research in Family Practice

COMMENTARY

THE papers and abstracts in this section have been greatly expanded to reflect the increasing vigor and quality of clinical research taking place in the field. The focus of this research ranges widely across the spectrum of illness in primary care, including the natural history of disease, diagnosis, management, prevention, and the interactions of psychosocial and environmental factors and illness. These studies and reports are based in the family physician's environment, and their results have direct clinical application.

Some of the papers reflect a community-wide role of the family physician beyond the scope of his direct care of families. A striking example is the excellent work carried out over many years by Jack Medalie in Israel involving the ongoing study of angina pectoris, myocardial infarction, diabetes mellitus, and their related psychosocial factors in 10,000 adult men.

The papers by Curtis Hames, a family physician in active practice and research for many years in a rural county of Georgia, provide an impressive illustration of the contributions that are possible through the systematic follow-up and study of an unselected patient population in a family practice setting. One paper describes the development of a long-standing collaboration with the School of Public Health at the University of North Carolina that made possible major population-based studies of cardiovascular and cerebrovascular disease in a rural county.

The Oral Contraception Study of the Royal College of General Practitioners is a continuing, long-term prospective study involving about 46,000 women of childbearing age in the United Kingdom. Started in 1968, this study involves about 1400 general practitioners and is an excellent example of a productive collaborative research effort by a specialty organization in this field. The study has provided solid documentation of markedly increased death rates in women who have used oral contraceptives compared to controls who have never used them. These important findings have deservedly received the widespread attention and concern of physicians around the world.

The papers and abstracts included in this section represent work carried out in the United States, Canada, the United Kingdom, Israel, and Australia. The commonalities of content, methods, problems, and application of research in family practice are far greater than the differences from one county to another. Much can be learned by sharing this experience among countries.

PAPERS

Now and Then*

David Morrell

In the first James Mackenzie lecture, William Pickles started with a quotation from Jane Austen:

> You must employ the material which lies closest to your hand; you must contrive your story out of the simplest everyday matters as a small bird builds its nest from the mosses and twigs of the tree it lives in.

How well Will's life lived up to the sentiments in this quotation! Reading the biography of Will Pickles of Wensleydale by John Pemberton (1970), one sees how in his clinical work he used every clue which came to hand in framing his diagnosis. During his 40 years in Aysgarth he came to know the individuals who made up his community, their personalities, their strengths, and their weaknesses. He studied the interactions in his community, their comings and goings. On the basis of this knowledge, he was able to respond to their requests for care and began to ask questions about the cause and spread of diseases. On the basis of the investigations he undertook in response to these questions, he became recognized throughout the world as an outstanding epidemiologist.

*Reprinted by permission from *Journal of the Royal College of General Practitioners*, 29:457–465, 1979.
The William Pickles Lecture was delivered at the Annual Spring Meeting of the Royal College of General Practitioners in Cardiff on Sunday, 22 April 1979.

Influences on Pickles

It is interesting to reflect on how Will Pickles first became stimulated to undertake his epidemiological work and how he acquired the skills necessary to carry out his studies, which he described simply as observing nature.

James Mackenzie

It is apparent from his biography that his interest in epidemiology did not start until he reached the age of about 40. It appears to date from the time when he first read William Budd's (1873) book on typhoid and James Mackenzie's (1916) book on the principles and diagnosis of heart affections. In this book, Mackenzie had written:

> The life of a general practitioner is not considered one that can help much in the advance of medicine. It is indeed regarded so lightly that no steps are ever taken to train one who intends to become a general practitioner in any branch that would enable him to undertake research work. As a result of my experiences, I take a very different view and assert with confidence that medicine will make but halting progress while whole fields essential to the progress of medicine will remain unexplored until the general practitioner takes his place as an investigator.

It seemed clear that this book fired Will Pickles' enthusiasm. He was not slow to see

3

the opportunities which were presented in his work. From his early years, he had apparently shown great enjoyment in observing the behaviour of birds and mammals. He now turned this training in careful observation to the human species.

Other Colleagues

Although we know that Will spent four weeks every year in attending refresher courses in London, there is no evidence that he spent any of this time in studying epidemiology or statistics. He did, however, have a number of informal contacts among epidemiologists. One of the earliest was Alison Glover, who introduced Will to a system of recording developed by the Medical Research Council for measuring the incidence of illness in boarding schools. Later he became acquainted with Dr Sylvest, who first described a new illness which presented on the Danish island of Bornholm and which Will also observed in Wensleydale. He was also a great friend of Major Greenwood at the London School of Hygiene and Tropical Medicine, where he became acquainted with Bradford Hill, and John Pemberton was, as we know, a great admirer of Pickles and no doubt very often an adviser.

It seems to me that his epidemiological skills were acquired by a close personal relationship with epidemiologists. The data which he subjected to analysis were acquired by his unique position as a general practitioner; his enthusiasm was derived from the work of such men as James Mackenzie, William Budd, and John Snow.

Lessons to be Learnt

We surely have some important lessons to learn from this. We, as general practitioners, are uniquely placed to collect information which will advance knowledge of medicine. To analyse and interpret these data we need to work closely with epidemiologists and statisticians. To bring the whole project to fruition, we need the sort of enthusiasm which can be seen in Budd, Mackenzie, and Pickles.

Will Pickles was a founder member of our College and expected great things from it. He would, I am sure, be gratified to see the development of academic general practice and vocational training, but I wonder if he would have been a little disappointed that with all the advantages of special training and organization, so many of the aspects described by Mackenzie as ripe for exploration by general practitioners have been left untouched; or to see that there is very little in the vocational training of general practitioners which prepares them to undertake research work. He might, indeed, look askance at the academic departments of general practice which often have sophisticated teaching programmes but have often initiated very little research; or at our College, which has inspired some large scale multicentre studies but largely failed to stimulate the man on the ground to produce more William Budds, Will Pickles, or James Mackenzies.

Population Base

I would like to reflect on this problem to see if it is possible to identify its aetiology, because if we fail to find the cause we will be unlikely to find the solution. Why has the epidemiology in general practice today failed to live up to the immense promise of yesterday? I will start where all epidemiological studies start and look for a moment at the population base.

When the National Health Service was introduced, many saw the registered population of the general practitioner as the ideal population base on which to carry out epidemiological investigations. In 1967, my colleagues and I demonstrated, however, that only 80 per cent of the patients for whom we held records in an Inner London practice were, in fact, resident within the practice area (Morrell et al., 1970). This figure has since been confirmed in many other studies, and population mobility, particularly in urban centres, presents a serious problem to a research worker.

This is a far cry from the situation which pertained at Bedale where Pickles held an assistantship before the first world war. He describes the incident as follows: "A gypsy woman driving a caravan into the village in the summer twilight, a sick husband in the caravan, a faulty pump at which she proceeded to wash her dirty linen, and my first and only serious epidemic of typhoid left me with a lasting impression of the unique opportunities of a country doctor for the investigation of infectious disease." If a gypsy woman drove her caravan into my practice in Lambeth I might indeed notice it, but our population does not move like this. Patients slip in and out of the practice. They make quite an impact when they are there, but disappear, not into the summer twilight, but into the night and we are unaware of their arrival or departure.

Mobility of Population

The fact that we do not have a stable denominator for our population studies in general practice today is in marked contrast to the experiences of Will Pickles and Will Budd. Both, of course, wrote of epidemiology in country practice, but there can be few country practices today which are as self-contained and so stable.

This mobility in the population which characterizes life today presents other problems, as we encountered in another study undertaken by my Department (Banks et al., 1975). This was concerned with following up a cohort of patients during a period of a year. The migration rate of this particular group aged 20 to 44 years exceeded 20 per cent in a year. This presents difficult problems for the general practitioner hoping to undertake studies in the natural history of diseases for which, theoretically, he is ideally placed. If he samples from his age/sex register, only 80 per cent of his sample will still be in his prac-

tice, and of those he identifies he is likely to lose by migration a further 10 to 20 per cent within one year. He finishes his study, if he is lucky, with 60 per cent of his original sample, from which it is difficult to draw any valid conclusions.

This is a problem Will Pickles did not encounter. It demands of those of us undertaking this type of research in general practice new methods of sampling with stringent methods for identifying the active members of the sample and vigorous follow-up. This inevitably adds to the cost of such projects, but with care it can be done.

In a recently reported study of three-year-old children in the London Borough of Lambeth followed up to the age of nine years, Pollak (1979) managed to trace 85 per cent of the original sample, but in so doing had to travel the length and breadth of the UK and employ detective skills of which the Missing Persons Bureau of Scotland Yard would be proud.

The instability of the population to which I have drawn attention is but one expression of the instability of the environment in which our patients live. The breakdown of family networks, the dispersal of the extended family, and mobility in housing and occupation are other factors. They all present problems for the epidemiologist. The classical description by Will Pickles of the incubation period of infectious hepatitis is in marked contrast,

> Having tracked down the source of infection to a village fête, he was left with one victim whose source of infection he could not elucidate. As he describes the situation: The infection in all these was easy to explain but in the fourth (M) it was not so clear. At last I tackled his sister, who gave him away quite shamelessly. Studies in epidemiology sometimes reveal romances. "Oh yes," she said, "He's very fond of E. He often goes in during the evenings and helps her to wash up."

Very few of us today have a captive population with this marvellous opportunity to watch the details of human relationships taking place before our eyes—although we sometimes call ourselves family doctors. Zander and colleagues (1978) in my Unit have shown how relatively ignorant we often are of our patients' family and social histories compared with their past medical histories. With the increased pace of life and the rapidity of change in social circumstances, we cannot hope to store this information in our memories. If we are to function effectively as family doctors and as family and community epidemiologists, we need new methods of recording information, and this most particularly includes new and better medical records.

Modern Research

Another feature of modern research in general practice which can be counterproductive to *good* research is the need for studies involving large populations and many observers. Dr Pickles and Dr Dunbar had a virtual monopoly of Wensleydale. We read that they met each day to plan their work, much of which took place in their patients' homes. I do not wish to labour this last point which caused the Editor of our College *Journal* so much unjustified criticism following his excellent James Mackenzie lecture last year (Pereira Gray, 1978), but it may have some relevance to the quality of research in general practice in terms of the information available.

What I do wish to stress is that the greater the number of doctors involved in a research project, the greater the difficulty of standardizing the information collected. To undertake high quality research in general practice, it is necessary to define clearly the information which is to be collected and to ensure that all those taking part abide by the definition and record information on all relevant occasions. We have shown repeatedly in my Department that the quality of information collected reflects the involvement of the doctors with the particular study. The doctor who writes the protocol and initiates the study will collect high quality data; the work of his partners reflects how far they have become involved in planning the study and are committed to its objectives.

Monitoring the Collection of Data

Will Pickles realized at an early stage that this difficulty which doctors experience in collecting high quality information in the hurly-burly of general practice can be overcome only by having constant supervision by a firm but persuasive monitor. For years his wife, Gertie, filled the role of monitor ensuring complete information collection and issuing repeated reminders. Later, his accountant's daughter, Madge Blade, took on this responsibility. John Pemberton comments in his biography, "Madge, like the computer, could store information, but she could return it flavoured with dry Yorkshire wit". In my Department, we have a Madge whose name happens to be Mary. Within 24 hours of each consultation, she checks the patient's medical record and woe betide the doctor who has not recorded his research information correctly! So much effort has gone into planning and conducting studies in general practice but without that crucial element of checking the accuracy and completeness of the information collected. Without this, Will Pickles was quick to realize that the information he collected would be incomplete and, without this, it is doubtful if he could ever have produced the quality of work and verified his deductions in the way we now applaud.

I have mentioned several factors which influence the sort of research which is possible in general practice today compared with the days of William Pickles. Perhaps the most telling factor, however, is the type of epidemiological enquiry which is relevant to the general practitioner of today. Will Pickles, like William Budd and John Snow, lived and worked in the days of infectious disease epidemiology. Certain events occurred which had certain characteristics in common. A search was then launched for their relationships to each other in place and time. If the research was well planned and conducted, this relationship was established and a common infective agent was suspected, be this the cholera vibrio, the typhoid bacillus or the coxsackie virus. The infecting agent itself was often not identified until years later, but the unitary causal hypothesis was clearly proven.

To a large extent, with advances in microbiology and virology, this field has now been gleaned and we are left with a large number of medical problems unlikely to be solved by identifying the single cause. Ischaemic heart disease is an example. We know its causation is multifactorial, but to establish this requires studies on a national and international scale far outside the scope of the ordinary general practitioner. Sorting out depression has occupied one outstanding investigator for more than a decade (Brown and Harris, 1978).

Does this then mean that the role of the general practitioner in advancing knowledge of disease is at an end? I believe that this is far from true, but I believe equally that it demands a re-orientation of our research effort and, in some cases, the development of far more rigorous and sophisticated techniques. Let me take you back to the original quotation of Jane Austen: "You must employ the material which lies closest to your hand".

Limitations of Morbidity Recording

Some 10 years ago, I first became interested in studying the patterns of illness in general practice. For several years, I persuaded my partners to record information about every consultation in our practice and during the same period we altered our methods of delivering primary medical care. We introduced an appointments system, we moved into new premises, and we started work in a primary care team with nurses and health visitors (Morrell and Kasap, 1972). It was in the course of these studies that I became aware of the limitations of recording morbidity in general practice. Morbidity studies in some way constrain the doctor to make a diagnosis. In the case of established chronic disease, this presents no problem.

In many of the illnesses seen in general practice, however, a mere labelling of a collection of symptoms with a diagnostic tag does not advance the solution of the problem and as a source of epidemiological information may be very misleading. A possible example of this is the apparent rise in the incidence of depression revealed in the Second National Morbidity Survey (RCGP et al., 1974) compared with the First (College of General Practitioners, 1968). It is highly questionable whether the incidence of depression has increased or whether this diagnostic tag is more often applied to mixed symptom complexes now that antidepressant drugs are available.

As a result of this disquiet, I started to look not at the diagnosis but at presenting symptoms. I related the presenting symptoms to the diagnosis recorded and compared the results with French's Index of Differential Diagnosis (Hart, 1973). As a result, I suggested (Morrell, 1971) that maybe the time had come to replace textbooks of differential diagnosis based on hospital experience with books based on data collected from general practice. Some five years later, I was happy to become associated with such a textbook of general practice based on presenting symptoms (Cormack et al., 1976).

Studies of Natural History

It was this work which brought home to me how little we really know about the natural history of the common symptoms presenting in general practice. This seems to me to offer enormous opportunities for studies. If general practice is an academic discipline, then it is concerned with advancing knowledge of those aspects of medicine which are peculiar to the work of the general practitioner. The interpretation of the presenting symptoms of illness at primary care level is surely one of these. At an interview in 1964 at the age of 79, Will Pickles talking of the opportunities for study in general practice commented: "We see disease in its early stages—very rarely a chance for the specialist—and we can follow it through from the beginning to the end of the illness." That there have been so few studies at this apparently simple level of research probably reflects that it is far less simple than it at first appears. In recording, it requires meticulous attention to definitions applied in the hurly-burly of the consulting room. How, for instance, do you define the presenting symptom and how do you rate and record secondary or tertiary symptoms? And how do you weight different symptoms and take into consideration their duration in reaching a diagnosis?

Studying the natural history of the symptoms demands rigorous follow-up procedures. Analysing the data requires methods which will deal not only with single symptoms but with symptom clusters. It is a challenging field of study for both the general practitioner and the statistician, and one which is very necessary if we are to take the next step and look at the effect of treatment on the symptoms we encounter in general practice.

Modern Problems

In treatment, we again differ from the general practice in the days of William Pickles. We are indeed more fortunate and have a variety of drugs available which he would have welcomed. I wonder, however, if he would have used them so recklessly and built up the sort of unrealistic expectations about our therapeutic potential which is a cause of so much over-prescribing by doctors and so much disappointment for patients. As a profession, we have in some ways been hypnotized by the technological and therapeutic revolutions of the last two decades. We have read of clinical trials carried out in hospital and seen them as applicable to general practice. The first piece of research I ever conducted in general practice was a randomized controlled trial of a monoamine oxidase inhibitor called 'Drazine' (McWhinney and Morrell, 1965). On the basis of hospital trials this drug was recommended particularly for depressed middle-aged ladies. I collaborated with Ian McWhinney, who at that time was still in Stratford, and we carefully defined the depressed women in the practice who could be entered in the trial. They then received either 'Drazine' or a placebo, the treatment being allocated at random by our receptionists. Within one month 70 per cent of the depressed women were better but so also were 70 per cent of the control group. This illustrated the very high placebo response in trials of drugs in mental illness. More importantly, however, it illustrated the danger of applying results of management in hospital patients to general practice, where illness is seen at a very different stage in its natural history.

Evaluation of Antibiotics

There are of course many illnesses that are seen almost entirely in general practice. It is perhaps surprising that only in recent years has the role of antibiotics in the management of acute respiratory illness been subjected to rigorous evaluation. The work of Howie (1976) in Aberdeen and Stott (Stott and West, 1976) in Cardiff are examples of high quality research in this field, and they have shown that these drugs have a limited role in managing these common conditions. I would, however, stress that such apparently simple studies must be meticulously planned and conducted. It is because in general practice we are called upon to manage ill defined collections of symptoms rather than clear-cut disease entities that it is so difficult to evaluate our management. I deprecate some drug trials in which general practitioners are persuaded to enter patients for the trial by a *per capita* payment for the number of patients entered, with little concern for defining precisely the type of patient entered or for checking the accuracy of the data recorded. It is difficult to see how this method of recruitment can fail to bias the results and to bring research in general practice into disrepute.

Common Clinical Problems

I have drawn attention to the natural history of the common presenting symptoms in general practice and their management. There is, however, another vast area open to the general practitioner who is prepared to undertake epidemiological studies. He may not be able to identify the cause of peptic ulcer or hypertension, but he can study the natural history of these and other related chronic diseases. Fry (1966) has set an example by keeping careful records over two decades. Nobody has challenged his findings that peptic ulcer and hypertension are relatively benign conditions in the majority of sufferers identified in general practice. Nobody has applied the same meticulous care to record keeping. He may be right but I am sure he will be the first to encourage others to repeat his work so that our decision making may be based on experience gained from a larger sample than he can study in his practice in Beckenham.

Epilepsy is a diagnosis which has important medical and social implications for the sufferer and has attracted some attention in the medical journals in the last year or so. It has been stated that the medical care for epilepsy is far from optimal. In order to examine this contention, we have reviewed in our practice all those patients labelled on our morbidity register as suffering from epilepsy. Of 54 such patients, nearly one third no longer have fits or drug therapy and yet the original diagnosis was made in almost all cases in hospital. We did not realize before that the prognosis of epilepsy is so good. Four of the patients in our practice are presenting serious problems in the control of their fits. They are the four patients whose care is currently shared between the hospital and the practice. I am not suggesting that it is the sharing of care which presents the problem; what I am indicating is that the 'difficult' patients are referred to hospital and that facts based on hospital populations of patients must not be extrapolated to the population at large.

Population Screening

Population screening for presymptomatic disease is another subject which has generated more heat than light. In America, the annual physical check-up occupies a large proportion of the general practitioner's time and it is interesting to note that in the New Charter proposed for general practice in this country it is recommended that it should attract an item-of-service payment (GMSC, 1979). And yet a randomized controlled trial in two general practices in South London carried out by my Department has not revealed any benefits in terms of mortality, morbidity, hospital use, or time off work over a follow-up period of five years (South East London Screening Study Group, 1977). Theoretically, population screening offers enormous benefits. In practice, as Sackett and Holland (1975) and Tudor Hart (1976) have suggested on the basis of well designed experiments, case finding in the course of the normal consultation may be far more cost effective.

Contributions by General Practitioners

I have given just three examples of ways in which general practitioners can contribute to the body of knowledge about general practice by research: the study of the natural history of symptoms, controlled trials of treatment, and studies of the natural history of chronic disease. There are many other topics of interest. There is the whole, wide, almost untouched subject of human behaviour in response to illness and the modification of behaviour by health education. For those more interested in the organization of the delivery of medical care, there are numerous experiments waiting to be carried out to measure the effect of changes in the method of delivering care on the outcome of care. All these fields of research can be exploited only by general practitioners and it is this fact that justifies the claim that general practice is an academic discipline. It contains within it a unique body of knowledge which must be developed and expounded by those who practise in this discipline.

I come back then to my original question: Why have so many of the topics described by Mackenzie as ripe for exploration by general practitioners been left almost untouched? I have tried to demonstrate the opportunities and at the same time to illustrate some of the difficulties. I would like to end by looking for a moment at the selection and training for general practice which I believe to be one of the most important reasons for the lack of progress in this area.

Today, probably more doctors enter general practice as a first career choice than at any time since the advent of the National Health Service. They choose this career for a variety of reasons. Some are disillusioned with technological medicine; others see the satisfactions of providing primary and continuing care for a community; others feel it has financial or social attractions or value the freedom it offers compared with a career in hospital medicine. Few enter general practice, however, because it offers an opportunity to carry out original research. This, I might say, was far distant from my mind when I settled in rural Hertfordshire 22 years ago. As I became involved in teaching, however, I felt the need for research because I became aware of the vast areas of ignorance concerning the subject which I was supposed to be teaching.

If we look at our vocational training schemes for general practice, few of these will evoke in the hearts of those taking part a burning desire to break new ground and add to the corporate body of knowledge required by general practitioners. In many

ways, they resemble reorientation courses. They are concerned with adapting the knowledge acquired in hospital to the primary care setting. The time of one year in general practice in a three-year course is little enough to achieve this adjustment and is totally inadequate to develop a research project.

If we look at continuing education, we find that with few exceptions this tends to be delivered by specialists and the general theme is keeping up to date with hospital medicine. Only rarely do we see a course designed to teach general practitioners research methods. What we desperately need are courses which question current therapy and provoke general practitioners to ask questions and develop research.

Academic Departments of General Practice

If we look at our academic departments, we find that most are financially underendowed and overstretched in satisfying demands for undergraduate education and patient care. Very few have continuing research grants. The senior members of these departments are, like me, converts from service practice and not trained in academic disciplines and the juniors are so poorly paid compared with their contemporaries in service practice that they can rarely sustain such a post for more than a few years.

In the College we tend to talk about the undergraduate departments of general practice as though teaching undergraduates was their entire responsibility. This is nonsense. In 1913, the Royal Commission on University Education in London (the Haldane Report) argued that academic units were essential for the systematic advancement of knowledge and practice and to provide for the whole profession an education designed to develop habits of critical thinking.

The functions of an academic unit were defined as: involvement in patient care at the highest possible standard; furtherance of the subject by research; and teaching with the twin purposes of encouraging a spirit of enquiry amongst undergraduates and of providing for the training and postgraduate development of future academic practitioners of the subject.

If exposing undergraduates to general practice is the sole occupation of academic departments of general practice, then they have no right to exist. Their role is to advance knowledge of general practice and to feed this into both undergraduate and postgraduate education in the discipline—and, dare I say it, to set standards in patient care. This is the role of academic departments in all other subjects and the College must encourage this role in the departments of general practice.

If we look at the departments of community medicine, we see in many cases very little collaboration between them and the emerging department of general practice. I think I have said enough to show that the type of research required in general practice is highly sophisticated. It presents problems of sampling, data collection in an uncontrolled and pressurized situation, and complex methods of data analysis. In this, the departments of community medicine have a great deal to offer us.

Preparation for Research

Those who enter general practice because they see this as an emotionally fulfilling career, and that applies to most of us, are ill equipped to undertake this work. There are a few who are so dedicated that they can acquire the requisite skills often at the expense of their wives, families, and even patients. For the majority, this is not possible.

If we are to see high quality research carried out in general practice, it will be necessary to develop research fellowships which will pay general practitioners to take time off from their practices to learn the skills which are necessary to undertake this type of work. In addition, courses must be developed to provide for their needs. There

was in existence an excellent course in epidemiology and statistics at the London School of Hygiene and Tropical Medicine but this demanded half daily attendance for six months and has now been discontinued. Very few general practitioners could attend such a course. What is required is more courses organized on perhaps a half-day per week basis, possibly spread over two years to respond to the needs of general practitioners interested in research. Such courses could incorporate project work for the doctor to undertake in his own practice, carefully designed and supervised by the course organizer. This seems to me the way to encourage high quality research in general practice.

I am very often asked to act as a referee for articles for medical journals describing research in general practice, or to referee applications to Trusts or the Department of Health and Social Security for research proposals. So often, the completed work or the proposal is so amateur that it cannot be supported. This saddens me because a great deal of work has often been carried out but it has been inadequately planned. This could be overcome if the type of training course which I have suggested could be developed. In addition, I think it is extremely important that those who undertake research in general practice should be in close contact with epidemiologists and statisticians. In theory, the reorganization of the National Health Service should have brought general practitioners into close relationships at district level with community physicians, who have such skills and resources available to them. Unfortunately, in practice, few community physicians have been able to take advantage of these opportunities which the administrative changes have theoretically placed at their disposal.

In this situation, I believe academic departments of general practice have a special part to play. They should be an integral part of the research effort of the school or university in which they are established and the district in which they work. They must accept some responsibility for giving an example in the quality of general practice care in that district and be provided with the resources from National Health Service funds to improve the quality of primary care services in their district, through relevant courses and relevant research.

Will Pickles

Will Pickles might be disappointed as he looks down on us from his eternal home, but I am sure he will understand if we look a little jealously on the opportunities for infectious disease epidemiology which were presented to him and feel that it is not really quite so easy today. At the same time, I am sure he will condemn us if we become so obsessed with the problems that confront us that we are afraid to take the first step into those unexplored fields which surround us. In concluding his Cutter Lecture at Harvard (1948), he said, referring to general practice:

> It may, of course, be a mere repetition of irksome tasks but this is probably the fault of the practitioner who, like Bunyon's man with the muck rake, rakes to himself the straws and sticks and dust of the floor and can look no way but downward regardless of the crown which is being held above his head.

I am happy to conclude my lecture with the same words.

REFERENCES

Banks, M. H., Beresford, S. A. A., Morrell, D. C., Waller, J. J. & Watkins, C. J. (1975). Factors influencing demand for primary medical care in women. International Journal of Epidemiology, 4, 189–195

Brown, G. W. & Harris, T. (1978). Social Origins of Depression. A Study of Psychiatric Disorder in Women. London: Tavistock Publications

Budd, W. (1873). Typhoid Fever, its Nature, Mode of Spreading and Prevention. London: Longmans Green and Co.

College of General Practitioners and General Register

Office (1958). Morbidity Statistics from General Practice. First National Study, 1955/56. London: HMSO

Cormack, J., Marinker, M. & Morrell, D. C. (Eds) (1976). Practice: A Handbook of Primary Medical Care. London: Kluwer-Harrap Handbooks

Fry, J. (1966). Profiles of Disease. Edinburgh: E & S Livingstone

Gray, D. J. Pereira (1978). Feeling at home. James Mackenzie Lecture 1977. Journal of the Royal College of General Practitioners, 28, 6–17

General Medical Services Committee (1979). Report of New Charter Working Group. London: British Medical Association

Hart, F. Dudley (Ed.) (1973). French's Index of Differential Diagnosis. 10th edition. Bristol: John Wight

Hart, J. Tudor (1976). General practice workload, needs and resources in the National Health Service. Journal of the Royal College of General Practitioners, 26, 885–892

Howie, J. G. R. (1976). Clinical judgement and antibiotic use in general practice. British Medical Journal, 2, 1061–1064

Mackenzie, J. (1916). Principles of Diagnosis and Treatment of Heart Affections. London: Frowde & Hodder & Stoughton

McWhinney, I. R. & Morrell, D. C. (1965). Treatment of mild endogenous depression with a monoamine oxidase inhibitor. Journal of the College of General Practitioners, 9, 95–99

Morrell, D. C., Gage, H. G. & Robinson, N. R. (1970). Patterns of demand in general practice. Journal of the Royal College of General Practitioners, 19, 331–342

Morrell, D. C. & Kasap, H. S. (1972). Effect of an appointment system on demand for medical care. International Journal of Epidemiology, 1, 143–151

Morrell, D. C. (1971). Expressions of morbidity in general practice. British Medical Journal, 2, 454–458

Pemberton, J. (1970). Will Pickles of Wensleydale. London: Geoffrey Bles

Pickles, W. N. (1948). Epidemiology in a country practice. Cutter Lecture. New England Journal of Medicine, 239, 419–427

Pickles, W. N. (1955). Epidemiology in the Yorkshire Dales. Practitioner, 174, 76–87

Pollak, M. (1979). In press

Royal College of General Practitioners, Office of Population Censuses and Surveys, and Department of Health and Social Security (1974). Morbidity Statistics for General Practice. Second National Study 1970/71. London: HMSO

Royal Commission on University Education in London

(1913). Haldane Report. Cmnd No. 6717. London: HMSO

Sackett, D. L. & Holland, W. W. (1975). Controversy in the detection of disease. Lancet, 2, 357–359

South East London Screening Study Group (1977). A controlled trial of multiphasic screening in middle age. International Journal of Epidemiology, 6, 357–363

Stott, N. C. H. & West, R. R. (1976). Randomised controlled trial of antibiotics in patients with cough and purulent sputum. British Medical Journal, 2, 556–559

Zander, L. I., Beresford, S. A. A. & Thomas, P. (1978). Medical Records in General Practice. Occasional Paper 5. London: Journal of the Royal College of General Practitioners

Second National Morbidity Survey*

Birmingham Research Unit of the Royal College of General Practitioners

The Second National Morbidity Survey began in November 1970. It was a joint enterprise involving the Royal College of General Practitioners (RCGP), Office of Population Censuses and Surveys (OPCS) and the Department of Health and Social Security (DHSS). For the first year it involved 115 general practitioners in 60 practices looking after about 292,000 patients. From November 1971 until October 1972 it involved 101 general practitioners looking after a population of about 256,000 patients. From November 1972 to October 1976, 33 of these doctors looking after a population of about 100,000 continued to record morbidity routinely. The first volume of morbidity statistics covered the first 12 months from November 1970 to October 1971 (RCGP *et al.*, 1974). In the second volume just published, covering the second 12 months' recording, the comparison of the results from the first and second years serves as a validation exercise; certain aspects of the data are considered in more detail, in particular the variability in rates between different practices.

The survey is about problems reported to general practitioners at face-to-face consultations and does not include indirect consultations over the telephone, consultations with relatives or friends, or with other staff. Patients consult general practitioners with problems and these problems do not always involve morbidity in the conventional sense. Consultations for prophylactic procedures and other medical examinations are considered separately, but consultations for other socio-economic problems unaccompanied by organic or psycho-emotional morbidity are not. The data

from this morbidity survey can therefore be used only indirectly as a measure of total workload in general practice. Work-load information can be better derived from supplementary studies, for example using practice activity analysis methods. With these provisos, morbidity surveys are the essential baseline for epidemiological research and academic teaching in general practice.

Method

The Second National Morbidity Survey was based on the standard College of General Practitioners (1963) disease index mainly because a group of geographically representative general practitioners was already maintaining this record system as a basis for the routine reporting of infectious and communicable diseases to the Birmingham Research Unit's weekly return service. The standard disease index had been designed for automated processing but it can also be the basis for a simplified form of morbidity tabulations in years between national surveys. The recording practices also used the standard age/sex register cards as the basis for the automated age/sex register which forms in its turn the basis for the six-monthly updated computer file of patient morbidity maintained by the OPCS. The OPCS was responsible for the data processing and production of final tabulations.

Age/Sex Baseline

The list of a doctor's patients maintained by the family practitioner committee (formerly executive council) may in time come to include the names of some patients who

*Reprinted by permission from *Journal of the Royal College of General Practitioners*, 30, 547–550, 1980.

are no longer going to consult him when they are ill (*selective list inflation*), the usual procedures to remove a patient's name having failed for one reason or another. Similarly, the number of patients on a doctor's list may be inaccurately low because at any one time it is not possible to estimate exactly the number of patients who have not yet registered but who will do so as soon as they fall ill; this, and other mistakes of underrecording are called *understatement*.

Both of these problems had to be taken into account in producing firm age/sex baselines for each practice population. The methods and the validation procedures used were described in the first volume and are further elaborated in the second volume. The implications are that in checking the original registers, the executive councils were more adept at rectifying excesses than omissions.

Results

Tabulations

The preliminary tabulations deal with the age/sex structure of the population and its comparability with that of the general population of England and Wales. Other tables deal with the frequency with which different patients consult in a year and in particular the numbers of those who do not attend at all.

The main tables deal with various rates for episodes, consultations, and patients consulting per 1,000 population at risk, by age and sex for each diagnosed condition and for reasons other than illness. Incidence rates are calculated separately. Other tables give similar rates by urban and rural distribution and by three main regional areas, North, South, and Midlands and South Wales. Inter-practice variability is so great that no further regional disaggregation is possible. Other tables deal with referrals to hospital for direct access investigations and to inpatient and outpatient departments, and referrals to local authority

services. Home visits for selected diagnoses are also given as a percentage of all consultations. These main tabulations are comparable with those of the first year's recording. In 28 out of the 43 practices, full International Classification of Diseases (WHO, 1957) recording of episodes was carried out in parallel with recording based on the College of General Practitioners (1963) classification of approximately 500 categories.

A comparison of rates in 1970/71 based on patients consulting with rates in 1971/72 based on episode data only was possible in four practices where total consultation recording was dropped in the latter period in favour of simple episode recording. This confirms that the absence of consultation recording has an adverse effect on the completeness of episode data.

Comparisons Between 1970/71 and 1971/72

There were slight changes in episode and consultation rates between the two years. There were small reductions in home visiting rates, a continuation of the trend noted when the first and second National Morbidity Surveys were compared (RCGP, 1976). This trend has also been found in the General Household Survey between 1971 and 1974 (OPCS, 1979). The consultation rates per person at risk per year are lower in the National Morbidity Survey (3.0) than in the General Household Survey (3.5).

The rates for referrals per 1,000 population at risk showed consistent small increases for all categories for both sexes at all ages, excluding only acute male in-patient admissions. The uniformity and consistency of results from the first compared with the second year of recording was also reflected in the rates for individual practices. This uniformity within the practices from one year to another is in marked contrast to the consistent and enormous range of variability between practices in all rates. Inter-practice variations are so large that a simple two-way analysis of variance indi-

cates that compared with the variation between practices within regions, the variation between regions is not sufficiently
large to be detected. It is for this reason that
regional disaggregation is limited to the
North, South, and Midlands and Wales.
The data cannot therefore be used as a basis
for estimating regional allocation of resources (DHSS, 1976).

Inter-Practice Variability

Consistent variations in clinical and administrative performance between practices
and between individual general practitioners as measured by referral rates to hospital
(RCGP, 1978a) use of diagnostic services
(RCGP, 1978b) and even episode and consultation rates (RCGP, 1973) have been
highlighted by the comparison of results
from the first two years of recording in the
Second National Morbidity Survey. In
Tables 1 and 2, consultations and referrals
in the Second National Morbidity Survey are
compared with data from other sources in
the form of rates, rank ordered from lowest
to highest and showing the intermediate
rates between each 20 percentile subgroup. For example, in Table 1 the first line
summarizes the consultation rates for the
general practitioners in the Second National Morbidity Survey during the year
1970–71. The first rate, 53 consultations

per week, is the lowest rate of all. The second rate, 118 consultations per week, is the
12th lowest rate, that is the rate for the general practitioner with the highest rate in the
first group of 12 practitioners, one fifth of
the total. Table 2 deals with referral rates
from the different practices in the same way.
Consultations rather than patients at risk
are used for the denominator in this table
because the practice activity analysis data,
with which the National Morbidity Survey
data are compared, are in this form. This is
a convenient way of showing a range of
rates particularly when they are not normally distributed.

The large range of referral rates to hospital (Table 2)—in this context a four-fold
difference between the lowest and the
highest rate—has particularly significance.
Ultimately the use of hospital services is
very largely determined by the primary referrals of general practitioners. These large
differences between the extremes for any
one rate cannot be attributed to differences
in the age and sex structure of the population. For example, age standardization of
the patient consulting rates for each sex results in a reduction of 10 per cent only in the
ratio of the 5th to the 95th percentile. Standardization for social class and occupational status will also be possible eventually
but it is likely that this will make only further marginal contributions to the variance.
These results are consistent with the

Table 1. *Average Number of Consultations per Doctor per Week. Comparison of 20 Percentile Rates for Second National Morbidity Study 1970/71 and 1971/72, and Royal College of General Practitioners Practice Activity Analysis Survey*

	Minimum Rate		Intervening Rates			Maximum Rate
National Morbidity Study 2 1970/71	53	118	144	159	199	339
	(12)	(12)	(12)	(12)	(12)	
National Morbidity Study 2 1971/72	89	121	148	181	219	337
	(9)	(9)	(9)	(9)	(9)	
Royal College of General Practitioners Practice Activity Survey	48	125	148	171	203	325
	(28)	(28)	(28)	(28)	(28)	

Figures in brackets are the number of doctors/practices in each 20 percentile group.

Table 2. *Referral Rates per 1,000 Consultations. Comparison of 20 Percentile Rates for Second National Morbidity Study 1970/71 and 1971/72, Royal College of General Practitioners Practice Activity Analysis Survey and Belgian Survey*

	Minimum Rate	Intervening Rates				Maximum Rate
NMS 2 1970/71	18.1	25.3	30.7	36.4	44.8	75.7
		(12)	(12)	(12)	(12)	(12)
NMS 2 1971/72	18.5	25.3	31.6	34.2	43.2	63.7
		(8)	(8)	(7)	(8)	(8)
Royal College of General Practitioners	16.8	30.9	38.0	46.0	57.0	98.1
Practice Activity Analysis Survey		(20)	(20)	(20)	(20)	(20)
Belgian Survey	13.0	25.0	29.5	38.0	52.0	127.0
(Fleming and Maes, 1980)		(8)	(7)	(7)	(7)	(8)

Figures in brackets are the number of doctors/practices in each 20 percentile group.

hypothesis that most of the inter-doctor variability is due to fundamental differences in the attitudes and values of individual doctors rather than differences in the characteristics of their patients and/or their clinical environment (Fleming and Maes, 1980). Studies of work-load must therefore be based on the experience of sufficient numbers of general practitioners to take account of this range of variability. This proviso can be mitigated somewhat by a complementary reduction in the quantity of patient-related data. These principles are in operation in the practice activity analysis programme of the Birmingham Research Unit (RCGP, 1977a).

The Denominator Problem

Registration of the population with general practitioners in the British National Health Service ensures a known population at risk (the denominator) for epidemiological research, as well as for information and planning purposes. In most other Western countries, registration does not occur and all primary health care statistics must be expressed in rates related to the patients who actually consult. Reliable methods for estimating the numbers of non-attenders and total populations at risk are therefore much

needed. It is ironic that the data from the National Morbidity Surveys in this country are one of the few sources of good data for statistical modelling of this problem.

Although the variations in the proportion of nonattenders in the different practice populations in the Second National Morbidity Survey are the smallest among all those variations studied, they paradoxically relate to fundamental, underlying problems. Patients and their doctors vary in what they understand by morbidity and illness and influence one another in these beliefs. Practices vary in the way that access to the practitioner is controlled; a particularly strong influence is the presence or absence of a repeat prescription system. It is also possible that 'non-attenders' in primary care are compensated for by those who use casualty departments and by direct internal referrals by one consultant to another hospital colleague (RCGP, 1977b). Although morbidity surveys alone cannot provide answers to these problems, they have brought them into the light of day.

Practice Profile

Each practice completed a profile of such characteristics as: the type of building(s) used; numbers of principals, assistants and trainees; appointment systems; shared use of rotas and deputizing services; access to hospital beds; special clinics in the practice; special diagnostic equipment in the practice; access to radiography and clinical biochemistry and pathology; and numbers of staff employed. The relationship of these characteristics to the various measured rates is explored. From an initial analysis of a great deal of data, the practice characteristics which seem to be most relevant to reported morbidity rates were location, size of partnership, doctor's age and availability of ancillary staff. However, the contribution to overall variations in morbidity rates was small. The details of all these measured variations have been sent to each practice as the basis for a programme of self-evaluation and audit.

Supplementary Studies

Continuous disease/index recording is the basis for this Second National Morbidity Survey and in turn it can support a variety of retrospective studies. These are all similar to the original retrospective Oral Contraception Study (RCGP, 1967) in which a significant correlation between thromboembolic morbidity and the use of oral contraceptives was first demonstrated. These supplementary retrospective studies include viral infections in pregnancy (Adelstein *et al.*, 1976); malignant hypertension (Bulpitt *et al.*, 1980); side-effects of pertussis vaccine; incidence of hypertension; gout (Currie, 1978a and b, 1979), long-term effects of whooping cough; diabetes and its associated morbidity; subsequent mortality rates in patients with psycho-neurotic diagnoses; pilot studies of glaucoma and beta-blockers and reserpine and breast cancer; long-term effects of hypoglycaemic agents; and long-term effects of beta-blockers. Some of these additional studies involve the use of standardized morbidity (episode) ratios, a technique developed for this purpose.

Six-Year Linked File

The data from approximately 85,000 patients followed for the full six years will be linked in one patient-based file. This will be the basis, using standardized morbidity (episode) ratios, for examining the positive and the negative relationships between different morbidities.

Socio-Economic Data

A file linking the morbidity experience of patients in the first year of the survey with a range of socio-economic variables will be available for comparison with similar data in the First National Morbidity Survey and in the General Household Survey.

Weekly Return System

Many of the practices involved in the Second National Morbidity Survey are also reporting to the Birmingham Research Unit a selection of communicable infectious and other diseases on a weekly basis.

Third National Morbidity Survey

It is hoped that a Third National Morbidity Survey will take place in 1981/82. In the meantime, the disease/index recording in the weekly return practices has been continuing since the end of the Second National Morbidity Survey recording in 1976. Non-automated processing of these indexes will produce simple basic tabulations to provide continuity between the years of national studies with their greater detail and range.

Conclusion

These reports in the series, *Morbidity Statistics from General Practice*, as the essential baseline for epidemiological research and teaching in general practice, should be available in the libraries of postgraduate centres to all general practitioners involved in academic study.

Acknowledgments

We are grateful to those general practitioners who participated in the National Morbidity Study, to the Office of Population Censuses and Surveys, and to the Department of Health and Social Security for providing the funding to enable the study to be undertaken.

REFERENCES

Adelstein, A. M., Donovan, J. W., Leighton, P. C. & Pike, M. C. (1976). Sequelae of virus infection in pregnancy. In Child Health-A Collection of Studies. Studies on Medical and Population Subjects No. 31. London: HMSO

Bulpitt, C. J., Bulpitt, P. F., Clark, P. B., Clifton, P., Lambert, P. & Dollerty, C. T. (1980). Malignant hypertension—a study of outcome and treatment in the National Morbidity Study. In preparation

College of General Practitioners Research Committee of Council (1963). A classification of disease. Amended version. Journal of the College of General Practitioners, 6, 207-216

Currie, W. J. C. (1978a). Diagnosis of gout in general practice. Current Medical Research and Opinion, 5, 714-719

Currie, W. J. C. (1978b). The gout patient in general practice. Rheumatology and Rehabilitation, 17, 205-218

Currie, W. J. C. (1979). Prevalence and incidence of the diagnosis of gout in Great Britain. Annals of the Rheumatic Diseases, 38, 101-106

Department of Health and Social Security (1976). Sharing Resources for Health in England. Report of the Resource Allocation Working Party (RAWP) London: HMSO

Fleming, D. M. & Maes, R. M. J. (1980). Facets of practice in the United Kingdom and Belgium. In press

Office of Population Census and Surveys (1979). General Household Survey 1977. London: HMSO

Royal College of General Practitioners Records Unit and Research Advisory Service (1967). Oral contraception and thromboembolic disease. Journal of the Royal College of General Practitioners, 13, 267-279

Royal College of General Practitioners, Office of Population Censuses and Surveys & Department of Health and Social Security (1974). Morbidity Statistics from General Practice. Second National Study 1970-1971. Studies on Medical and Population Subjects No. 26. London: HMSO

Royal College of General Practitioners (1973). Present State and Future Needs of General Practice. 3rd edn. Report from General Practice 16. London: Journal of the Royal College of General Practitioners

Royal College of General Practitioners Birmingham Research Unit (1976). Trends in National Morbidity. Occasional Paper 3. London: Journal of the Royal College of General Practitioners

Royal College of General Practitioners Birmingham Research Unit (1977a). Self-evaluation in general practice. Journal of the Royal College of General Practitioners, 27, 265-270

Royal College of General Practitioners Birmingham Research Unit (1977b). Total care usage of a defined population. Journal of the Royal College of General Practitioners, 27, 306-314

Royal College of General Practitioners Birmingham Research Unit (1978a). Practice activity analysis No. 5. Referrals to specialists. Journal of the Royal College of General Practitioners, 28, 251-253

Royal College of General Practitioners Birmingham Research Unit (1978b). Practice activity analysis No. 3. Investigations. Journal of the Royal College of General Practitioners, 28, 60-62

World Health Organization (1957). International Classification of Disease. Geneva: WHO

The "Iceberg" of Illness and "Trivial" Consultations*

D. R. Hannay

The medical symptom 'iceberg' and 'trivia' were defined in terms of people's own perceptions of their symptoms and their subsequent referral behaviour. The data were collected by household interviews of patients registered at a health centre and included information on personal and environmental characteristics. Bivariate and multivariate analysis was used to explore associations between those who were part of the symptom 'iceberg' or 'trivia', and factors which might have caused such incongruous referral behaviour.

Introduction

Research has been carried out in Glasgow into the prevalence of symptoms and referral behaviour in the community. In this context the term 'referral behaviour' is used to describe the behaviour of patients; it is this referral behaviour which is poorly understood and has led to conflicting points of view.

For instance, morbidity surveys carried out in the community indicate that much ill health does not reach medical attention, and the term 'illness iceberg' has been used to describe this phenomenon (Last, 1963). The size of the iceberg depends on whether presymptomatic conditions are included, but several studies suggest that only about one third of those with symptoms refer themselves for medical advice, irrespective of the primary care system (Pearse and Crocker, 1943; Butler, 1970; Wadsworth *et al.*, 1971). These findings do not fit with studies of general practice in the United Kingdom (Cartwright, 1967; Mechanic,

*Reprinted by permission from *Journal of the Royal College of General Practitioners*, 30, 551–554, 1980.

1968), which show that many doctors complain about being bothered about what they perceive as unnecessary 'trivia'.

The conflict of expectations between family doctors and patients was studied and an attempt made to define the concepts of the iceberg and trivia more precisely. This was done by interviewing in their own homes a random sample of patients registered with a health centre. The questionnaire included a checklist of symptoms, and each positive symptom was graded by the patient for pain, disability, and perceived seriousness. In addition, the patient was asked what action he or she had taken for each symptom and the replies were graded into a ranking scale of one for no referral, two for an informal or lay referral, and three for a formal or professional referral. A lay referral was an informal referral to a relative, friend, or acquaintance which did not primarily involve a professional role.

In this way patients' own perceptions of their symptoms were used as a basis for deciding whether their referral behaviour was explicable in terms of these perceptions or not, without imposing external value judgements about appropriateness. A symptom was defined as part of the medical iceberg if the referral was none or lay, when either the pain or disability was severe, or the symptom was considered to be serious. Conversely, those symptoms which were referred for professional advice, when there was no pain or disability and the symptom was not thought to be serious, were defined as part of the medical trivia. The number of medical symptoms which were part of the iceberg and trivia for each patient was calculated as an incongruous referral score—one score for the iceberg and another for the trivia (Hannay, 1979).

In this context, the medical iceberg refers

only to subjective symptoms and not to pre-symptomatic conditions which could be detected only by objective screening tests. It was found that 26 per cent of those with medical symptoms were part of the medical symptom iceberg and 11 per cent were part of the trivia (Hannay and Maddox, 1975). In view of the extent of these incongruous referrals, computer programmes were used to explore associations between factors which might be predictors of the tendency for people to be part of the symptom iceberg or trivia. This paper presents the results of this further analysis.

Method

Random monthly samples without replacement were drawn from the computer file of a health centre during the course of a year. The age/sex distribution of the sample was similar to the population in general, except that young adults tended to be under-represented because of high mobility in an area of urban redevelopment (Hannay and Maddox, 1977). A total of 1,344 interviews were completed, representing 3.1 per cent of the mean list size for the health centre for that year. Only three per cent of the sample refused to be interviewed. Most of these were elderly people and the main reason given was ill health. For children of 15 years and under the questions were answered by a parent or guardian.

Each patient was asked about a checklist of medical symptoms, which included 44 physical symptoms (Hannay, 1978), with eight mental symptoms for adults derived from a psychiatric screening test (Foulds and Hope, 1968), and four behavioural problems for children based on presenting problems at a child psychiatry clinic (Stone, F. H., 1971; personal communication). The questions were phrased in simple language and referred to the previous two weeks only. The patients were asked what they did about their symptoms, which were also graded subjectively as indicated above.

In addition to symptoms and referral be-haviour, the survey included information on personal characteristics and environmental factors such as housing, mobility, and employment. Personality was assessed using the shorter Maudesley Personality Inventory (Eysenck, 1958), and intelligence measured with questions from the shorter 16PF personality test (Cattell et al., 1970). Computer programmes for bivariate and multivariate analysis (Nie et al., 1970) were used to explore associations between variables which might be causal to referral behaviour, and the tendency for people to be part of the medical symptom iceberg or trivia, as reflected in their incongruous referral scores.

Results

Three hundred and six (23 per cent) of those interviewed had at least one medical symptom which was part of the symptom iceberg, and 126 (nine per cent) patients contributed to the symptom trivia. The maximum number of symptoms with an incongruous referral for any one patient was 15 for the iceberg, and five for the trivia. Of those interviewed, 1,183 (88 per cent) had one or more medical symptoms with an average of five per person. When expressed as a percentage of all those with positive symptoms, the size of the iceberg and trivia becomes 26 per cent and 11 per cent respectively (Hannay and Maddox, 1975).

The two incongruous referral scores were correlated with a wide range of independent variables, about half of which gave significant results. However, many of these associations may have been due to intervening factors not directly associated with referral behaviour.

Females were more likely than males to be part of the medical symptom iceberg, especially the middle aged (Figure 1). Those who were unemployed, who had no higher education or active religious allegiance, and those in social classes 3 and 4, were significantly more likely to be part of the medical symptom iceberg.

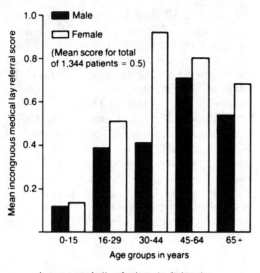

Incongruous medical lay referral score (medical symptom iceberg) the number of medical symptoms per patient for which the referral was none or lay, when either the pain or disability was severe, or the symptom was considered to be serious

Fig. 1. Age/sex distribution of the medical symptom iceberg.

Conversely, owner occupiers and those living in larger dwellings were significantly less likely to contribute to the medical symptom iceberg. People living in the worse rented accommodation and with frequent moves within the city were the most likely to be part of the iceberg, whereas those from overseas were the least likely. It is interesting that it was the more neurotic and less intelligent who did not trouble their doctor when perhaps they should have done, rather than the other way round. A long walk to the health centre, preference for the doctor's previous surgery, and lack of a telephone all seemed to discourage medical referral. The tendency to be part of the medical symptom iceberg increased with the prevalence of both medical and social symptoms, and also with the numbers of previous illnesses and medicines taken, both prescribed and unprescribed.

The tendency to refer trivia for medical advice increased with age and for women (Figure 2). It was also significantly higher for the retired, separated or divorced, unemployed, and those who had left school early. There was a social class gradient, with those in social class 5 being the most likely to refer trivia, but the differences were not significant. Medical symptom trivia were least likely amongst owner occupiers, and significantly more likely for those living in one room or in households of one or two people only. Those living on the top floors of high rise flats had three times the amount of trivial referrals as those on the lower four floors. The tendency to refer medical symptom trivia also increased with the prevalence of symptoms and poor self-estimates of past and present health. There was no clear relationship between trivial referrals and measures of personality, doctor preference, or access to the health centre.

Some of these significant correlations may have been due to interaction effects, and in order to allow for this, those variables which might be causal for the tendency to be part of the medical symptom iceberg or trivia were used in multivariate analysis. There were two of these regression equations, one for the iceberg scores and one for the trivia scores.

Twenty-eight variables were entered into a regression equation as possible predictors of the tendency to be part of the medical symptom iceberg. Of these variables, six had significant regression coefficients in the following order of importance.

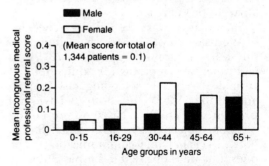

Incongruous medical professional referral score (medical symptom trivia) = the number of medical symptoms per patient for which the referral was professional, when the pain and disability were none, and the symptom was not thought to be serious.

Fig. 2. Age/sex distribution of the medical symptom trivia.

1. Neuroticism score
2. Number of previous illnesses
3. Self-estimate of previous health (poor)
4. Age
5. Number of moves
6. Sex (female)

Of these, only the variable for female sex was not significant on simple correlation.

Twenty-eight variables were also entered into a regression equation as possible predictors of the tendency to refer medical symptom trivia. Of these variables, nine had significant regression coefficients in the following order of importance:

1. Number of present illnesses
2. Separation or divorce
3. Age
4. Poor experience of doctors and hospitals
5. Few years in present residence
6. Difficulty in contacting doctor
7. Number of short hospital stays
8. Sex (female)
9. Number of long hospital stays

Three of these variables were not significant on simple correlation, namely—recent moves, difficulty in contacting a doctor, and few long hospital stays.

Discussion

There have been many surveys of morbidity in the community, some of them cross-cultural (White and Murnaghan, 1969), but none of which have really defined which symptoms or 'illnesses' were appropriate for medical referral, and certainly not by reference to the subjective perceptions of the patients themselves. In the same way, there have been studies of workload in primary medical care from a number of countries (McFarlane and O'Connell, 1969; Bernstein and Dolan, 1972; Ridley-Smith, 1973), but none of these seemed to take into account the quality of demand. One study of health referral patterns in America (Cauffman et al., 1974) reported that eight per cent of medical referrals were 'inappropriate', and a follow-up of patients in Germany (Wesiack, 1971) concluded that 11 per cent of the conditions seen were 'trifling', but the criteria used to reach these decisions did not seem to assess the perceptions of patients. A similar criticism could be made of a recent study in the United Kingdom of 'minor' illnesses in general practice (Marsh, 1977), in which a minor illness seemed to be defined by the doctor without apparent reference to the patients' views on the matter.

As referral behaviour is motivated by the person who has the symptoms, it seemed sensible to use the patients' own assessments of their symptoms to define whether the action taken was explicable in terms of their own perceptions. If the referral behaviour could not be explained in terms of these perceptions then it seemed reasonable to call such behaviour incongruous and so define those who were part of the medical symptoms iceberg and trivia.

The preponderance of women in the 30 to 44 year age group may have been due to mothers with growing families being less able to seek professional advice for their symptoms. Studies from America support the impression from the present survey that low socioeconomic status is associated with a tendency not to seek medical care (Ludwig and Gibson, 1969; Hyman, 1970). Those with a high mobility in the worst housing in Glasgow were most likely to be part of the medical symptom iceberg, and as these were also the characteristics of nonresponders, it is likely that the survey results underestimated the extent of the iceberg.

One study of general practice (Jacob, 1969) also reported a preponderance of the divorced and widowed amongst those making greater demands, as in the present survey, but other studies have found no personal or social differences between patients considered in need of treatment and those who were not (Thomas, 1974). The significant correlation between the medical symptom trivia and social symptoms underlines the fact that there are often latent reasons for apparently unnecessary referrals. A survey of general practice in Holland (Brouwer and Touw-Otten, 1974) concluded that the majority of adults had some other reason for seeking medical advice than the presenting complaint. Another study of people labelled as 'problem patients' by their doctor found that such patients considered themselves to be more ill, and had more interpersonal and social difficulties (Fabrega et al., 1969).

It was the more neurotic and those with poor estimates of past and present health who emerged on regression analysis as being most likely to be part of the medical symptom iceberg, which was also associated with increasing age, mobility, and females. Low intelligence scores and a long bus journey to the health centre were also more common amongst those in the medical symptom iceberg, but the regression coefficients for these factors were not significant.

It is not surprising that those who referred medical symptom trivia should have considered that they had a number of illnesses and that they tended to be older and female. The associations with separation and divorce or a recent move suggest that psychosocial problems may have been the reason for trivial referrals. The contrasting significance of short and long hospital stays on regression analysis is hard to interpret; but the variables for difficulty in contacting a doctor and poor experience of doctors and hospitals suggest a result rather than a cause of referral behaviour.

The results of this study perhaps produce more questions than answers, but the questions raised are based on a rational definition of the symptoms iceberg and trivia, which have tended previously to be vague value judgements. Inevitably, attempts at the quantitative analysis of large amounts of sociographic data will result in the over-simplification of complex situations. For instance, about seven per cent of those in the medical symptom iceberg also referred medical trivia, which indicates that even for

one person different types of referral behaviour may coexist, depending on the symptoms involved. However, the fact that there was no overlap between the iceberg and trivia for the great majority of patients suggests that there are distinctive patterns of referral behaviour. Many of the major correlates of this referral behaviour which emerged on multivariate analysis were not unexpected. However, what was surprising, apart from the size of the medical symptom iceberg compared with trivia, was the fact that it was the more neurotic who were most likely to be part of the iceberg, rather than the trivia as many might have expected.

Acknowledgments

This study was made possible by a grant from the Social Science Research Council. I would like to thank the general practitioners at the Woodside Health Centre for permission to interview their patients, Mr E. J. Maddox, Mrs MacLaren, Mrs Scobbie, and Mrs Wyllie for their help as interviewers, and Mrs Robertson for secretarial assistance.

REFERENCES

Bernstein, J. M. & Dolan, L. J. (1972). Annual reports from general practice, 1970: Manchester. Update 4, 993–1004

Brouwer, W. & Touw-Otten, F. (1974). Analysis of the pre-medical period. Huisarts en Wetenschap, 17, 3–15

Butler, J. R. (1970). Illness and the sick role; an evaluation of three communities. British Journal of Sociology, 21, 241–261

Cartwright, A. (1967). Patients and their Doctors: A study of General Practice. London: Routledge and Kegan Paul

Cattell, R. B., Eber, H. W. & Tatsuoka, M. M. (1970). Handbook for the 16 Personality Factor (Form C-1963). USA: Institute for Personality and Ability Testing

Cauffman, J. G., Lloyd, J. S., Lyons, M. I. et al. (1974).

A study of health referral patterns. American Journal of Public Health, 64, 331–356

Eysenck, H. J. (1958). A short questionnaire for the measurement of two dimensions of personality. Journal of Applied Psychology, 42, 14–17

Fabrega, H., Moore, R. J. & Strawn, J. R. (1969). Low income medical problem patients: some medical and behavioral features. Journal of Health and Social Behaviour, 10, 334–343

Foulds, G. A. & Hope, K. (1968). Manual of the Symptom Sign Inventory. London: University of London Press Ltd.

Hannay, D. R. (1978). Symptom prevalence in the community. Journal of the Royal College of General Practitioners, 28, 492–499

Hannay, D. R. (1979). The Symptom Iceberg: A Study of Community Health. London: Routledge & Kegan Paul

Hannay, D. R. & Maddox, E. J. (1975). Incongruous referrals. Lancet, 2, 1195–1197

Hannay, D. R. & Maddox, E. J. (1977). Missing patients on a health centre file. Community Health, 8, 210–216

Hyman, M. D. (1970). Some links between economic status and untreated illness. Social Science and Medicine, 4, 387–399

Jacob, A. (1969). The social background of the 'artificial practice'. Journal of the Royal College of General Practitioners, 17, 12–16

Last, J. M. (1963). The iceberg: completing the clinical picture in general practice. Lancet, 2, 28–31

Ludwig, E. G. & Gibson, G. (1969). Self perceptior of sickness and the seeking of medical care. Journal of Health and Social Behaviour, 10, 125–133

McFarlane, A. H. & O'Connell, B. P. (1969). Morbidity in family practice. Canadian Medical Association Journal, 101, 259–263

Marsh, G. N. (1977). 'Curing' minor illness in general practice. British Medical Journal, 2, 1267–1269

Mechanic, D. (1968). Medical Sociology. New York: Free Press

Nie, N. H., Bent, D. H. & Hull, C. H. (1970). Statistical Package for the Social Sciences. New York: McGraw-Hill

Pearse, I. H. & Crocker, L. H. (1943). The Peckham Experiment. London: Allen and Unwin

Ridley-Smith, R. M. (1973). Why the patients came. New Zealand Medical Journal, 76, 240–246

Thomas, K. B. (1974). Temporarily dependent patients in general practice. British Medical Journal, 1, 625–626

Wadsworth, M. E. J., Butterfield, W. J. H. & Blaney, R. (1971). Health and Sickness; The Choice of Treatment. London: Tavistock Publications

Wesiack, W. (1971). Problems and methods of follow-up examinations in practice. Munchener Medizinische Wochenschrift, 113, 1023–1028

White, K. L. & Murnaghan, J. H. (1969). International Comparisons of Medical Care Utilizations. Washington: US Department of Health, Education and Welfare

Screening for Hypertension: Case Finding*

K. V. Rudnick

A 13-year-review of a Hamilton, Ontario, family practice resulted in the detection of 607 hypertensive patients through case finding. By using a series of simple strategies, the measurement and recording of patients' blood pressures increased from 41% in 1965 to 98% in 1977. Team members now consistently measure and record the blood pressures at virtually all encounters of patients at risk and are convinced that case finding is the only method of detection of hypertension which is at all logical economical and practical.

In Screening for any condition, certain criteria must be satisfied before initiating mass screening programs. These criteria have been well described previously.[1-4]. They can be summarized into four points as developed by the World Health Organization (after Sackett[5]).

1. The therapy for the condition must favorably alter its natural history, not simply by advancing the point in time at which diagnosis occurs, but by improving survival, function or both.
2. Available health services must be sufficient both to ensure diagnostic confirmation among those whose screening is positive and to provide longterm care.
3. Compliance among asymptomatic patients in whom an early diagnosis has been achieved must be sufficient to alter the natural history of the disease in question.
4. The burden of disability for the condition in question—disease frequency, distribution, severity, alternate approaches to its detection and control—must warrant action.

Hypertension is the only disease complex for which screening is of value according to these criteria. However, recent accumulation of evidence indicates that several problems must be solved before mass hypertension screening programs can be instituted. At least 50% of those screened have already had their blood pressures checked; also, patient and physician compliance among hypertensives is low.[6-10]

One other point made by Wilson and Jungner[3] is that case finding, if a continuous process, is the detection method of choice. Nowhere is case finding as appropriate as in a family physician's office because the patients are unrestricted by age, sex, anatomy, occupation, education or complaint. Providing easy accessibility, availability and continuity with some enthusiasm and concern, the family physician can detect through case finding during office visits for other problems a reservoir of symptomless hypertensive patients. Diligent and sustained effort to measure and record the blood pressure at each clinical encounter must be maintained to achieve a high detection rate, for if the attention wanes, the detection rate falls.[11]

Wilson and Jungner[3] further recommended that case finding be economical. Case finding does not increase the cost appreciably if the patient is visiting the family physician for another reason. If case finding *does* include prescriptive screening, then the cost can be appreciable. Nevertheless, the cost of case finding in the family

*Reprinted by permission from *Canadian Family Physician*, 25: 1170-1172, Oct. 1979.

physician's office would still be considerably lower than other methods of detection, evaluation and treatment.

Objectives

The primary objective of a screening program is to identify those citizens who would benefit from diagnosis and consequent therapy for a disorder. Some screening programs have actually created more harm than good because no therapy is available for the condition identified, e.g. sickle cell trait.

Sackett and Holland reason that the series on "Screening for Disease"[13] in *Lancet* incited a heated exchange of letters to the editor due to disagreement over the proper function for screening. They further point out that the continuing confusion between screening, case finding and epidemiological surveys is largely a matter of terms and definitions. To ease the confusion, the objectives of this paper should be clearly specified:

1. To illustrate that case finding is the method of choice in the detection of hypertension.
2. To demonstrate that the family physician is best suited to attempt case finding.
3. To describe simple strategies for detecting hypertension that are valid in any family physician's office.

Definitions

The application of discriminating or sorting procedures to populations, whole or selected, has a long and rather unsatisfactory history, and chaos has arisen over the interpretation of terms.

Whitby[2] defines "screening" as "the presumptive identification of unrecognized disease or defect by the application of tests, examinations, or other procedures which can be applied rapidly." He further adds that screening can be conducted on the whole population or a major subgroup—e.g. all adults—when it is called "mass screening", or it can be carried out on selected subgroups of the population when it is called "selective screening."

Hart[14] describes "medical screening" as the discovery of a disorder by using certain tests, examinations or procedures. He stipulates that it is not diagnostic, it merely discriminates the afflicted, yet apparently well, from those who do not have the disorder.

Hart defines prescriptive screening as being undertaken to detect, evaluate and treat a specific disorder.

Adler[15] distinguishes between "screening" and "case finding" in that screening is instigated by the doctor who invites the patient to attend for a test, an examination or a procedure; case finding is concerned with identifying a disease or defect when the patient, as opposed to the doctor, initiates the consultation. "Case finding" is used in this sense in this paper. Fuller definition, purposes and properties of the terms used are available in Sackett and Holland's paper.

Methods

A few simple strategies were devised in an attempt to increase the detection of hypertensive patients. These include such simple methods as verbal agreements of team members to take blood pressures and record them in the chart. The next maneuver was to ask each team member to record blood pressure readings on every patient 16 years and over on a "blood pressure day sheet". This sheet containing the patient's name and blood pressure was posted daily in an obvious place near the door leading to the work room where the charting was done. The next strategy was to attach a sign on the blackboard immediately near the door, at eye level, so that this acted as a reminder as team members left the work room to see the patient in the examining room. A further method was a chart review at the end of the day. The introduction of a red label pasted on the right hand corner of the chart with spaces for dates and blood pressure readings was attempted to provide higher team member compliance. A green label pasted on the left upper corner of the chart with the letters "HT" was attempted to encourage blood pressure recording. Finally, a somewhat comical poster, pasted on walls and doors of examining rooms, was directed at the patient asking the question, "Have you had your blood pressure taken?" This was meant to remind the patient to ask the health care professional to check his/her blood pressure.

Results

Table 1 reveals that over the 13 year period 63.6% of the at risk population (16 and over) had their blood pressures taken and recorded and 607 new hypertensive patients were detected. The rate increased from 41% in 1965 to 69% in 1973, merely by continually reminding each other to measure and record blood pressures. In 1974, by posting a "blood pressure day sheet" the rate of measurement and recording rose to 87%. In 1975, the attention waned and the rate fell to 73%, but rose to 76% in 1976. With a renewed interest and a

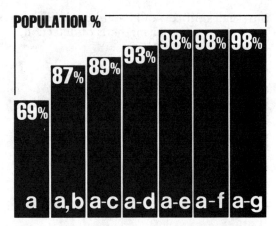

Fig. 1. Strategies and results of case-finding. Strategies employed: a = verbal contract; b = BP daysheet; c = blackboard notice; d = chart review; e = blood pressure label; f = hypertensive label; and g = notice to patients.

few simple strategies the rate increased as in Figure 1. This figures shows that the blackboard notice increased the rate of blood pressure measurement and recording by two percent. The chart review at the end of the day yielded a further increase to 93%. The red blood pressure label increased the measurement and recording a further five percent. The green hypertensive label and the poster in the waiting room failed to increase the rate of blood pressure measurement and documentation.

Table 1. *Detection of Hypertensive Patients by Case Finding*

	1965	1966	1967	1968	1969	1970	1971	1972	1973	1974	1975	1976	1977	Totals
Population at risk	3831	3970	4177	3990	3914	4073	3138	2093	2699	2322	1643	2086	1788	39,724
Patient visits	7035	7091	6952	6817	6744	6392	6505	3871	3988	3635	3276	3162	3055	68,523
Visits when BP recorded	2884	3474	4073	4172	4295	4237	4429	2330	2751	3162	2391	2406	2944	43,599
Percent of visits when BP recorded	41.0	48.9	58.6	61.2	63.7	66.3	68.1	60.2	69.0	87.0	72.9	76.1	98.0	63.6
Number of hypertensives newly detected	28	43	129	106	99	29	31	24	75	13	6	8	16	607

Conclusions

The renewed interest in screening depends upon three new factors. One is the new technology that permits rapid, inexpensive and accurate measurements of many variables in patients. The second is the experience of the new breed of epidemiologists who have become experts in using and evaluating the techniques in large population surveys. The third factor, though not strictly new, is the resurgence of the family doctor as the collector of data, which really puts the information into true perspective. This last component is crucial to the essence of medical screening.

A further important contribution to screening for hypertension, and particularly case finding, is an understanding of the criteria for evaluation of screening. Without these criteria, screening becomes an exercise in futility—a collection of data which, in fact, may do more harm than good. Case finding, which best fits the criteria of Wilson and Jungner[3] has already linked the patient to a source of care and virtually ensured evaluation, treatment and control of hypertension. As a result of recent evaluations in the control of hypertension, Canadian task forces have recommended detection of hypertension in primary care rather than the community based hypertension programs and supermarket screening.[19,20] As proposed previously, only in the family physician's office can this succeed.

A recent paper[11] has emphasized that for the control of hypertension six steps are necessary: detection of the hypertensive individual; linkage to a source of care; an appropriate diagnostic workup; initiation of proper therapy; compliance with treatment, and provision of lifelong follow up. Sackett[12] re-emphasizes the same points. Haynes et al[21] point out the dangers of labelling hypertensive patients; this only strengthens the concept of the six essential steps for the control of hypertension.

Programs for detecting hypertension have been stimulated by several developments. One was the identification of hypertension as a major risk factor in stroke, congestive heart failure and coronary heart disease; another was the demonstration in the trials by the Veterans Administration Cooperative Study Group that treatment of hypertension could lower morbidity and mortality. A public health program directed against hypertension which would include detection, evaluation and treatment would then be of high priority. But many[14-16] have asked the question, "Are they worth it?" According to Wilson and Jungner's criteria[3] such a public health program is doomed to failure, as is selective screening.

Again, hypertension is the only disease complex that fits the previously suggested guidelines for screening. Keeping in mind the problems encountered, case finding is the only method of detecting hypertension which is at all logical, economical and practical. It is linked with a source of care, a simple method of evaluation and work-up, a plan of proper treatment, an understanding of medication compliance, accessibility, continuity and compliance. Consequently, case finding is the method of choice for detecting hypertension.

REFERENCES

1. Sackett DL: Screening for early detection of disease: To what purpose? Bull NY Acad Med 51:39-52, 1975
2. Whitby LG: Screening for disease: Definitions and criteria. Lancet 2:819-821, 1974
3. Wilson JMG, Jungner G: Principles and Practice of Screening for Disease. Geneva, World Health Publication, Health Paper 34, 1968, p. 14
4. Cochrane AL, Holland WW: Validation of screening procedures. Br Med Bull 27:3-8, 1971
5. Sackett DL: Screening for disease: Cardiovascular disease. Lancet 2:22-24, 1974
6. Wilber JA, Barrow JD: Hypertension—A community problem. Am J Med 52:653-663, 1972
7. Schoenberger JA, Stamler J, Shekelle RB, et al:

Current status of hypertension control in our industrial population. JAMA 22:559–562, 1972

8. Gibson ES, Mishkel M, Gent M, et al: Epidemiology of Cardiovascular Disease. Paper read at American Heart Association Conference on Cardiovascular Epidemiology, Tampa, Florida, 1972

9. Silverberg DS: Long-term follow-up of a hypertension screening program. Can Med Assoc J 114:425–428, 1976

10. Sackett DL, Haynes RB: Compliance with Therapeutic Regimens. Baltimore, Johns Hopkins University Press, 1976

11. Rudnick KV, Sackett DL, Hirst S, et al: Hypertension: The family physician's role. Can Fam Physician 24:477–484, 1978

12. Sackett DL: The detection and treatment of hypertension in Canada: Changing recommendations from recent research. Clin Invest Med 1:171–174, 1978

13. Sackett DL, Holland WW: Controversy in the detection of disease. Lancet 2:357–362, 1975

14. Hart CR: Screening in General Practice. Edinburgh, Churchill Livingston Press, 1975

15. Adler, MW: Detection of blood pressure in general practice: Screening or case finding? J R Coll Gen Pract 26:171–176, 1976

16. Baitz T, Shimizu A: Blood pressure surveys: Are they worth it? Can Fam Physician 23:70–73, 1977

17. Genest J, Kuchel O, Leduc G, Granger P, et al: Screening programs for hypertension. Can Med Assoc J 111:147–149, 1974

18. Shapiro M, Bleho J, Curran M, et al: Problems in the control of hypertension in the community. Can Med Assoc J 118:37–40, 1978

19. Report of the Ontario Council of Health: Hypertension. Toronto, Ontario Council of Health, 1977

20. Report of the Hypertension Study Committee of the Canadian Heart Foundation and Canadian Cardiovascular Society, Ottawa, 1978

21. Haynes RB, Sackett DL, Taylor DW, et al: Increased absenteeism from work after detection and labelling of hypertensive patients. N Engl J Med 229:741–744, 1978.

The Once and Future Hypertensive*

M. F. D'Souza

It is unsatisfactory to describe uncomplicated hypertension as a disease. Evidence from the Framingham (Kannel *et al.*, 1969) and other longitudinal studies such as the Build and Blood Pressure Study (Society of Actuaries, 1959) has shown that all levels of blood pressure have a calculable risk for future strokes and heart attacks. There is no level at which things suddenly become risky. The higher the blood pressure, the greater the risk.

As a result it can be argued that we should look upon raised blood pressure simply as a risk factor, and treat it according to our clinical judgement in each individual, particularly where there are associated diseases. It seems best, however, in uncomplicated cases, to use data from group measurements in controlled trials to determine levels of blood pressure at which treatment on average produces benefit, and to treat people above these thresholds as hypertensive. There is no evidence as yet that antihypertensive treatment produces benefit in women or in those over 70 years of age. The Veterans Administration Study (1970) has, however, shown that there is a significant likelihood of benefit in treating middle-aged men with a diastolic blood pressure greater than 104 mm Hg (phase five).

In this paper, therefore, I am going to assume that a diastolic pressure ≥ 105 mm Hg represents the best available definition of 'hypertension' for both men and women, and examine how many remain 'diseased' using this criterion, if repeated measurements are taken over a five-year period.

*Reprinted by permission from *Hypertension in Primary Care*. An Occasional Paper published by *The Journal of the Royal College of General Practitioners*. July, 1980.

The Study

As part of a larger study to evaluate the effects of multiphasic screening for chronic disease in the middle-aged, blood pressure was measured in samples from two general practices in South-East England (Trevelyan, 1973). All patients aged 40 to 64 years in each practice were identified with their spouses, yielding a total of 7,229 people who were allocated randomly by family into two groups of similar size designated 'screening' and 'control' (Figure 1). Only the screening group will be examined in this paper.

Method

In each patient the blood pressure was taken twice under controlled conditions (using a random-zero sphygmomanometer on the left arm with the patient seated). All information was passed to the patient's general practitioner who was especially alerted if the diastolic pressure was 100 mm Hg or more (phase five). He then took the final decision about whether or not to treat.

Results

At the initial screening of 2,420 patients in 1967/68, there were 537 people who had at first reading a diastolic pressure of ≥ 90 mm Hg (phase five), of whom 99 had a diastolic pressure of ≥ 105 mm Hg (Table 1). Fifty of these 99 were known to have had raised pressure before screening of whom 21 were on antihypertensive therapy already. Seventeen were started on treatment after this screening. A further five were started on treatment after a repeat screening in 1969/70. Comparison with the con-

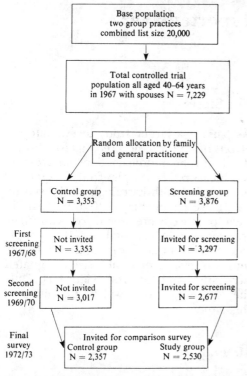

Fig. 1. Study population and design. N is the total number present at a particular point in time, the loss being due to deaths or departures from the area, or administrative difficulties.

trol group in 1973 revealed no significant differences in population blood pressures suggesting that screening had resulted in no benefit. Furthermore, it was found that individual men who had raised blood pressure and who, owing to decision or oversight, were not treated showed just as big a fall after five-year follow-up as those who were treated. These and other figures from this study suggested that the antihypertensive treatment had little effect (D'Souza *et al.*, 1976). It is for this reason that in the analysis given below the treated and untreated have been grouped together.

The Stability of Categories of Blood Pressure Over Time

Table 1 shows the stability of each of four groups of blood pressure categories when the same individuals are measured again immediately. As can be seen, at either end of the blood pressure distribution there is very little stability. Table 2 shows the same exercise when five years separates the two readings. Similar instability is observed for high and low blood pressure categories, though 36.4 per cent were lost to follow-up.

Table 1. *Group Concurrence of Two Immediately Consecutive Diastolic Readings 1967/68. (Percentages in Brackets.)*

Blood Pressure Group Initial Reading	Blood Pressure Group Second Reading				Missing Data
	'Low'	Normal	Raised	High	
'Low'					
<60 mm Hg	36 (50.7)	35 (49.3)	0	0	0
N = 71 (2.9)					
Normal					
60–89 mm Hg	35 (1.9)	1,656 (91.4)	119 (6.6)	1 (0.06)	1
N = 1,812 (74.9)					
Raised					
90–104 mm Hg	0	89 (20.3)	326 (74.4)	21 (4.8)	2 (0.5)
N = 438 (18.1)					
High					
≥105 mm Hg	0	2 (2.0)	30 (30.3)	67 (67.7)	0
N = 99 (4.1)					
Totals 2,420 (100)	71 (2.9)	1,782 (73.6)	475 (19.6)	89 (3.7)	3 (0.1)

Table 2. *Group Concurrence of Readings after Five Years' Follow-Up. (Percentages in Brackets.)*

Group of Initial Reading	Lost to Follow-Up	Available	Group of Five-Year Follow-Up Readings (Percentage of Those Available in Each Group in Brackets)			
			'Low'	Normal	Raised	High
'Low' <60 mm Hg N = 71	23 (32.4)	48	11 (22.9)	30 (62.5)	6 (12.5)	1 (2.0)
Normal 60–89 mm Hg N = 1812	647 (35.7)	1165	56 (4.8)	983 (84.4)	118 (10.1)	8 (0.7)
Raised 90–104 mm Hg N = 438	168 (38.4)	270	3 (0.6)	131 (48.5)	111 (41.1)	25 (9.3)
High ≥105 mm Hg N = 99	43 (43.4)	56	0 (0.0)	9 (16.1)	32 (57.1)	15 (26.8)
Totals N = 2,420	881 (36.4)	1539	70 (4.5)	1,153 (74.9)	267 (17.3)	49 (3.2)

Discussion

Each clinical recording of the blood pressure is not only a measure of the pressure at that moment, but can also be considered to be an 'estimate' of the patient's average daily blood pressure. However, if at the moment of measurement the pressure recorded is a poor estimate, that is, is far removed from that individual's mean pressure, subsequent readings will only rarely be similar to it. This phenomenon is known statistically as regression towards the mean. Thus, any classification of an individual into blood pressure categories (be they hypertensive or hypotensive) on the basis of just one reading is liable to considerable error.

From a clinical point of view, it is clear from this study that if one creates a category of either hypotension (low) or hypertension (high) based on only one reading, less than half those so categorized are really 'residents' in their categories over time (assuming that treatment had little effect and that those lost to follow-up were not important).

Closer examination of the data does reveal, however, that some measure of 'tracking' occurs over time: even though an individual does not remain in the same category he is much more likely to move up or down only one step. Thus, a single pressure recording may be used as a predictor of vague blood pressure grouping at either the high or low end of the spectrum but is very suspect for precise categorization. This makes for serious difficulties in clinical decision-making, if the start of treatment or more particularly adjustment of existing therapy were to be based on a single clinical reading.

Many papers have reported similar observations before. Armitage and Rose (1966) suggested that one third of patients are misclassified as hypertensives. John Fry (1975) provided documentary proof with a 15-year follow-up showing that 30 per cent of 'hypertensives' show a fall in pressure and that 58 per cent of them remain alive and well without treatment. Miall and Chinn (1974) have carried out a similar, though much more detailed, exercise to that shown in this paper, taking age and sex into account in trying to determine a screening policy. They showed that only one third of those with initial pressures ≥ 110 mm Hg (phase four) remained in this category over time.

The problem remains as to what to make

of such findings. On the one hand it is clear that some people who would benefit from clinical treatment of hypertension are not being detected or treated. On the other hand, there must be many people who are healthy yet who are being put on drugs and labelled as unhealthy.

Current recommendations to take three separate recordings of pressure on three different days during the first month of diagnosis will go some way to eliminating this problem, but evidence from this study suggests that changes occur over much longer periods of time. One is drawn to the conclusion that we must be wary of viewing the diagnosis of 'hypertension' as a life sentence. Instead, we should be ready to withdraw treatment from previously diagnosed 'hypertensives', albeit under close surveillance. On the other hand it might also be argued that where there is evidence of target organ damage such as retinopathy or renal disease, we should consider anti-hypertensive therapy regardless of the level of blood pressure.

Author's Update

The recent U.S. Hypertension Detection and Follow-up Program[1] and the Australian Therapeutic Trial in Mild Hypertension[2] both would lead one to take the level at which therapeutic intervention was now advisable as $\geqslant 100$ mm Hg phase 5 rather than the level $\geqslant 105$ suggested in this paper.

A well documented case of "a once and future hypertensive" was reported by the author at the Royal Society of Medicine (13th March, 1981). He is a 68 year old male patient with marked and sustained hypertension (many diastolic levels $\geqslant 130$ mm Hg measured over a period of four years) who was potentially cured by giving up alcohol abuse. His diastolic pressure

settled to $\leqslant 85$ mm Hg without treatment for a period of three years (BP measured monthly). Recently he has resumed drinking and his diastolic BP has risen to 90 mm Hg.

1. Hypertension Detection and Follow-up Program Cooperative Group (1979). Five year findings of the hypertension detection and follow-up program: 1. Reduction in mortality of persons with high blood pressure, including mild hypertension. JAMA, 242, 2562–77
2. The Australian Therapeutic Trial in mild hypertension. Report by the Management Committee (1980). Lancet, i, 1261–7

REFERENCES

Armitage, P. & Rose, G. A. (1966). The variability of measurements of casual blood pressure. A laboratory study. Clinical Science, 30, 325–335

D'Souza, M. F., Swan, A. V. & Shannon, D. J. (1976). Screening for hypertension in general practice: The results of a long-term controlled trial. Lancet, 1, 1228–1232

Fry, J. (1975). Long-surviving hypertensives—a 15-year follow-up. Journal of the Royal College of General Practitioners, 25, 481–486

Kannel, W. B., Castelli, W. P., McNamara, P. M. et al. (1969). Some factors affecting morbidity and mortality in hypertension. Milbank Memorial Fund Quarterly, 67, 116–142

Miall, W. E. & Chinn, S. (1974). Screening for hypertension: some epidemiological observations. British Medical Journal, 2, 278–294

Society of Actuaries (1959). Build and Blood Pressure Study. Chicago Society of Actuaries. Vol 1

Trevelyan, H. T. (1973). Study to evaluate the effects of multiphasic screening within general practice in Britain. Preventive Medicine, 2, 278–294

Veterans Administration Co-operative Study Group (1970). Effects of treatment on morbidity in hypertension. Results in patients with diastolic blood pressure averaging 90 through 114 mm Hg. Journal of the American Medical Association, 213, 1143–1152

Natural History of Hypertension: A Case for Selective Non-Treatment*

John Fry

Over a period of twenty years, 704 hypertensives have been diagnosed in a London suburban general practice. This is a rate of 162 per 1000 for adults aged thirty years and over. In males the rate was 138 per 1000 and in females it was 187 per 1000. In 28 percent the hypertension was mild, 58 percent moderate, and in 14 percent it was severe. During the period of observation specific hypotensive therapy was used rarely and therefore this survey may represent the natural history of high blood-pressure. The observed/expected (O/E) mortality-rate was 1.85 (3.01 in males and 1.62 in females), but most of this excessive mortality affected those hypertensives who were less than sixty years of age at first diagnosis. The O/E mortality-rates were inversely related to age. The initial height of the diastolic blood-pressure was a prognostic factor in the under-sixties, mortality increasing with the rising diastolic pressure. However, there were no increasing mortality-rates with rising pressure in the over-sixties. The conclusions are that specific hypotensive therapy is indicated for those hypertensives who are under sixty years, in males more than in females, and particularly in the younger hypertensives with high diastolic blood-pressure. There is no strong case for hypertensives first diagnosed over the age of sixty to be treated with specific hypotensives, and such therapy is less necessary in females than in males. Since half of all diagnosed hypertensives are over the age of sixty, a policy of selective non-treatment of high blood-pressure would result in considerable saving of medical manpower and financial resources.

*Reprinted by permission from *The Lancet*, 431–433, August 24, 1974.

Introduction

The nature and outcome of high blood-pressure are not clear. There may be distinct types of hypertension with a variety of causes and as many possible courses with different prognoses.

Current opinion[1] suggests that high blood-pressure leads to increased morbidity and mortality, and that control of even moderate or mild hypertension results in improvement compared with no treatment.[2,3] However, these opinions may be unrepresentative in that they have tended to be based on selected populations and exclusive age-groups. The populations generally have been those that have attended specialist hospital units, and most interest has been paid to the young and middle-aged male hypertensives. Groups in London and Cardiff[4] have carried out small short-term trials; Stuart et al.[5] have undertaken longer surveillance on a small rural population in Jamaica; and a World Health Organisation pilot programme is in progress in a number of centres observing a wide range of the general population.[6] Nevertheless, there are no major large studies completed yet that can help us decide whether all persons with raised blood-pressure should be treated intensively for the rest of their lives in order to reduce complications and to prolong life.

Ultimately a compromise is likely, because no system of health care can screen whole populations regularly and undertake long-term management of hypertensives with drugs for many years. We will need to agree on some clinical factors that will enable us to select those persons with raised blood-pressures who seem to be most vulnerable to complications and death.

This study is an attempt to define such

factors of vulnerability in a general-practice population observed over twenty years.

Material and Methods

Over many years long-term records have been kept of all patients in this practice, and a disease index and register have made it possible to pick out those patients diagnosed as having certain specific conditions. Being a National Health Service practice it has been possible to have a regular age and sex distribution of the population at risk.[7,8]

During the twenty-year period (1949 to 1969) separate records have been kept of all persons diagnosed as having high blood-pressure. These hypertensives have all been followed up for five years or more unless they died or moved out of the practice. It has not been possible to maintain contact with those patients who moved away. The follow-up records noted the patients' progress, any complications, and the causes of deaths.

The criterion for a diagnosis of hypertension was a diastolic blood-pressure of 100 mm. Hg or more recorded in a sitting position on at least three separate occasions.

During the period of the study (1949 to 1969) my policy in the management of hypertension was not to use specific hypotensive drugs, because of the absence of any definite proof of benefits from them for the mild and moderate uncomplicated type of cases that are seen in general practice. Unless there were definite indications or advice by a specialist, my patients with raised blood-pressure did not receive specific hypotensive therapy. For the purposes of this review all those who are or have been on long-term hypotensive therapy have been excluded, but there were only 35 of these patients. To avoid any bias, however, all deaths in those under review, including those who had received hypotensive drugs, have been included in the analysis.

To assess the outcome of these non-treated hypertensives, their observed mortality rates were compared with the expected mortality of the population, as shown in the life-tables for 1951, 1961, and 1971, prepared by the then General Register Office (now the Office of Population Censuses and Surveys). It was not possible over the long period of observation to obtain matched non-hypertensive controls from the practice, and I considered it reasonable to compare the outcome in terms of mortality with national rates. I appreciate, however, that contributing to the national rates of mortality there may have been some hypertensives both treated and untreated, especially in the older age-groups. Despite such possible errors it seems reasonable to present this series as representative of the natural history of high blood-pressure as seen in a London suburban practice.

Results

During the twenty years, 704 patients (256 males and 448 females) in the practice have been diagnosed as having hypertension. The population at risk at the midpoint of period of observation (1960) was 5500.

Table 1. *Age and Sex Specific Incidence of High Blood-Pressure Seen in a 20-Year Period*

| Sex | No. of New Cases of Hypertension in 20 Yr. per 1000 Population Aged: | | | | | |
	30–39	40–49	50–59	60–69	≥70	All Ages
Males	18	106	148	320	225	138
Females	35	107	254	382	221	187
All persons	28	107	200	360	222	162
No. of hypertensives	*28*	*113*	*190*	*233*	*140*	*704*

Table 1 shows the age and sex specific incidence of the hypertension during the 20-year period. Hypertension is a condition associated with ageing, but the incidence falls in the over-seventy age-group.

More than half of all the hypertensives diagnosed were over the age of sixty, but this is not the group on which most research and therapeutic trials have been conducted. Most published reports relate to young and middle-aged hypertensives, usually male. It may be incorrect to apply such selective findings to elderly hypertensives.

The point prevalence of known hypertension in adults (over thirty) in the practice has averaged 62 per 1000 (males 42 and females 76 per 1000) during the twenty-year period of study.

Degree of Hypertension

As measured by the level of diastolic blood pressure at diagnosis there was a preponderance of mild and moderate cases. In more than half (53 percent) the diastolic blood-pressure was less than 120 mm. Hg (Table 2). Hypertension in general practice is largely a problem of management of these mild and moderate cases.

There was no notable rise in diastolic blood-pressures with age. For successive decades from thirty to seventy or more the average levels at diagnosis were 111, 121, 112, 118, and 111 mm. Hg.

General Outcome

During the period of observation the general outcome in these hypertensives was shown in Table 3. Almost a half died, but

Table 2. *Diastolic Blood-Pressures at Diagnosis*

Diastolic Blood-Pressure (mm. Hg)				All Hyper-tensives
100–109	*110–119*	*120–129*	*130 and Over*	
196	247	160	101	704
(28%)	(35%)	(23%)	(14%)	

Table 3. *General Outcome in Hypertensives (%)*

	No Ill-Effects (Symp-tomless)	Compli-cations	Death	Moved	All
Male	22	10	54	14	100
Female	30	9	41	20	100
All persons	27	9	46	18	100
No.	*186*	*68*	*322*	*130*	*704*

since many of these were elderly it is important to relate observed deaths with those expected. The removal-rate of 18 percent is unfortunate but inevitable in a mobile suburban society. If those who moved are excluded, the general picture is that 33 percent of these hypertensives are symptom-free and unaffected, 11 percent have some complications related to their high blood-pressure, and 56 percent are dead.

The periods of follow-up and observation ranged up to twenty years but were not less than five years, except when death occurred earlier.

The chief causes of death were cardiac (50 percent of all deaths) and cerebrovascular (25 percent). Likewise most complications were also cardiac (45 percent of all complications) and cerebrovascular (40 percent).

Observed and Expected Deaths

From life-tables it was possible to compare the expected death-rates with those that were actually observed (320) in the 669 hypertensives (35 on hypotensive therapy were excluded).

The observed/expected death-rates (O/E) are shown in Table 4. These hypertensives had an increased O/E ratio of 1.85. The ratio was 3.01 for males and appreciably lower (1.62) for females. The O/E death-rates were higher in males in all but one of the age-groups.

The O/E death-rates were inversely related to age. The highest ratios were for those aged thirty to thirty-nine; the ratio

Table 4. *Observed Expected (O/E) Death-Rates in Hypertension at Different Ages (Corrected for Length of Follow-Up)*

	Age					
	30–39	*40–49*	*50–59*	*60–69*	*70+*	**Total**
Males	12.0	4.13	2.54	1.35	0.98	3.01
Females	6.21	5.10	1.91	1.12	0.80	1.62
All persons	7.51	4.91	2.22	1.15	0.87	1.85

was little greater than 1 for the decade sixty to sixty-nine, and was actually less than 1 in the over-seventies.

The practical applications of these findings are that the risks to life of high blood-pressure vary with the age at which hypertension was first observed. Over the age of sixty there seem to be no extra risks, whereas in young hypertensives the risks to life are appreciable.

The Effects of Blood-pressure Levels on Outcome

In the group as a whole, the death-rates increased with the diastolic blood-pressure levels. In those with an initial diastolic blood-pressure between 100 and 109 mm. Hg the mortality-rate during the period of observation was 38 percent, at 110–119 mm. Hg it was 43 percent, at 120–129 mm. Hg it was 50 percent, and at 130 mm. Hg and over it was 54 percent.

Relating the initial diastolic blood-pressure levels with age and sex, it was found that at all ages the death-rates were higher in males than in females. Death-rates were related closely to the initial diastolic blood-pressure levels in the younger hypertensives, but in the over-sixties there were no relationships between the diastolic blood pressure and the observed mortality-rates.

It appears that height of diastolic blood-pressure was of serious import in younger and middle-aged hypertensives, and especially so in males. This was not the case in those in whom high blood-pressure was diagnosed first at the age of sixty years and over.

Discussion

If these observations are taken as a guide, then there are probably some 2½ million people with known high blood-pressure in the United Kingdom, and possibly almost as many unknown hypertensives as yet undiagnosed. Put another way, the British general practitioner with an average-size practice may expect to diagnose and manage about 600 hypertensives in his professional lifetime.

Such numbers of a disease represent an enormous amount of potential professional effort for general practitioners and for hospital physicians and their teams. If it is accepted that all diagnosed hypertensives require specific hypotensive drugs for the rest of their lives, then this will require a considerable amount of financial and other resources.

The decisions on how best to manage high blood-pressure cannot be arrived at satisfactorily without a sound and accurate knowledge of the disease (hypertension), its course, and its response to specific and non-specific measures. This paper attempts to show the outcome of high blood-pressure, untreated by specific drugs.

The results suggest that high blood-pressure is a condition associated with ageing, and half the hypertensives were diagnosed when they were aged sixty years or more. The levels of the diastolic blood-pressures at diagnosis were such that 28 percent could have been said to have been "mild", 58 percent "moderate", and 14 percent "severe". Analysis of the observed death-rates compared with those expected shows that there were some definite factors associated with extra risks. The outlook generally was worse in males than in females; mortality-rates varied inversely with age (i.e., they were much greater than expected in young adults but no more, and even less in the over-seventies, than expected in the elderly). The higher levels of diastolic blood-pressure were a bad prognostic factor in those under sixty, but did not seem to have much influence on the outcome in the older hypertensives.

If such findings can be applied to our system of management, then large numbers of hypertensives may be selected for non-treatment. Hypotensive therapy may be non-beneficial in over-seventies and may be less indicated in females than in males at all ages. If these suggestions are followed up, then about half of hypertensives may not require expensive, long-term, and potentially unpleasant forms of treatment. On the other hand, the younger the hypertensive the more urgent and intensive should be his investigation and specific treatment to reduce the raised blood-pressure, especially in males.

REFERENCES

1. Hlth Bull. 1971, 29, 33
2. United States Veterans Administration. J. Am. med. Ass. 1967, 202, 1028
3. United States Veterans Administration, ibid., 1971, 213, 1143
4. Br. med. J. 1973, iii, 434
5. Stuart, K. L. Desia, P., Lalsingh, A. ibid. 1974, ii, 195
6. W.H.O. Chron. 1972, 26, 451
7. Fry, J. Profiles of Disease, Edinburgh, 1966
8. Fry, J. Common Diseases. Lancaster, 1974

Introduction To
Evans County Cardiovascular and
Cerebrovascular Epidemiologic Study*

Guest Editor: John C. Cassel

Curtis G. Hames

This brief introduction will include a short historical note concerning the development of the Evans County study, a description of the study site, its physical and racial structure, an overview of its accomplishments and hopes for its future.

The Epidemiological Study of Cardiovascular Disease developed in Evans County, Georgia, from the clinical observation that coronary heart disease appeared to occur less frequently among blacks than whites, even though hypertension was obviously more common in blacks and they consumed a higher animal fat diet. In addition there was no difference in coronary mortality by sex in the blacks although such a difference did occur in whites.

The study was, therefore, basically designed to answer two questions: First, were these clinical observations valid? That is, does coronary heart disease really occur more commonly among whites than blacks living in Evans County, and, if so, what was the extent of the differences? Second, presuming a positive answer, what were the reasons for the observed differences?

At about the time these observations were being made in 1956–1967, James Watt, MD, was head of the National Heart Institute. Following a mandate from Congress to expand the base for medical research he envisioned a program to include not only the Institute of Health's own research, the academic and university research, the clinical and laboratory research, facilities of the

Veterans Hospitals, and other government agencies, industrial and private research laboratories but also research at the grass roots level where he felt there was a tremendous opportunity for the collection of epidemiological data. Epidemiological research at the comminity level could provide invaluable information concerning the natural history of many diseases, studies in genetics, delivery of health care systems to name but a few possibilities. In many instances data of these types could not be collected under any other circumstances. He envisioned such a program of research functioning through the local health departments in conjunction with the local practicing physicians. It was at this time, at the suggestion of Jeremiah Stamler, MD, that a small grant had been submitted to the National Institutes of Health for support of such a community study in Evans County.

Dr. Watt became aware of the application and visited this county and its health departments as one of several sites for possible pilot study areas. He subsequently was greatly instrumental in nurturing the development of the project; ie, by expanding the concept of its usefulness, providing the administrative machinery for funding and support through the local health department, the assignment of US Public Health Officers for examination of the population and requiring that we seek adequate statistical design and assistance. This was obtained through the support of departments of epidemiology and biostatistics at the University of North Carolina School of Public Health. Dr. Watt had hoped this

*Reprinted by permission from *Archives of Internal Medicine*, 128(6): 883–886, December 1971.

project might serve as a stimulus for the development of other community based research projects over the entire county; however, the Evans County study is the only black-white epidemiological study in the United States, and it and the Tecumseh study are the only two total community epidemiological studies.

The following brief description of the study site characteristics will give the reader some general feeling for the population under surveillance.

Evans County is located on the coastal plains, about 60 miles inland from the port city of Savannah, Ga. The county is 19 miles at its greatest diameter and consists of flat or slightly rolling terrain of red clay and sandy soil. Much of the county is covered by pine forests which are harvested for pulpwood, turpentine, and lumber. Only small industry is present: fruitcake is manufactured and a local sewing factory employs some 500 people, mostly females. The basic economy continues to be agriculture. However, in recent years there has been a gradual shift to employment at the nearby Fort Stewart under government civil service or to more industrial jobs reached by commuting to Savannah.

The population has been fairly stable as indicated by the fact that the Evans County official population in 1960 was 6,952 and 7,290 in 1970 or a 4.9% increase in ten years. There are approximately 4,847 whites (66.5 percent) and 2,434 blacks (33.5 percent). Only nine persons of other races were enumerated. The black-white ratio has remained almost constant in ten years, showing a surprisingly stable population composition at the time of unusually great black outmigration in other areas of the south. There are 664 children at the age of 5 years, 2,166 ages 5 to 17 years, 3,697 ages 18 to 64, and 763 ages 65 and over. From age 14 and above 3,300 were married, 486 widows, 129 divorced, 1,199 never married. A total of 36.6 percent are living in incorporated areas while 63.4 percent are living in a completely rural setting. Households number 2,174, including 324 one person

households; in addition, 17 persons are living in group quarters. There are 2,364 housing units in Evans County, 1,348 occupied by owners, 826 occupied by tenants and 190 vacant, mostly for seasonal use by agricultural workers. The proportion of home owners has increased from 49.2 percent in 1960 to 57 percent in 1970. In addition to the 2,023 single family units there are now 186 government housing units and 148 trailers or mobile home units. A percentage of occupied units with more than one person per room has decreased from 18.6 percent in 1960 to 12.6 percent in 1970. Of all the occupied housing units 1,701 have piped water, toilets, and bath while 473 lack some or all plumbing. The median rent paid by tenants in 1970 was approximately $30 per month.

The original study was launched in this county in 1960 when 100 percent of all residents over age 40 and a 50 percent sample of those between 15 and 39 were given a complete physical examination together with a battery of laboratory tests. In addition samples of serum from each individual were frozen and retained for future studies. Since that time the population has been carefully and systematically followed, and survivors reexamined during the period 1967-1969. The results of this follow up and reexamination insofar as cardiovascular and cerebrovascular disease are concerned are reported in the succeeding papers of this issue.

During the period 1960-1970, the availability of a well documented total population under careful surveillance, with frozen serum dating from 1960, has been utilized by numerous academic institutions from various parts of the world as well as by government agencies for a wide variety of research purposes. These studies have extended from molecular biological investigations through clinical research to large scale epidemiological and ecological studies.[1-45] In all such endeavors the principal investigator has served as an interlocutor between the people and the various scientists maintaining rapport and reducing undue confusion or disturbance on the part of the citizens. On numerous occasions it has been demonstrated that such a function is essential for public relations if this delicate balance so vital for the success of any research study in a free living population is to be maintained.

While many of these research projects are not necessarily related to cardiovascular disease, brief comments on a few of them are made here to illustrate the potentialities that can be derived from a close liaison between a practicing physician and academic institutions. The development and supervision of the basic research design by the Department of Epidemiology at the University of North Carolina has made it possible to draw any type of random sample or matched case-control series for purposes of such studies. Further the principal investigator, as a native to the study site, has an unique vantage point, in that he has had direct contact with as many as three to five generations of families and has been able to observe them over time. Such a vantage point displays the potential role of genetics in many diseases in much clearer focus and has lent direction to the research effort. Such effort brought Baruch S. Blumberg MD, PhD, and W. Thomas London, MD, and other geneticists[4,7-9,12,13,23,29,36] to Evans County to utilize the available resources of the study. In a search for the Australian antigen among over 2,000 serum samples from Evans County, Drs. Blumberg and London found a patient with the Australian antigen who also had severe hepatitis. His hepatitis was well documented and served as one of the two original clues to linking the Australian antigen with viral hepatitis. Cardiovascular epidemiology correlates, ie, height, weight, body build, blood pressure, diet, exercise, and social status; levels of triglycerides, cholesterol, γ-globulins, lipoproteins, plasma renin, urinary sodium potassium, carbohydrates, catecholamines; hematocrit value; and numerous clotting factors including platelet stickiness, have been determined in these population groups living side by side where gross differences from coronary heart disease and hypertension exist.[14-22,24-27,30-35,39-44] Studies are also now under way to determine the prevalence of hyperlipoproteinemias as classified by Fredrickson along with the correlation of morbidity and mortality with all the various lipid fractions determined in these patients both chemically and by ultracentrifugation. Geneticists from the University of Oslo in Norway and Florence, Italy, are using known genetic markers for possible correlation also with the various same fractions. The computer analysis of electrocardiographic data has been collected to better understand the significance of ST segment elevation in the blacks and its possible relationship to membrane chemistry. A total of 11,000 virus antibody determinations have been made for their possible correlation with congenital heart disease as well as coronary heart disease. The possible relationship of glucose 6-phosphate dehydrogenase deficiency to increased hypertension and decreased CHD as reported by Long and associates,[45] has been determined in the Evans County population. Alpha 2 antitrypsin deficiency was found to occur in about 2 percent to 3 percent of the population and its possible relationship to predisposition to develop emphysema has been determined.[12,29] Some 1,400 family aggregations have been characterized in the population. The natural history of transitory ischemic attacks and cerebrovascular accidents are being monitored on a long-term basis. The effects of migration on health is being studied among individuals who have migrated from the study site since 1960. Personality type, incidence of new disease, motivation, social achievement and many other factors are included in the study. No other known southern community has data of this type available for study. The community has also served as a base for training medical students as well as ancillary personnel. The early development of an intensive coronary care unit in the local 42-bed hospital was achieved several years before it became widely utilized even in much larger hospitals.[38]

Our new goals for the future lie not only in the observation of the natural history of disease but also in the area of genetics and ultimately in the utilization of such a well-defined population for preventive intervention studies; ie, with over 1,000 cases of hypertension defined a hypertensive control program could ideally be developed here as a model for use in all parts of the country.

Because of the wealth of data and information that can be obtained from such epidemiological studies other communities should set up similar basic studies where many questions concerning health care and the long-term observation of chronic disease can be answered in the natural environment.

Acknowledgment

This investigation was supported by Public Health Service research grant HE-03341.

REFERENCES

1. Hames, CG: An atherogenic profile. J Med Assoc Georgia 49:188-191, 1960
2. A Report of Selected Characteristic Evans and Bulloch Counties, Ga. 1960, Public Health Service
3. Hames CG, Greenberg BG: A comparative study of serum cholesterol levels in school children and their possible relation to atherogenesis. Amer J Public Health 51:374-385, 1961
4. Parker WC, Bearn AG: Haptoglobin and transferrin variation in human and primates: Two new transferrins in Chinese and Japanese populations. Ann Hum Genet 25:227-241, 1961
5. McDonough JR, Hames CG, Greenberg BG, et al: Observations on serum cholesterol levels in the twin population of Evans County, Georgia. Circulation 25:962-969, 1962
6. McDonough JR, Hames CG, Stulb SC, et al: Cardiovascular disease field study in Evans County, Ga. Public Health Rep 78:1051-1059, 1963
7. Robinson JC, Blumberg BS, Pierce JE, et al: Studies on the inherited variants of blood proteins: II. Familial segregation of transferrin $B_{1-2}B_2$. J Lab Clin Med 62:762-765, 1963
8. Cooper AJ, Blumberg BS, Workman PL, et al: Biochemical polymorphic traits in a U.S. white and Negro population. Amer J. Hum Genet 15:420-428, 1963
9. Workman PL, Blumberg BS, Cooper AJ: Selection, gene migration and polymorphic stability in a U.S. white and Negro population. Amer J Hum Genet 15:429-437, 1963
10. McDonough JR, Garrison GE, Hames CG: Blood pressure and hypertensive disease among Negroes and whites: A study in Evans County, Georgia. Ann Intern Med 61:208-228, 1964
11. Brewer GJ, Gall JC, Honeyman MS, et al: Inheritance of quantitative expression of G-6-PD deficiency in heterozygous Negro females: A twin study. Clin Res 13:265, 1965
12. Kueppers F, Briscoe WA, Bearn AG: Hereditary deficiency of antitrypsin. Science 146:1678-1679, 1964
13. Blumberg BS, Workman PL, Hirschfeld J: Gamma globulin, group specific and lipoprotein groups in a U.S. white and Negro population. Nature 202:561-563, 1964
14. Hames CG, McDonough JR, Elliott JL: Hypertension in identical twins. Lancet 2:585, 1964
15. McDonough JR, Hames CG, Stulb SC, et al: Coronary heart disease among Negroes and whites in Evans County, Ga. J Chronic Dis 18:443-468, 1965
16. Lichtman MA, Hames CG, McDonough JR: Serum protein electrophoretic fractions among Negro and white subjects in Evans County, Ga Amer J Clin Nutr 16:492-508, 1965
17. Stulb SC, McDonough JR, Greenberg BG, et al: The relationship of nutrient intake and exercise to serum cholesterol levels in white males in Evans County, Ga. Amer J Clin Nutr 16:238-242, 1965
18. McDonough JR, Hames CG, Garrison GE, et al: The relationship of hematocrit to cardiovascular states of health in the Negro and white population of Evans County, Ga. J Chronic Dis 18:243-257, 1965
19. Lichtman MA, Hames CG, McDonough JR: Serum gamma globulin levels among Negroes and whites in Evans County, Ga. Clin Res 13:30, 1964
20. Ibrahim MA, Jenkins CD, Cassel JC, et al: Personality traits and coronary heart disease. J Chronic Dis 19:255-271, 1966
21. Garrison GE, McDonough JR, Hames CG, et al: Prevalence of chronic congestive heart failure in

the population of Evans County, Georgia. Amer J Epidem 83:338–344, 1966

22. Skinner JC, Benson H, McDonough JR, et al: Social status, physical activity and coronary proneness. J Chronic Dis 9:773–783, 1966

23. Berg K, Bearn A: An inherited X-linked serum in man: The XM system. J Exp Med 123:379–397, 1966

24. Hames CG, McDonough JR, Stulb SC: Physical activity and ischemic heart disease among Negroes and whites in Evans County, Ga, in Raab W (ed): Prevention of Ischemic Heart Disease: Principles and Practice. Springfield, Ill, Charles C Thomas Publisher, 1966

25. McDonough JR, Hames CG: Influence of race, sex and occupation on seasonal changes in serum cholesterol. Amer J Epidem 83:356–364, 1967

26. Lichtman MA, Vaughan JH, Hames CG: The distribution of serum immunoglobins, anti-gamma-G globulins ("rheumatoid factors") and antinuclear antibodies in white and Negro subjects in Evans County, Georgia. Arthritis Rheum 10:204–215, 1967

27. McDonough JR, Garrison GE, Hames CG: Blood pressure and hypertensive disease among Negroes and whites in Evans County, Ga, in Stamler J (ed): Epidemiology of Hypertension, New York, Grune & Stratton Inc, 1967

28. Brewer GJ, Gall JC, Honeyman M, et al: Inheritance of quantitative expression of erythrocyte glucose-6-phosphate dehydrogenase activity in the Negro: A twin study. Biochem Genet 1:41–53, 1967

29. Kueppers G, Bearn AG: An inherited A4 antitrypsin variant. Humangenetik 4:217–220, 1967

30. Lichtman MA, McDonough JR, Hames CG: Serum gamma globulin concentration in related and non-related subjects. Human Biol 39:307–315, 1967

31. Williams OD, Grizzle JE: Analysis of longitudinal data: An investigation of the relationship among systolic blood pressure, diastolic blood pressure, serum triglyceride, and serum cholesterol, abstracted. Circulation 38 (suppl 6):207, 1968

32. Jenkins CD, Hames CG, Zyzanski SJ, et al: Psychological traits and serum lipids: I. Findings from the California Psychological Inventory. Psychosom Med 31:115–128, 1969

33. Hames CG: An epidemiological study of platelet stickiness, in Schettler G (ed): Platelets and the Vessel Wall-Fibrin Deposition: Symposium of the European Atherosclerosis Group. Stuttgart, Germany. Georg Thieme Verlag, 1970, pp. 129–143

34. Heyden S, Bartel AG, Hames CG, et al: Elevated blood pressure levels in adolescents, Evans County, Georgia: Seven year follow-up of 30 patients and 30 controls. JAMA 209:1683–1689, 1969

35. Hames CG: Coronary heart disease and smoking: A reducible risk factor. J Med Assoc Georgia 58:440, 1969

36. Kueppers F: Studies on the Xh antigen in human serum. Humangenetik 7:98–103, 1969

37. Hames CG: Stress and heart disease. J Med Assoc Georgia 59:194–195, 1970

38. Bartel AG, Hames CG: Intensive coronary care in a 42-bed rural hospital. J Med Assoc Georgia 59:285–289, 1970

39. Simpson MT, Hames CG, Olewine DA, et al: Physical activity, catecholamines and platelet stickiness, in Myocardiology: Recent Advances in Studies on Cardiac Structure and Metabolism. Baltimore, University Park Press, to be published

40. Hames CG: The correlation of ischemic heart disease with social class among whites and blacks in a total community epidemiological study. Lex et Scientia 7:53–62, 1970

41. Heyden S, Bartel AG, Hames CG, et al: Elevated blood pressure levels in adolescents, Evans County, Ga, in Braunwald E (ed): Year Book of Cardiovascular Medicine and Surgery. Chicago, Year Book Medical Publishers Inc, 1970

42. Grim CE, McDonough JR, Dahl LK, et al: On the higher blood pressure of blacks: A study of sodium and potassium intake and excretion in a biracial community, abstracted. Clin Res 18:593, 1970

43. Grim CE, McDonough JR, Dahl LK, et al: Dietary sodium, potassium, and blood pressure. Three hundred Racial Differences in Evans County, Georgia, abstracted. Circulation 62 (suppl 3):85, 1970

44. Karp H, Heyman A, Heyden S, et al: Incidence and Risk Factors of Stroke Among the Biracial Population in Evans County, Georgia, abstracted. Circulation 62(suppl 3):93, 1970

45. Long WK, Wilson SW, Frenkel EP: Associations between red cell glucose-6-phosphate dehydrogenase variants and vascular diseases. Amer J Hum Genet 19:35–53, 1967

Cardiovascular Mortality in Transient Ischemic Attacks*

Siegfried Heyden, Gerardo Heiss, Albert Heyman, Alfred H. Tyroler, Curtis G. Hames, Ulrich Patzschke, and Christian Manegold

Statistical analyses were made of the mortality of persons diagnosed as having definite TIA in an epidemiologic survey of a biracial Southern community. None of the usual risk factors associated with this illness such as heart disease, hypertension or diabetes appears to account for the excess deaths observed in a 10 year period of follow up.

The Mortality Rate of patients with transient cerebral ischemic attacks (TIA) has been found to be considerably greater than that of the general population of comparable age and sex.[1,2] Although the increase in mortality in TIA is usually attributed to the presence of associated factors such as hypertension, diabetes or heart disease, there have been few attempts to quantify the relative significance of these conditions. The purpose of the present paper is to determine by means of statistical analyses which, if any, of these concomitant risk factors contribute to the high death rate from TIA.

Patients and Methods

The study population consists of residents of Evans County, Georgia, a small rural community in the high stroke belt of the Southeastern United States.[3] The initial survey of this community comprising approximately 60 percent White and 40 percent Black population was carried out in 1960 and included all residents 40 years of age or older and a 50 percent sample of those 15 to 39 years of age. A follow up survey was made between July, 1967, and July, 1969, to determine the 7 to 9 year incidence of vascular disease in this population. The present report is based on the 2471 stroke-free survivors who were reexamined at that time. Twenty-eight of them gave a history of having had definite focal manifestations of TIA with sudden onset of transient limb paralysis, sensory loss, visual defects or speech disorders lasting for 24 hours or less and clearing without significant deficit.† Seven of thse 28 persons were Black, 21 White. An additional 51 persons were diagnosed as having uncertain TIA with a history of non-focal neurologic episodes such as alteration in consciousness, dizziness or drop attacks. The neurologic complaints in these people were often vague and could not be differentiated from anxiety or emotional disturbances. Forty-two of these 51 persons were White, 9 Black. None of the 79 persons with definite or uncertain TIA had evidence of a completed stroke in the period between 1960 and 1967–69.

From the time of the second survey examination to December 31, 1978, a follow up period averaging 10 years, a surveillance was carried out to determine the frequency and cause of death. Death certificates were obtained from all persons dying from any cause. In 1978, a physical examination and electrocardiogram was made of all survivors who had a diagnosis of definite or

*Reprinted by permission from *Stroke*, 11(3):252–255, May–June 1980.

†This represents a heterogeneous group of patients with respect to time of occurrence of neurologic manifestations, between the first and the second examination, i.e., 1960 through 1967/69.

45

uncertain TIA at the second survey examination. Survivorship analyses were carried out employing the Mantel-Haenszel life table method which is free of distributional assumptions and uses the logrank test for hypothesis testing.[5]

Results

Table 1 shows the frequency of vascular disease appearing among the survivors of the 79 persons with symptoms of TIA. Eleven of the 28 persons with definite TIA were alive at the end of the follow up period. Three of them developed myocardial infarction during this time, 3 had a completed stroke and 6 had angina, congestive heart failure and other evidence of vascular disease. Of the 51 persons with uncertain TIA, 35 survived. Four of them developed infarction, 4 had a completed stroke and 14 had other manifestations of vascular disease.

Table 2 shows the number and cause of death in the 3 population groups observed in the 9 to 10 year period from the 1967–69 survey to the end of 1978. Seventeen or 61 percent of the 28 persons with definite TIA died during this interval as compared to only 16 or 31 percent of the 51 persons with uncertain TIA. Of the 2392 persons remaining, only 52 or 20 percent died. As would be expected, the deaths in each of these 3 groups were due chiefly to vascular

Table 1. *Vascular Illness Occurring Among Survivors of 28 Persons with Definite and 51 with Uncertain TIA*

Types of Vascular Disease*	11 Survivors with Definite TIA	35 Survivors with Uncertain TIA
Myocardial infarction	3	4
Completed stroke	3	4
Other cardiac conditions (angina, congestive failure, etc.)	6	14
Hypertension (BP ≥ 160/90)	6	17
No evidence of heart disease	3	14
Unknown	1	—

*Categories not mutually exclusive.

diseases. The mean age of persons with definite and uncertain TIA were approximately the same (59 and 61 years respectively), but was greater than that of the remaining population free of stroke or TIA (52 years).

Life table analyses were used to contrast the mortality during the 10 year follow up period. The comparison of the mortality experience of each of the 3 population groups takes into consideration the person-years of follow up contributed by

Table 2. *Number and Causes of Deaths in Persons with Definite and Uncertain TIA and in Stroke-Free Population from 1967–69 to 1978*

	Definite TIA	Uncertain TIA	Stroke-Free Population
Number of persons	28	51	2392
Mean age at time of 1967 survey	59	61	52
Total deaths during followup observation	17 (61%)	16 (31%)	478 (20%)
Cause of death			
Ischemic heart disease	3 (11%)	3 (6%)	138 (6%)
Stroke	4 (14%)	5 (10%)	75 (3%)
Other vascular illness	1	3	50
Miscellaneous causes	8 (29%)	5 (10%)	207 (9%)
Unknown	1	0	8

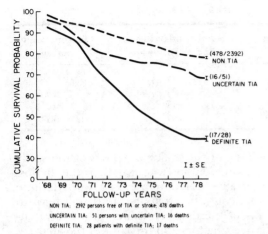

NON TIA: 2392 persons free of TIA or stroke; 478 deaths
UNCERTAIN TIA: 51 persons with uncertain TIA; 16 deaths
DEFINITE TIA: 28 patients with definite TIA; 17 deaths

Fig. 1. Survivorship of persons with definite TIA, uncertain TIA and those free of stroke or TIA during 10 year follow up observation.

each person until death or termination of the study (see Fig. 1). As shown in the figure, deaths occurred almost uniformly during this 10 year period. The logrank test of the survival probabilities showed the 3 groups to be significantly different from each other ($\chi^2 = 22.9$; $p < 0.00001$). The age standardized mortality rate ratio was 2.15 for definite TIA compared to uncertain TIA;

and 2.90 and 1.30 respectively for definite TIA and uncertain TIA compared to the stroke and TIA-free population.

Discriminant function analyses were performed to assess the risk factor attribute for TIA, adjusting simultaneously for the other risk factors of mortality. Using a stepwise procedure, the following variables (as determined in 1967–69) were entered into the model: age, smoking status, diabetes, diastolic blood pressure, electrocardiographic abnormalities, serum cholesterol and diagnosis of TIA. With the exception of serum cholesterol, each of these variables was a significant independent predictor of total mortality ($p < 0.00001$). Thus, with all other risk factors present in the discriminant function, the diagnosis of TIA per se was a significant predictor of mortality.

This information is summarized in Table 3 as relative risks, i.e., mortality rate ratios, both unadjusted and adjusted for all other risk factors in the model. The risk factors are ranked by the magnitude of their adjusted rate ratios. The strongest predictor of mortality in this population was age, followed by major electrocardiographic abnormalities (normal vs any major abnormality) at the time of the 1967–69 survey. A

Table 3. *Relative Risk of Mortality During 10 Years of Follow Up for TIA and Other Cardiovascular Risk Factors*

	Unadjusted Rate Ratios	Adjusted Rate Ratios*	95% Lower Limit for the Adjusted Rate Ratios
Age	3.30	3.16	2.75
Major electrocardiographic abnormalities†	2.53	2.33	1.74
Definite TIA vs TIA & stroke-free population	3.62	2.29	1.64
Current cigarette smoking	1.92	1.61	1.40
Diastolic blood pressure (>90 mm Hg)	1.66	1.44	1.30
Diabetes	1.36	1.21	1.19
Cholesterol	1.47	1.19	0.98
Uncertain TIA vs TIA & stroke-free population	2.31	1.03	0.10

*Major ECG abnormalities were defined as any one of the following Minnesota Codes: All 1-1; 3-1, 3-2; 4-1, 4-2; 5-1, 5-2; 6-1, 6-2, 6-4; 7-1, 7-2, 7-4; 9-2.
†Adjusted for all other variables.

Table 4. *Mortality in Persons with TIA During 5 to 15 Year Period of Observation*

Study Location	Years of Followup	Total Number TIA Cases	Number of Deaths at End of Followup	Percent Deaths per Year
Winston-Salem (6)	5.5	225	82	6.5
Framingham (2)	8	85	31	4.1
Evans County	10	28	17	6.1
Rochester (1)	15	199	187	6.1

diagnosis of definite TIA ranked third as a prognostic factor of death in this multivariable analysis. The diagnosis of uncertain TIA, however, was no longer a significant risk factor for death once adjusted for the other risk factors. Cigarette smoking (current smoker vs non-smoker), diastolic blood pressure (< 90 mm Hg vs ≥ 90 mm Hg) and diabetes (definite or probable vs non-diabetic) each carried significant additional risk of mortality ($p = 0.05$). The level of serum cholesterol (< 240 mg/dl vs ≥ 240 mg/dl) by contrast, was not predictive of death after adjustment for the other variables.

Discussion

This study of mortality of persons with TIA is based on an epidemiologic investigation of cerebrovascular disease in a biracial community in which survivorship following the diagnosis of TIA was monitored for approximately 10 years. Our analyses were primarily concerned with mortality of persons diagnosed as having either definite or uncertain TIA as compared with that of the general population free of TIA or stroke. The mortality (61 percent) found in persons with definite TIA was significantly higher than that (31 percent) found in persons with uncertain TIA or than that (20 percent) of the stroke and TIA-free population. The number of persons in this study with definite TIA was small and one must, therefore, be cautious in making generalizations. Nevertheless, these observations are of interest in the prediction of TIA outcome.

One of the major purposes of the study was to demonstrate whether the higher mortality noted in persons with definite TIA could be attributed to their age or to any of the usual concomitant cardiovascular risk factors. On the basis of the analyses described above, neither age nor hypertension, diabetes, major electrocardiographic abnormalities, smoking or hypercholesterolemia could account solely for the excess number of deaths in this group of individuals. Thus, it would appear that the diagnosis of definite TIA carried with it a mortality risk by mechanisms which are not yet clear.

The excess mortality associated with TIA has been reported in other studies.[1,2,6,7] As shown in Table 4, the annual mortality found in 4 studies of TIA are remarkably similar to rates of approximately 6 percent per year. These studies on the relationship of risk factors and the outcome of TIA usually compare various groups of patients with this illness and do not contrast the prognosis of TIA with similar cohorts who are free of cerebrovascular disease. The results of this epidemiologic study of a biracial community, however, indicate that persons with definite TIA have an excess mortality for reasons outlined above.

REFERENCES

1. Cartlidge NE, Whisnant JP, Elveback LR: Carotid and vertebral-basilar transient cerebral ischemic attacks: A community study. Rochester, Minnesota. Mayo Clin Proc 52:117–120, 1977
2. Wolf PA, Dawber TR, Colton T, Thomas HE, Jr.,

Kannel WB: Transient cerebral ischemic attacks and risk of stroke: The Framingham Study. Presented at the AHA Conference on Cardiovascular Epidemiology at San Diego, CA, March 7-9, 1977

3. Heyman A, Karp HR, Heyden S, Bartel A, Cassel JC, Tyroler HA, Cornoni JC: Cerebrovascular disease in the biracial population of Evans County, Georgia. Arch Int Med 128:949-955, 1971

4. Karp HR, Heyman A, Heyden S, Bartel A, Tyroler HA, Hames CG: Transient cerebral ischemia: Prevalence and prognosis in a biracial rural community. JAMA 225:125-128, 1973

5. Peto R, Pike MC, Armitage P, Breslow NE, Cox DR, Howard SV, Mantel N, McPherson K, Peto J. Smith PG: Design and analysis of randomized clinical trials requiring prolonged observation of each patient: II. Analysis and examples. Br J Cancer 35:1-39, 1977

6. Toole JF, Yuson CP, Janeway R, Johnston F, Davis C, Cordell AR, Howard G: Transient ischemic attacks: A prospective study of 225 patients. Neurology (Minneap) 28:746-753, 1978

7. Whisnant JP, Cartlidge NEF, Elveback LR: Carotid and vertebral-basilar transient ischemic attacks: Effect of anticoagulants, hypertension and cardiac disorders on survival and stroke occurrence—A population study. Ann Neurol 3:107, 1978

Major Factors in the Development of Diabetes Mellitus in 10,000 Men*

Jack H. Medalie, Cheri M. Papier, Uri Goldbourt, and Joseph B. Herman

The average annual incidence of diabetes among 8,688 adult men followed up for five years was 8.0/1,000 with Asian, African and Israeli-born having higher rates than European-born.

Multivariate analysis of the findings suggested the following: the most significant variables associated with the development of diabetes are overweight and peripheral vascular disease; the high incidence of diabetes in immigrants from Asia and Africa might be an example of Neel's "thrifty genotype" or failure of adaptation to relatively rapid environmental changes; serum cholesterol level, blood pressure, uric acid level, and education were important also; and the probability of developing diabetes within five years rises from 17/1,000 (when the major variables are low or absent) to 450/1,000 (when they are high and present). This has important clinical implications.

Diabetes mellitus, despite being recognized since antiquity[1] and having been the focus of attention of many distinguished scientists, still poses many unanswered problems. To aid in the elucidation of some of these, a five-year prospective study was undertaken among Israeli men. A mul-

*Reprinted by permission from *Archives of Internal Medicine,* 135:811–817, June 1975.

Received for publication May 16, 1974; accepted Jan 27, 1975.

From the Department of Family Medicine, Tel Aviv University Sackler School of Medicine, Tel-Hashomer, Israel.

Reprint requests to Building 130, Tel-Hashomer Hospital, Chaim Sheba Medical Center, Tel-Aviv, Israel (Dr. Medalie).

tivariate analysis of the factors associated with the development of diabetes in this study group is presented.

Previous reports provide background information for the study.[2,3] Briefly, approximately 10,000 male Israeli government and municipal workers, age 40 years and older, were examined three times during the period 1963 to 1968 in the context of the Israeli Ischemic Heart Disease Project. The examinations, which experienced less than a 5 percent drop-out rate during the entire period, encompassed clinical, biochemical, behavioral, genetic, biographic, and psychosocial factors. They were conducted in Tel Aviv, Jerusalem, and Haifa. Selection of subjects was based on differential sampling ratios varying from 25 percent to 100 percent in order to include a minimum of 1,000 men from each of six areas of birth—Israel, eastern Europe, central Europe, southeastern Europe, Asia, and north Africa.

Methods

Approximately 120 independent variables were tested against the development of diabetes from 1963 to 1968 among 10,000 adult males. The incidence rates as well as the significantly associated variables (from the univariate analysis) have been reported elsewhere.[4] These significant variables as well as a few others were used to calculate a multiple logistic function in respect of the incidence of diabetes using the methods of Cornfield et al[5] and Truett et al.[6] (Specifically, the rates of diabetes incidence in tertiles of the variables produced a slope over assigned scores 0, 1, and 2 that, when divided by their standard errors, exceeded the two-sided .05 level for a normal deviate. For attribute variables, there was a significant departure, also at the .05 level, from independence of incidence rates on the different categories of the variable.)

Subjects at Risk for the Incidence Study

In 1963, all subjects were examined and those found to have a casual blood sugar level of 130 mg/100 ml or more (Somogyi-Nelson method) or who gave a history of diabetes were identified as suspects. After follow-up, those suspects with a normal glucose tolerance test (GTT) or with less than 120 mg/100 ml in three successive tests and without a confirmed history were classified as negative. These, together with the original group of negatively screened persons (nonsuspects), were considered "at risk" for diabetes incidence.

The method of determining the diabetic incidence cases has been described in detail elsewhere. The incidence data reported here relate to an observation period of approximately five years and are based on 8,688 subjects (of the original 9,494) at risk for diabetes for whom all measurements included in the variables of the multiple logistic were known. (The two-year incidence study was based on 8,369 subjects only, because it excluded subjects who at that time were classified as "unknown" but who were subsequently followed up and classified.)

Results

Diabetes incidence rates by area of birth are shown in Table 1. It shows an overall average annual incidence of 8.0/1,000, with Asia, north Africa, and Israel showing much higher rates than the three areas in Europe.

As expected, Table 2 shows that the means of seven numeric variables were higher in the diabetic than in the nondiabetic group. The two nonnumeric or attribute variables show that the diabetic group had fewer people born in Europe and a lower educational level than the nondiabetic group.

In Table 3, a satisfactory "fit" is observed between the expected and observed number of diabetes incidence cases in the top and bottom deciles as well as percentile groups inside the 10 percent to 90 percent span. The two bottom lines reflect the contribution of the multivariate risk model to classification of future cases as "high risk." If future cases were randomly dispersed in the sample, regardless of the values of the "risk factors," all rates in those lines would be close to 1.

Comparing the incidence ratio of the top decile of the population (obtained by ranking the subjects according to their theoretical probabilities) to the average (overall incidence rate) shows a 2.3 times greater incidence of diabetes for subjects in the upper decile. The incidence ratio of subjects in the

Table 1. *Five-Year Incidence of Diabetes Mellitus by Birthplace*

Birthplace	No. at Risk	No. of Cases	Age-Adjusted Rate/1,000	Average Annual Incidence/1,000
Israel	1,337	56	42	8.4
Asia	2,225	116	56	11.2
North Africa	1,151	47	42	8.4
Eastern Europe	1,817	57	28	5.6
Central Europe	1,315	37	28	5.6
Southeast Europe	1,649	60	35	7.0
Total	9,494	373	40	8.0

Table 2. *Means and Standard Deviations for 1963 Variables in Multiple Logistic Risk Function (1963–1968)*

Variable*	Age 40–49 yr			Age 50–59 yr			Age >60 yr			Total		
	Diabetic Incidence Cases (Mean)	Nondiabetics (Mean)	Pooled Standard Deviation	Diabetic Incidence Cases (Mean)	Nondiabetics (Mean)	Pooled Standard Deviation	Diabetic Incidence Cases (Mean)	Nondiabetics (Mean)	Pooled Standard Deviation	Diabetic Incidence Cases (Mean)	Nondiabetics (Mean)	Pooled Standard Deviation
Age in 1963	44.4	43.9	2.9	54.3	53.8	2.7	62.3	62.3	2.1	51.2	48.9	6.8
Wt/ht², gm/sq cm	2.69	2.54	0.33	2.73	2.58	0.32	2.65	2.56	0.34	2.70	2.56	0.33
PVD-IC, 0-1	0.042	0.017	0.13	0.058	0.032	0.18	0.114	0.049	0.22	0.058	0.025	0.16
Cholesterol, mg/100 ml	211	205	40	220	212	39	227	215	40	217	208	40
SBP, mm Hg	135	130	17	142	138	22	151	147	24	140	134	20
Uric acid, mg/100 ml	5.12	4.73	0.93	4.94	4.78	0.97	4.90	4.86	1.01	5.01	4.76	0.95
Hemoglobin, mg/100 ml	15.1	15.0	1.2	15.3	14.9	1.3	14.9	14.8	1.3	15.5	15.0	1.2
Born in Europe, 0-1	0.31	0.43	0.45	0.50	0.58	0.49	0.52	0.63	0.49	0.42	0.50	0.50
Education, 0-low, 9-high	3.83	4.29	2.1	4.08	4.72	2.38	4.18	4.58	2.48	3.99	4.46	2.25
No. of subjects with all measurements known	144	4,703	⋯	156	2,929	⋯	44	712	⋯	344	8,344	⋯
Total	4,847			3,085			756			8,688		

*Wt/ht² is weight/height²; PVD-IC, peripheral vascular disease-intermittent claudication; SBP, systolic blood pressure.

Table 3. *Goodness of Fit and Degree of Discrimination of Multiple Logistic Risk Function*

	Age, yr							
	40–49		*50–59*		*>60*		*Total*	
Percentile Group	*Observed*	*Expected*	*Observed*	*Expected*	*Observed*	*Expected*	*Observed*	*Expected*
0–9	2	3.5	1	4.1	0	1.5	5	8.8
10–24	7	8.5	10	10.3	3	3.3	20	21.1
25–49	21	21.4	31	26.2	9	7.5	52	53.7
50–74	43	34.5	43	39.6	15	10.9	95	84.5
75–89	31	33.4	32	35.1	6	9.5	92	78.6
>90	40	45.4	39	40.8	11	12.0	80	101.5
Total	144	146.6*	156	156.2*	44	44.6*	344	348.2
Incidence Ratio, top decile†/average	2.8		2.5		2.5		2.3	
Incidence Ratio, top-quartile/bottom quartile	7.9		6.5		5.7		6.9	

*Differs from sum of table by 0.1 due to rounding off.
†Top decile obtained when population ranked according to expected incidence.

Table 4. *Standardized Beta Coefficients* of the Multiple Logistic Risk Function*

Variables	40–49	50–59	>60	Total†
	Age, yr			
Age in 1963	0.16‡	0.19		0.31
Wt/ht², gm/sq cm	0.33	0.38	0.27	0.36
PVD-IC, 0-1	0.17	0.14	0.32	0.18
Cholesterol, mg/100 ml		0.16	0.29	0.15
SBP, mm Hg	0.22			0.10
Uric acid, mg/100 ml	0.28			0.13
Hemoglobin, mg/100 ml		0.22		
Born in Europe, 0-1	−0.26			−0.20
Education, 0-low to 9-high	−0.22	−0.26		−0.22

*Coefficient of the estimated logistic risk function, discriminant analysis multiplied by the standard deviation of the population in the particular age group.
†Calculated by a discriminant analysis on the total data.
‡Coefficients 2.327 times (or more) their SE are in bold face type, corresponding to approximate .01 level of significance (one-sided). Coefficients between 1.645 and 2.327 times their SE are in roman type, corresponding to approximate .05 level of significance (one-sided). Coefficients less than 1.645 their SE are (ie, not significantly different from 0) are not included.

top quartile compared to those in the bottom quartile declines with age and ranges from 7.9 in the 40 to 49 age group to 5.7 in the 60 and older group with an overall ratio of top to bottom quartiles of 6.9.

The standardized beta coefficients of the multiple risk function are shown in Table 4. The significant variables at the .01 level are (1) age; (2) weight/height² (wt/ht²); (3) peripheral vascular disease-intermittent claudication (PVD-IC); (4) total serum cholesterol level; (5) born outside Europe (ie, in Asia, north Africa, or Israel); and (6) low educational level. The significant variables at the .05 level are (7) systolic blood pressure and (8) uric acid level. (The assumption is that these coefficients are approximately normally distributed with a mean of 0 [under the hypothesis of no association] and one-side single-comparison levels are used. The latter point is important because significance is "too easily" determined, in the case of a multiple-comparison situation.)

Figure 1 shows the effect or the theoretical possibility of developing diabetes in five years by multiple combinations of raising one or more of these six major risk factors 1.645σ above the average (equal 95th percentile) level for this population. If all eight factors are average, then the probability of developing diabetes is 32/1,000. With any one of these factors raised above average, the rate will rise. For example, the presence of PVD-IC brings the rate up 90/1,000. When more than one is elevated, the risk rises still higher (eg, with wt/ht² raised to the 90th percentile point and PVD-IC present, the rate goes up to 151/1,000). With six variables elevated, the rate rises to 408/1,000 (13 times the average). On the other hand, a reduction of the same six to 1.645σ below the average (equal 5th percentile) reduces the probability of developing diabetes to 17/1,000.

An overweight and peripheral vascular disease were the two factors most highly associated with the development of diabetes,[7] the probability or risk of developing the condition in five years by different

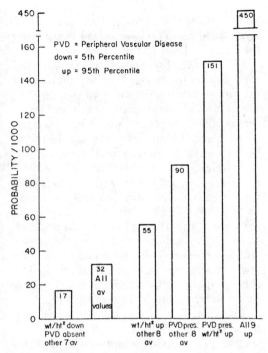

Fig. 1. Probability of developing diabetes mellitus within five years, based on overweight, PVD-IC, and other major variables.

categories of these two variables was examined. Table 5 shows a rise for each, independently of the other, within age groups, and a proportionately higher rise when both are high.

Comment

The term "diabetes mellitus" is used in different contexts to denote different things. Does it, for example, refer to a disease entity or to "hyperglycemia" or "glucose intolerance"? Is there any difference between hyperglycemic people with and without clinical signs and symptoms? Should the term "diabetes mellitus" be confined only to people with hyperglycemia and clinical signs and symptoms?[3] The vast literature on this subject suggests the existence of various types of diabetes, viz:

1. Potential—eg, a child whose parents are diabetics or the identical twin of a diabetic individual.
2. Latent—those with an abnormal GTT under conditions of stress, eg, during pregnancy, infections, or obesity, but whose GTT often returns to normal on improvement of the condition.
3. Asymptomatic, chemical, or subclinical—those with a diabetic response to a GTT but with no clinical signs or symptoms.
4. Prediabetes—the period in the life of a diabetic before clinical signs and symptoms are discovered (some authors in-

Table 5. *Five-Year Incidence by Peripheral Vascular Disease Intermittent Claudication, Weight/Height Index, and Age*

Age, yr	PVD-IC Absent		PVD-IC Present		Total	
	No.	Rate/ 1,000	No.	Rate/ 1,000	No.	Rate/ 1,000
40–49						
Wt/ht²*	1,775	15	28	36	1,803	15
Wt/ht²†	1,741	29	39	51	1,780	30
Wt/ht²‡	1,603	45	24	125	1,627	46
50–59						
Wt/ht²*	1,002	31	36	0	1,038	30
Wt/ht²†	1,112	46	38	79	1,150	47
Wt/ht²‡	1,158	67	44	159	1,202	71
>60						
Wt/ht²*	265	42	16	(125)§	281	46
Wt/ht²†	288	52	16	(0)	304	49
Wt/ht²‡	261	65	16	(188)	277	72
Total						
Wt/ht²*	3,042	22	80	38	3,122	23
Wt/ht²†	3,141	37	93	54	3,234	38
Wt/ht²‡	3,022	55	84	155	3,106	58

*Wt/ht² indicates values of 2.417 or less.
†Wt/ht² indicates values between 2.417 and 2.703.
‡Wt/ht² indicates values above 2.703.
§( ) indicates rates based on small numbers.

clude "potential" and "latent" diabetics in this category).

5. Abnormal but not diabetic GTT with or without clinical features—among adults, about 25 percent developed diabetic GTT curves within two years.[9]

6. Clinical diabetic patients with hyperglycemia and clinical signs and symptoms. This category may be divided into two large groups: a group with clinical signs and symptoms attributable to a deranged metabolism of foodstuffs and with moderate to severe changes in glucose tolerance, and a group with abnormal vascular changes and abnormal responses to GTT but whose hyperglycemia per se is mild or moderate. The severity of the vascular changes is not usually reflected in the severity of the "glucose intolerance."[10]

The question whether the middle-aged and elderly who are asymptomatic but have abnormal responses to an oral GTT should be called diabetic is a difficult one. The aging process itself results in a diminished tolerance to orally administered glucose and a diminution in the renal clearance.[8] This suggests that, if people lived long enough, the vast majority would perhaps develop hyperglycemia as currently defined. On the other hand, a majority of asymptomatic hyperglycemics at GTT become overtly diabetic with symptoms during the subsequent five to ten years.[8] For the purposes of the present study," diabetes mellitus" included all subjects with hyperglycemia or glucose intolerance who adhered to our definition regardless of any other clinical symptoms or signs.

Looking at mortality and morbidity, we note that the mortality attributed to diabetes in Israel is 3.6/100,000 population and is near the lower end of the 1964 international scale that varies from a high in Malta (43.0/100,000) to a low 1.6 in Iceland.[11] These figures, however, must be accepted with caution, due to national differences in medical care, classification, and notification. Morbidity varies even more, from a low of 0.3/1,000 among the Eskimos of Greenland[11] to a fantastic 450/1,000 among the Pima Indians of the United States.[12]

The results of this study have confirmed the fact that overweight is the major factor in the development of diabetes among men.[13] (An ideal index of overweight is one that is highly correlated with weight but not with height. The index wt/ht^2 was found to be the one that best satisfies these criteria.[7]) Overweight may be of two types. The common type is characterized by excessive weight gain early in life that reaches a peak in early adult life and remains more or less constant thereafter. This pattern is paralleled by the cellularity of the fat deposits, which increase in size until early adult life and thereafter remain constant.[14] The other type is characterized by relatively rapid weight gain during middle-age.

The fact that "total calories" (reflecting usual current diet) was not found to be associated with the development of diabetes might suggest that most of the overweight subjects were of the first type. However, whichever type is referred to, the overweight diabetics exhibit not only hyperglycemia but also hyperinsulinemia as shown by abnormal insulin curves during GTT.[9,13,15] This would indicate that there is a relative ineffectiveness of the circulating insulin,[13,15] regardless of the actual site of the anti-insulin effect.[15]

An interesting theory based on animal experiments[13] and results of studies in various parts of the world[16-19] has been developed by Neel.[19] He suggested that, in a population with an excessive prevalence of inappropriate hyperglycemia, the major environmental event may have been a relatively sudden change. From the conditions existing through many generations that required hard physical work, with overall restricted and irregular availability of food, they changed to conditions of essentially unrestricted food availability throughout the year and greatly decreased need for physical activity. In other words, overweight diabetics might represent the detrimental aspect of a "thrifty genotype" unmasked by an environmental change characterized by unrestricted availability of food. Put in another way, obese diabetics might represent "failures of adaptation" to the relatively rapid transition to a sedentary existence combined with a relatively high caloric intake.[19] This might partly explain the very high prevalence of diabetes and obesity among the Indians in South Africa,[16] the Maoris in New Zealand,[18] the North American Pima Indians,[17] and some black people in the United States.

This theory of "thrifty genotype" or "failure of adaptation" might have some relevance to the study population born in Africa or Asia (relatively underdeveloped areas) who then immigrated to a somewhat more developed country (Israel). Although the food supply in Israel has not always been unrestricted, nor is their existence a sedentary one, generally speaking more food is available and less exercise is experienced than in countries of origin. Similar changes have occurred within Israel itself as it has moved from an underdeveloped to a developed status. The type of food available is also different, but there is no evidence to confirm the theory that diabetes is due only to excess of sugar ingestion.[20] Animal experiments further show that many rodent species transferred from their wild environment to caged living conditions tend to become obese. This is particularly pronounced when the normal habitat is the desert or semidesert, arid regions. Thus, diabetes is most severe in animals directly transferred and in the first generation raised in the laboratory. The hyperglycemic syndrome then tends to become milder and disappear in the subsequent laboratory-raised generations.[13]

The present study[4] showed a rise in diabetes incidence in the first generation born in Israel, but there was no drop in the second as postulated earlier. This might mean, however, that, whereas in these small laboratory animals it took only two generations to adapt to the new conditions, in man it might take longer.

Peripheral vascular disease in various forms has traditionally been regarded as a complication of diabetes. There is no doubt that it is a frequent accompaniment of diabetes, but a few unusual features have been recognized in the last few years. These are the following: (a) "the great majority of diabetic patients with peripheral occlusive arterial disease display a mild form of diabetes, as defined by minimal or even no insulin requirements",[10] (b) many patients with peripheral vascular disease are found to have abnormal GTT results or develop abnormal responses to GTT with the passage of time; and (c) the evidence that "good control" of diabetes prevents, delays, or even diminishes the signs or effects of vascular disease is very tenuous.[21]

These facts make it "impossible at this time to state whether insulin failure and vascular disease arise from a common cause or from different causes, or whether they are interdependent."[21]

This has turned the attention of many to changes in the basement membrane, particularly with respect to the mode of action of insulin and other hormones, as well as the development of vascular abnormalities in long-term diabetes.[22]

Electron microscopic studies of capillaries of the eyes, kidneys, and muscles, suggest that, in the majority of new juvenile diabetics, the basement membrane changes occur secondarily to the onset of the disease. There is no evidence that this is the case in maturity-onset diabetes; but as the latter develop during a period of many years probably from a state of prediabetes, it is still not certain from microscopic studies, if the basement membrane changes of the blood vessels occur primarily or secondarily to the disease process.[22]

It looks, therefore, as if the possibilities regarding the metabolic and vascular changes are (1) interrelated and interdependent, which raises the question of which is more basic and preceded the other; (2) not related but are both associated with an end result termed "glucose intolerance"; or (3) interrelated but not interdependent, ie, they may develop independently but, once present, often affect, aggravate, and even lead to the other. Our results show that signs of peripheral vascular disease can and do precede the development of glucose intolerance (with or without other metabolic effects) by some years. This does not mean that there were no metabolic changes affecting the basement membrane of the peripheral vessels even before an obvious change in glucose intolerance was noticed. Combining the results of this study with clinical experience suggests that the third possibility most closely fits known facts. That is, the metabolic and vascular changes can and evidently do develop independently of each other.

Previous publications have shown an association between the group means of area of birth and Quetelet index (wt/ht^2)[7]; African- and Israeli-born have the highest indexes. There is a similar association between area of birth and educational level. African- and Asian-born have proportionately many more subjects in the lower education categories. In the multivariate analysis, however, these variables are independently associated with the development of diabetes. The relationship does not seem to be mediated through diet. None of the many dietary variables investigated, including total calories, total carbohydrates, and sugar consumption, were found to be significantly associated with the incidence of diabetes.

Blood pressure and cholesterol levels, two of the major factors associated with manifestations of atherosclerosis in the brain, heart, and limbs[23,24] are associated too with diabetes incidence in this study. This might suggest that blood pressure and cholesterol are implicated in the production of peripheral vascular disease, which is a precursor of diabetes. This, however, would be an oversimplification, as overweight is also associated with high levels of blood pressure and lipids, suggesting a type of relationship as depicted in Fig. 2.

The role of uric acid level is another perplexing subject, and the theory that it is involved in the prediabetic state with a subsequent fall after the onset of diabetes due to a "competition" in the tubular excretion of uric acid and glucose is an intriguing one.[25,26]

Most experienced clinicians are well aware that stressful situations can cause alterations in the blood and urinary glucose levels of their diabetic patients. This has been confirmed experimentally by Hinkle and Wolf[27] and Wolff and Thomas.[28] It was therefore disappointing not to find any significant associations between psychosocial factors (as reported by the subjects) and development of diabetes. Only one area (brooding when hurt by family members or their bosses) was associated, but as there was no hypothesis regarding this, it could well be a chance finding from the multitude of variables tested.

The findings from this multivariate analysis have implications for the clinician and are as follows:

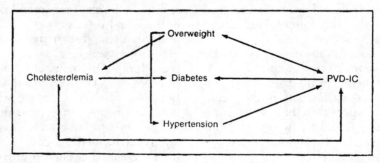

Fig. 2. Relationship between blood pressure, lipid levels, and overweight.

1. They provide the clinician with the major factors that need to be considered for the prevention or early detection of adult onset diabetes.
2. They have reaffirmed the extreme importance of overweight.
3. They point to the importance of the probably independent role of peripheral vascular disease.
4. They suggest that this type of diabetes is probably the end result of a number of different paths of changes, affecting and affected by both metabolic and vascular changes.
5. They suggest that, since neither diet nor smoking were implicated in the development of diabetes, the relationship with atherosclerosis might be via processes that are associated with overweight, blood pressure, and cholesterol increase.
6. They provide a scale of probability of risk for diabetes. The suggested risk function enables one to rank (in Israel, at least) any group of males of this age group in approximate order of risk for diabetes.

Statistical Analysis

The main issue of the analysis in this report is to relate five-year incidence of diabetes simultaneously to antecedent measurements, among which certain correlations exist. Some adjustment needs to be made for these intercorrelations. Obviously, by breaking the data down into different subgroups, it is not possible to stay within adequate cell sizes. An alternative logistic multivariate approach has been provided by Cornfield et al[5] for the bivariate case. Truett et al[6] generalized that approch for a number of variables exceeding two. Kahn et al.,[3] performing a multivariate analysis on two-year diabetes incidence data from this study, have already provided detailed discussion of the logistic multivariate model. Briefly, the model requires that the two matrices of covariance be identical in the eventually diabetic ("ill") portion of the population and in the eventually nondiabetic ("well") portion of it, viz, all others except patients with abnormal GTT results not classified as diabetics and the sum of

$$\alpha + \sum_{i=1}^{n} \beta_i \chi_i$$

have a univariate normal distribution, where β ($i = 1 \ldots n$) are the risk coefficient in the logistic function, dependent on the means and the common covariance matrix, and α is a function of the two latter magnitudes as well as of the sizes of the "ill" and "well" population. The α and the β, appear in the multiple logistic function in the following form: P (probability to develop diabetes in five years)

$$= 1/[1 + \exp(-\alpha - \sum_{i=1}^{n} \beta_i \chi_i)],$$

where χ_i, $i = 1 \ldots n$ are the values of n "predicting variables" for an individual whose theoretical probability we are estimating.

Since it is possible to summarize such probabilities over arbitrary percentiles of a sample, one can compare them to the actual number of incidence cases within these groups, thereby obtaining an estimate of the "degree of fit" between expected and observed incidence. A usual χ^2 test goodness-of-fit does not apply here, hence the "eyeball" character of this comparison.[29] Apart from the matter of "a good fit," viz, close agreement between observed and expected values in percentiles, a second measure is of interest. That measure relates to "the degree of discrimination" or the sharpness of the "risk gradient."[30,31] The latter property can be absent despite the presence of a good "fit" and vice versa. It could be expressed in several ways, eg, ratio of the incidence observed in the top theoretical decile (or quartile) to that observed in the bottom decile (or quartile) or to the overall incidence.

Prior to employing the multiple risk function, a linear regression was run where the dependent variable equals 1 for diabetes incidence cases and 0 for others. The "independent" variables (ie, on the right side of the regression equation) were those found statistically significant in the univariate analysis, excluding the subset described above.

These variables were age; born in Europe or elsewhere; educational level; marital status; wt/ht^2; systolic blood pressure; systolic blood pressure lability; PVD-IC; left axis deviation on resting electrocardiogram; angina pectoris; pulse rate; total serum cholesterol value; uric acid level; hemoglobin value; smoking; "brooding"; total calories; and total carbohydrates.

It can be shown that coefficients obtained using such a linear regression are approximately proportional to those of the multiple logistic function. We then picked the nine variables still significant at .05 for the overall population, or at .01 for at least one age group, and computed multiple three logistic functions for each of the age groups. The standardized risk coefficients (β_i times the standard deviation of variable i) are shown in Table 4.

Acknowledgment

This study is a collaborative project between the National Heart and Lung Institute, Bethesda, Md, the Hadassah Medical Organization, and the Ministry of Health, Jerusalem, Israel, and is supported by PL480 Counterpart Funds, Research Agreement 375,106.

REFERENCES

1. Major RH: Classic Descriptions of Disease, ed 3. Springfield, Ill, Charles C Thomas Publisher, 1955
2. Groen JJ, Medalie JH, Neufeld HN, et al.: An epidemiologic investigation of hypertension and ischemic heart disease within a defined segment of the adult male population of Israel. Isr J Med Sci 4:177-194, 1968
3. Kahn HA, Herman JB, Medalie JH, et al.: Factors related to diabetes incidence: A multivariate analysis of two years observation on 10,000 men. J. Chron Dis 23:617-629, 1971
4. Medalie JH, Papier C, Herman JB, et al.: Diabetes mellitus among 10,000 adult men: I. Five-year incidence and associated variables. Isr J Med Sci 10:681-697, 1974
5. Cornfield J, Gordon T, Smith WW: Quantal response curves for experimentally uncontrolled variables. Bull Int Stat Inst 38:97-115, 1961
6. Truett J, Cornfield J, Kannel W: A multivariate analysis of the risk of coronary heart disease in Framingham. J Chron Dis 20:511-524, 1967
7. Goldbourt U, Medalie JH: Weight-height indices: The choice of the most suitable index and its association with selected variables among 10,000 adult males of heterogeneous origin. Br J Soc Prev Med 28:116-126, 1974
8. Jackson WPU, Vinik AI: Hyperglycemia and diabetes in the elderly, in Ellenberg M, Rifkin H (eds): Diabetes Mellitus: Theory and Practice, New York, McGraw-Hill Book Co Inc, 1970
9. Herman JB, Medalie JH, Rabin D: The problem of abnormal glucose tolerance. Isr J Med Sci 8:915, 1972
10. Haimovici H: Peripheral arterial disease in diabetes mellitus, in Ellenberg M, Rifkin H (eds): Diabetes Mellitus: Theory and Practice. New York, McGraw-Hill Book Co Inc, 1970
11. McDonald GW: The epidemiology of diabetes, in Ellenberg M, Rifkin H (eds): Diabetes Mellitus: Theory and Practice. New York, McGraw-Hill Book Co Inc, 1970
12. Sievers ML: Disease patterns among Southeastern Indians. Pub Health Rep 81:1075-1085, 1966
13. Renold AE, Stauffacher W, Cahill JFG: Diabetes mellitus, in Stanbury JB, Wyngarden JB, Fredrickson DA (eds): The Metabolic Basis of Inherited Disease, ed 3. New York, McGraw-Hill Book Co Inc, 1972
14. Hirsch JL, Knittle JL, Salans LB: Cell lipid content and cell number in obese and non-obese human adipose tissue. J Clin Invest 45:1023, 1966
15. Mirsky IA: Certainties and uncertainties in diabetes mellitus in Ellenberg M, Rifkin H (eds): Diabetes Mellitus: Theory and Practice. New York, McGraw-Hill Book Co Inc, 1970
16. Campbell G: Diabetes in Asians and Africans in and around Durban. S Afr Med J 37:1195-1208, 1963

17. Genuth SM, Bennett PH, Miller M, et al: Hyperinsulinism in obese diabetic Pima Indians. Metabolism 16:1010–1015, 1967
18. Prior IAM, Davidson F: The epidemiology of diabetes in Polynesians and Europeans in New Zealand and the Pacific. NZ Med J 65:375–383, 1966
19. Neel JV: Diabetes mellitus: A "thrifty" genotype rendered detrimental by progress. Am J Hum Genet 14:353–362, 1962
20. Cohen AM: Prevalence of diabetes among different Jewish groups in Israel. Metabolism 10:50–58, 1961
21. Knowles HC: Control of diabetes and the progression of vascular disease, in Ellenberg M, Rifkin H (eds): Diabetes Mellitus: Theory and Practice. New York, McGraw-Hill Book Co Inc, 1970
22. Hanson RO, Lundback K: The basement membrane morphology in diabetes mellitus, in Ellenberg M, Rifkin H (eds): Diabetes Mellitus: Theory and Practice. New York, McGraw-Hill Book Co Inc, 1970
23. Gordon T, Kannel WB: Predisposition to atherosclerosis in the head, heart and legs. JAMA 221:661–666, 1972
24. Medalie JH, Kahn HA, Neufeld HN, et al: Five-year myocardial infarction incidence: II. Association of single variables by age and birthplace. J Chron Dis 26:329–349, 1973
25. Herman JB, Mount FW, Medalie JH, et al: Diabetes prevalence and serum uric acid: Observations among 10,000 men in a survey of ischemic heart disease in Israel. Diabetes 16:858–868, 1967.
26. Herman JB, Keynan A: Hyperglycemia and uric acid. Isr J Med Sci 5:1048–1052, 1969
27. Hinkle LE Jr, Wolf S: Studies in diabetes mellitus: Changes in glucose ketone, and water metabolism during stress. Proc A Res Nerv Ment Dis 29:338–389, 1950
28. Wolff HG, Thomas C: Stress and Disease. Springfield, Ill, Charles C Thomas Publisher, 1953
29. Halperin M, Blackwelder WC, Verter JI: Estimation of the multivariate logistic risk function: A comparison of the discriminant function and minimum likelihood approaches. J Chron Dis 24:125–158, 1971
30. Kleinbaum DG, Kupper LL, Cassel JC, et al: Multivariate analysis of risk of coronary heart disease in Evans County, Georgia. Arch Intern Med 128:943–948, 1971
31. Goldbourt U, Medalie JH, Neufeld HN: Clinical myocardial infarction over a five-year period: III. A multivariate analysis of incidence. J Chron Dis, 28:217–237, 1975

A Randomized Controlled Trial of Aspirin in the Prevention of Early Mortality in Myocardial Infarction*

P. C. Elwood, W. O. Williams

A randomized controlled trial is reported in which a single dose of aspirin (300 mg) was given to patients with myocardial infarction on first contact with a general practitioner. A total of 1,705 patients with confirmed infarction were studied, and survival ascertained. There was no evidence of benefit from the aspirin.

Introduction

There is growing evidence about the beneficial effect of aspirin on mortality from myocardial infarction, presumably through its inhibitory effect on platelet aggregation (Verstraete, 1976). No trial has yet reported results which are statistically significant, yet the available data show remarkable consistency. Thus a 24 percent reduction in mortality by aspirin during the year after infarction was reported by Elwood and colleagues (1974) and subsequent trials have reported reductions of 30 percent (Coronary Drug Project Research Group, 1976) and 42 percent (Breddin et al., 1977).

All this evidence relates to prevention, albeit secondary prevention. There are reasons, however, which make an effect on early mortality following infarction possible. These reasons relate to three possible mechanisms. First, an early dose of an antiplatelet drug could reduce the eventual size of the thrombus in the coronary circulation. Secondly, there is evidence that infarction can precede thrombosis (Warren, 1973) and in patients in whom this is the sequence, early aspirin could inhibit or limit

thrombosis. Thirdly, Hughes and Tonks (1968) have described intravascular platelets clumping in experimental animals, and Haerem (1974) has described platelet aggregates and micro-thrombi in the intramyocardial vessels in fatal coronary disease in humans. While Haerem postulates that this may be a mechanism in sudden death from arrhythmia, it could be that an early dose of an anti-platelet drug could reduce further platelet aggregation and hence either reduce the eventual size of an infarct or reduce the risk of arrhythmia.

For these reasons we decided to set up a trial to test the hypothesis that a dose of aspirin given soon after the onset of symptoms of myocardial infarction would reduce mortality.

Method

We wrote to all the members of the Royal College of General Practitioners. The trial was described and cooperation invited. Those who agreed to help were sent six sealed envelopes, each containing two capsules of either aspirin 300 mg or matching placebo, at random. These were to be given on first contact with any patient who it was believed might have suffered a myocardial infarct. A short record form was enclosed, with a stamped addressed envelope for its return, asking for identification details and a few clinical details. One month after the admission of a patient to the trial we wrote to the general practitioner to find out whether the patient had died or survived. In addition we asked the doctor whether or not any evidence confirming infarction had

*Reprinted by permission from *Journal of the Royal College of General Practitioners* 29:413–416, 1979.

become available after the initial record had been sent in. Confirmatory evidence was sought at several levels of certainty and this was indicated in the enquiry, but we did not ask for fine detail. We accepted any evidence judged by the doctor himself to have confirmed the occurrence of infarction. This included the course of the illness, the opinion of a hospital consultant physician, and ECG or enzyme changes judged to indicate infarction.

The certified cause of death was not ascertained for all deaths though it was given for many by the doctor. We assumed that deaths from causes other than coronary thrombosis were very few, which seems a reasonable assumption with regard to very early deaths.

Results

Of the 2,530 patients admitted to the trial, no confirmatory evidence of myocardial infarction was later reported in 825 (422 were given aspirin, 403 placebo). Thus the analysis was based on 1,705 patients (about 67 percent), 1,279 males and 426 females.

Table 1 sets out the mortality in males and Table 2 in females. There is no evidence of benefit in either sex. Tables 3 and 4 set out the same analysis for patients who

Table 1. *Cumulative Mortality in Males during the 28 Days Following the Giving of 300 mg Aspirin or Matching Placebo (Percentages are Given in Brackets)*

	Given Aspirin	Given Placebo
Number of Confirmed Myocardial Infarctions	608	671
Cumulative deaths		
Same day	48 *(7.9)*	53 *(7.9)*
Same day +1	56 *(9.2)*	68 *(10.1)*
Same day +2	67 *(11.0)*	76 *(11.3)*
Same day +3	73 *(12.0)*	80 *(11.9)*
Same day +28	114 *(18.8)*	129 *(19.1)*

Table 2. *Cumulative Mortality in Females during the 28 Days Following the Giving of 300 mg Aspirin or Matching Placebo (Percentages are Given in Brackets)*

	Given Aspirin	Given Placebo
Number of Confirmed Myocardial Infarctions	219	207
Cumulative deaths		
Same day	18 *(8.2)*	15 *(7.2)*
Same day +1	23 *(10.5)*	21 *(10.1)*
Same day +2	25 *(11.4)*	22 *(10.6)*
Same day +3	27 *(12.3)*	25 *(12.1)*
Same day +28	45 *(20.5)*	43 *(20.8)*

Table 3. *Cumulative Mortality in Males who had Received Treatment within Four Hours of the Onset of Symptoms (Percentages are Given in Brackets)*

	Given Aspirin	Given Placebo
Number of Confirmed Myocardial Infarctions	329	404
Cumulative deaths		
Same day	33 *(10.0)*	41 *(10.1)*
Same day +1	39 *(11.9)*	51 *(12.6)*
Same day +2	45 *(13.7)*	56 *(13.9)*
Same day +3	47 *(14.3)*	58 *(14.4)*
Same day +28	70 *(21.3)*	88 *(21.8)*

Table 4. *Cumulative Mortality in Females who had Received Treatment within Four Hours of the Onset of Symptoms (Percentages are Given in Brackets)*

	Given Aspirin	Given Placebo
Number of Confirmed Myocardial Infarctions	124	118
Cumulative deaths		
Same day	11 *(8.9)*	8 *(6.8)*
Same day +1	14 *(11.3)*	12 *(10.2)*
Same day +2	15 *(12.1)*	13 *(11.0)*
Same day +3	16 *(12.9)*	13 *(11.0)*
Same day +28	23 *(18.5)*	26 *(22.0)*

Table 5. *Cumulative Mortality in Patients who had Had an Initial Blood Pressure of 100 mm Hg Systolic or Less*
(Percentages are Given in Brackets)

	Males		Females	
	Given Aspirin	Given Placebo	Given Aspirin	Given Placebo
Number of Confirmed Myocardial Infarctions	77	85	23	24
Cumulative mortality				
Same day	10 (*13.0*)	11 (*12.9*)	3	1
Same day +1	12 (*15.6*)	18 (*21.2*)	0	0
Same day +2	16 (*20.8*)	20 (*23.5*)	0	0
Same day +3	17 (*22.1*)	22 (*25.9*)	0	0
Same day +28	26 (*33.8*)	31 (*36.5*)	9	2

had been seen initially, and who had received treatment within four hours of the onset of symptoms. Again there is no evidence of benefit from aspirin.

Based on the assumption that a low blood pressure indicates a serious infarct, Table 5 set out the deaths in patients who had had a blood pressure on first examination of 100 mm Hg systolic or less. The numbers are small, especially in females, but again there is no evidence of benefit.

Discussion

These results give no encouragement to the use of aspirin in the early treatment of myocardial infarction. There are, however, several limitations to the study.

Although only a small dose of aspirin was used, it was about three times the dose found effective in preventing platelet aggregation. It has been shown repeatedly that doses of aspirin over about 100 mg have a profound effect on platelet aggregation (Rowan et al., 1976). The effect occurs as early as 15 minutes after an oral dose (Stuart, 1970) and can be detected for at least two days subsequently (Burch et al., 1977).

We decided to use a 300 mg dose of aspirin in this trial because it would probably not only be ethically acceptable to most doctors but also large enough to have the desired effect on platelets. It is possible that this dose, while sufficient to affect platelet aggregation in a normal person, may not be sufficient to suppress gross aggregation heralding an infarction. However, recent discussions on aspirin have noted an effect on the vessel wall which may not be beneficial, and the use of a low dose at infrequent intervals has been strongly recommended (Moncada and Vane, 1978).

A beneficial effect of aspirin in myocardial infarction has not been established beyond all reasonable doubt. Nevertheless, the evidence available to us when we proposed the trial was highly suggestive and since then further confirmatory evidence has been reported. This is all consistent with a preventive effect and comes from trials in patients who have already had one infarct.

The possibility remains that a drug which has a direct anti-arrhythmic effect might be of value in the acute situation following an infarct. It would be reasonable to consider the possibility of conducting a similar study using a drug with an anti-arrhythmic effect.

Acknowledgments

We are grateful to the staff at the headquarters of the Royal College of General Practitioners for their help in contacting members of the College, and we are most grateful to the members who co-operated in the trial. Nicholas Research Laboratories kindly supplied capsules of aspirin and placebo and Mr M. P. Mitchell and Mr C. M. Kloosterman of Whitchurch Hospital Pharmacy film-packed these.

REFERENCES

Breddin, K., Oherla, K. & Walter, E. (1977). German-Austrian Multicenter two years' prospective study on the prevention of secondary myocardial infarction by ASA in comparison to 'Phenprocounon' and placebo. Report of German Austrian Study Group. Sixth International Congress on Thrombosis and Haemostasis. Thrombosis Haemostasis, 38, 168(A)

Burch, J. W., Standford, N. & Majerus, P. W. (1977). Inhibition of platelet cyclo-oxygenase by oral aspirin. Clinical Research, 25, 513(A)

Coronary Drug Project Research Group (1976). Aspirin in coronary heart disease. Journal of Chronic Diseases, 29, 625–642

Elwood, P. C., Cochrane, A. L., Burr, M. L., Sweetnam, P. M. et al. (1974). A randomized controlled trial of acetyl-salicylic acid in the secondary prevention of mortality from myocardial infarction. British Medical Journal, 1, 436–440

Haerem, J. W. (1974). Platelet aggregates and mural micro-thrombi in the early stages of acute fatal coronary disease. Thrombosis Research, 5, 243–249

Hughes, A. & Tonks, R. S. (1968). Lung and heart lesions from intravascular platelet clumping and its sequelae. Journal of Pathology and Bacteriology, 95, 523–526

Moncada, S. & Vane, J. R. (1978). Unstable metabolites of arachidoric acid and their role in haemostasis and thrombosis. British Medical Bulletin, 34, 129–135

Rowan, R. M., McDonald, G. A., Renton, R. L. & Corne, S. J. (1976). Inhibition of platelet release reaction by acetyl-salicylic acid. Postgraduate Medical Journal, 52, 71–75

Stuart, K. (1970). Platelet function studies in human beings receiving 300 mg of aspirin per day. Journal of Laboratory and Clinical Medicine, 75, 463–471

Verstraete, M. (1976). Are agents affecting platelet functions clinically useful? American Journal of Medicine, 61, 897–914

Warren, J. V. (1973). A revolution in coronary artery disease. Journal of Chronic Diseases, 26, 547–551

Mortality Among Oral-Contraceptive Users*

Royal College of General Practitioners'
Oral Contraception Study†

In a large prospective study carried out in the United Kingdom, the death-rate from diseases of the circulatory system in women who had used oral contraceptives was five times that of controls who had never used them; and the death-rate in those who had taken the pill continuously for 5 years or more was ten times that of the controls. The excess deaths in oral-contraceptive users were due to a wide range of vascular conditions. The total mortality-rate in women who had ever used the pill was increased by 40 per cent, and this was due to an increase in deaths from circulatory diseases of 1 per 5000 ever-users per year. The excess was substantially greater than the death-rate from complications of pregnancy in the controls, and was double the death-rate from accidents. The excess mortality-rate increased with age, cigarette smoking, and duration of oral contraceptive use.

Introduction

The Oral Contraception Study of the Royal College of General Practitioners is a continuing long-term prospective study of approximately 46,000 women of childbearing age in the United Kingdom. It began in 1968 and is designed to evaluate the effects of oral contraceptives on health.

*Reprinted by permission from *The Lancet,* October 8, 1977, pp. 727–731.
†Principal author: Dr. VALERIE BERAL, department of medical statistics and epidemiology, London School of Hygiene and Tropical Medicine, WC1. Director: Dr. CLIFFORD R. KAY, R.C.G.P. Research Unit, Manchester.

Women were recruited by 1400 general practitioners who have recorded all new episodes of illness reported by the study population. A comprehensive account of the illnesses in those using oral contraceptives continuously ("takers"), those who stopped using them during the course of the study ("ex-takers"), and those who had never used them ("controls") was published in May, 1974.[1] This paper discusses the deaths recorded during the follow-up period until June, 1976, which covers some 200,000 women-years of observation.

Methods

The study design, methods of data collection, analytical techniques, and the potential sources of bias have already been discussed in detail.[1] In summary, 23,000 current takers and 23,000 controls who were matched by age and marital status to the takers, were recruited over a 14-month period. Controls who later became oral-contraceptive users were included in the "taker" category from the time of change. Ex-takers who resumed oral-contraceptive use were thereafter excluded from the present analyses. At 6-monthly intervals the general practitioners report on the occurrence of illness, pregnancy, or death and on the details of oral-contraceptive use in the study population. For all deaths the general practitioners report the cause of death in the same format as is required for the death certificate. The underlying cause of death was coded by C. R. K. using the 8th revision of the International Classification of Diseases (I.C.D.) and checked by V.B.

The deaths in the takers, ex-takers, and

controls are related to the respective cumulative calendar-months of observation in each group and expressed as rates per 100,000 women-years. In certain analyses the takers and ex-takers are grouped together as "ever-users". Mortality-rates are standardised by the indirect method,[1] using the total population rates as standard. Seventeen women who died from conditions which had been diagnosed before their recruitment have been excluded from these analyses.

Results

Table 1 compares the mortality-rates from various causes in ever-users of oral contraceptives with those in controls. The number of deaths, mortality-rates, and women-years of observation are shown in Table 1a when all periods of pregnancy and related deaths are excluded, and in table 1b when they are included. When pregnancy is excluded, the total women-years of observation is similar in the ever-users and the controls. The controls have double the pregnancy-rate of the ex-takers, thus, when pregnancy is included the periods of observation are greater in the controls than the ever-users. Irrespective of the inclusion or exclusion of pregnancy, however, there is a 40 per cent increase in total mortality-rate among the ever-users. This is because the increase in the women-years of observation in the controls was accompanied by only 2 additional deaths from complications of pregnancy. (There is no program to standardise the rates for age, parity, smoking, and social class; but standardisation for these factors when pregnancy was excluded had no appreciable effect on the comparisons between the two groups.) Since the inclusion of pregnancy does not alter the

Table 1. *Mortality-Rate per 100,000 Women–Years from Various Causes by Oral-Contraceptive Use*
     (a) excluding pregnancy (standardised for age at entry, parity, social class, and smoking).
     (b) including pregnancy (unstandardised rates).

I.C.D. Code	Cause	Mortality-Rate (No. of Deaths)		Ratio of Rate in Ever-users to Controls
		Ever-users	*Controls*	
(a) 140–209	*All cancers*	15.8 *(14)*	21.1 *(20)*	0.8
390–458	*All diseases of the circulatory system*	25.8 *(24)*	5.5 *(5)*	4.7*
	Non-rheumatic heart-disease and hypertension	10.4 *(11)*	2.5 *(2)*	4.0†
430–438	Cerebrovascular disease	13.2 *(10)*	2.8 *(3)*	4.7†
E800–999	*Accidents and violence*	17.1 *(16)*	10.0 *(9)*	1.7
E800–949; E980	Accidents	9.5 *(9)*	7.6 *(7)*	1.3
E950–999	Suicide	5.3 *(5)*	2.2 *(2)*	2.4
	Other causes	3.0 *(2)*	7.8 *(9)*	0.4
	Total	63.6 *(56)*	46.0 *(43)*	1.4
	Women-years of observation	91,880	91,521	
(b) 630–678	*Complications of pregnancy, childbirth, and puerperium*	0.0	1.8 *(2)*	—
	Total	58.0 *(56)*	40.9 *(45)*	1.4
	Women-years of observation	96,624	110,065	

*p<0.01.
†p<0.05.
Because the rates for each cause are standardised separately there are small discrepancies between the sum of the individual rates and the "total" rates.

comparisons of death-rates in ever-users and controls, and for consistency with earlier reports,[1] all periods of pregnancy and associated deaths are excluded from the subsequent analyses. Table 1a shows that the standardised mortality-rate from the circulatory diseases in ever-users is 4.7 times that of controls, from non-rheumatic heart disease and hypertension it is 4.0 times that of controls, and from cerebrovascular disease it is 4.7 times the control rate. The excess total mortality in ever-users can be accounted for by the excess deaths from circulatory diseases.

Table 2 details the causes of death by oral-contraceptive use. The diversity of circulatory diseases among the oral-contraceptive ever-users is notable, although the number of deaths from any single disease is small.

Table 3 shows the standardised mortality-rates from certain diseases of the circulatory system by contraceptive use at the time of death. The mortality-rate from all circulatory diseases in the takers is 4.9 times that of the controls and in the ex-takers is 4.3 times that of the controls. A review of the records of the 8 ex-takers who died from circulatory diseases revealed that 2 had discontinued oral-contraceptive use when they were found to be hypertensive, and later died of malignant hypertension.

Table 2. *Cause of Death by Oral-Contraceptive Use*

		No. of Deaths	
I.C.D. Code	**Cause**	*Ever-Users*	*Controls*
0,00–090	Infections (1 septicaemia, 1 hepatitis)	0	2
140–209	Malignant disease*	14	20
288	Agranulocytosis	0	1
340	Multiple sclerosis	1	1
400	Malignant hypertension	2	0
410	Acute myocardial infarction	7	2
411	Acute myocardial insufficiency	1	0
425	Cardiomyopathy	1	0
430	Subarachnoid hæmorrhage	9	0
431	Cerebral hæmorrhage	1	2
432	Cerebral thrombosis	0	1
444.2	Mesenteric-artery thrombosis	2	0
450	Pulmonary embolus	1	0
560	Abdominal hernia (postoperative)	0	2
563	Ulcerative colitis	0	1
571	Cirrhosis of liver	1	0
582	Chronic nephritis	0	1
630–678	Complications of pregnancy, childbirth and the puerperium	0	2
796	Ill-defined causes	0	1
E800–949	Accidents	8	6
E950–959	Suicide	5	2
E960–999	Homicide	2	0
E980	Poisoning—reason unknown	1	1
	All causes	56	45

*Cancer deaths in ever users: 1 large intestine; 1 rectum; 1 pancreas; 2 lung; 1 connective tissue; 1 melanoma; 3 breast; 1 cervix; 1 kidney; 1 brain; 1 leukæmia. Cancer deaths in controls: 1 œsophagus; 1 stomach; 1 large intestine; 1 rectum; 1 peritoneum; 2 lung; 6 breast; 3 ovary; 1 vulva; 1 Hodgkin's disease; 2 leukæmia.

Table 3. *Mortality-Rate per 100,000 Women-Years from Various Diseases of the Circulatory System by Contraceptive Use at Time of Death (Standardised for Age at Entry, Parity, Social Class, and Smoking)*

I.C.D. Code	Cause	Mortality-Rate (No. of Deaths)			Ratio of Rate to That of Controls	
		Takers	*Ex-takers*	*Controls*	*Takers*	*Ex-takers*
400–429	*Non-rheumatic heart-disease and hypertension*	12.1 *(8)*	7.6 *(3)*	2.6 *(2)*	4.7*	3.0
400	Malignant hypertension	0.0	3.8 *(2)*	0.0	0.0	..
410	Acute myocardial infarction	8.1 *(6)*	3.3 *(1)*	2.5 *(2)*	3.2	1.3
430–438	*Cerebrovascular disease*	12.4 *(6)*	14.7 *(4)*	2.8 *(3)*	4.4	5.3
430	Subarachnoid hæmorrhage	9.3 *(5)*	15.9 *(4)*	0.0	..*	..*
431–432	Cerebral thrombosis and hæmorrhage	2.6 *(1)*	0.0	2.8 *(3)*	0.9	0.0
440–458	*Other vascular diseases*	2.5 *(2)*	2.9 *(1)*	0.0		..
390–458	*All circulatory diseases*	*26.8 (16)*	*23.9 (8)*	*5.5 (5)*	*4.9†*	*4.3†*

*p < 0.05.
†p < 0.01.

The other 6 ex-takers stopped using oral contraceptives for non-medical reasons. None of the 4 who died of subarachnoid hæmorrhage had been reported to be hypertensive.

Table 4 compares the standardised mortality-rates from circulatory and total diseases in ever-users of oral contraceptives and controls according to the women's cigarette consumption at recruitment into the study. The ratio of the mortality-rate in ever-users to controls is 4.7 to 1 for non-smokers, and 4.4 to 1 for smokers. Because of the small number of deaths in the non-smokers, only the excess deaths in smokers is statistically significant.

Table 5 compares the mortality-rates from circulatory and total diseases in ever-users of oral contraceptives and controls by the women's age at the time of death. The rates increase with age, but at all ages they are higher in ever-users than in controls. When these data were re-analysed, classifying women by their age at entry into the study, a similar increase in each age-specific mortality-rate was noted among the ever-

Table 4. *Mortality-Rate per 100,000 Women-Years from Diseases of Circulatory System (I.C.D. 390–458) and Total Deaths by Smoking Habit at Entry and Oral-Contraceptive Use (Standardised for Age at Entry, Social Class, and Parity)*

Cigarette Smoking at Entry	Cause of Death	Mortality-Rate (No. of Deaths)		Ratio of Rate in Ever-users to Controls
		Ever-users	*Controls*	
Non-smokers	Circulatory	13.8 *(5)*	3.0 *(2)*	4.7
	Total	49.8 *(20)*	36.3 *(23)*	1.4
Smokers	Circulatory	39.5 *(19)*	8.9 *(3)*	4.4†
	Total	76.8 *(36)*	57.9 *(20)*	1.3

†p < 0.01.

Table 5. *Mortality-Rate per 100,000 Women-Years from Diseases of Circulatory System (I.C.D. 390–458) and Total Deaths, by Age at Death (Unstandardised)*

Age	Cause of Death	Mortality-Rate (No. of Deaths) Ever-users	Controls	Ratio of Rate in Ever-users to Controls
15–24	Circulatory	7.5 (1)	0.0	..
	Total	14.9 (2)	11.8 (1)	1.3
25–34	Circulatory	8.8 (4)	4.4 (2)	2.0
	Total	37.5 (17)	24.4 (11)	1.5
35–44	Circulatory	42.6 (12)	9.6 (3)	4.5*
	Total	88.8 (25)	73.4 (23)	1.2
45–49	Circulatory	140.9 (7)	0.0	..*
	Total	241.5 (12)	119.5 (8)	2.0

*p < 0.05.

users; standardisation for smoking, parity, and social class made no important difference to the rates. At present there is no program to standardise the data in Table 5 for these factors, but it is unlikely that the procedure would materially alter the comparisons between ever-users and controls.

Table 6 shows the mortality-rate from circulatory diseases by duration of oral-contraceptive use. The analysis is confined to women who had been using oral contraceptives continuously up to the time of death (takers). With increasing duration of use there is a striking increase in the ratio of the age-standardised mortality-rate of ever-users to that of controls. Those who had taken the pill for 5 years or more experienced a rate which was 9.7 times that of controls. All the deaths in women with a duration of use of 5 years or longer occurred at age 35 or older. As yet there are only small numbers of women under the age of 35 who have taken the pill continuously for this length of time, so their risk cannot be assessed separately.

The relationship of mortality to the type and dose of œstrogen and progestagen was examined. Because of the large number of preparations, the secular trends in œstrogen content of oral contraceptives, and the

Table 6. *Mortality-Rate per 100,000 Women-Years from Diseases of Circulatory System (I.C.D. 390–458) by Duration of Continuous Oral-Contraceptive Use*

Duration of Oral-Contraceptive Use (Mo.)	Mortality Rate (No. of Deaths) Age (at Time of Death) 15–34	35–49*	Age Standardised*	Ratio of Age-Standardised Rates to That of Controls
0	3.7 (2)	7.9 (3)	5.2 (5)	1.0
1–59	8.5 (3)	33.0 (4)	17.5 (7)	3.4
60+	0.0	113.8 (9)	50.5 (9)	9.7

*Tests for linear treands, p < 0.01.

small number of deaths, no clear pattern emerged.

It is also very unlikely that diagnostic biases have occurred in the broad I.C.D. groupings used for these analyses. If the excess deaths from circulatory disease among the oral-contraceptive users were a diagnostic artefact, then it would be expected that the death-rate from all other causes would be correspondingly reduced in ever-users. But the difference in death-rate between ever-users and controls from other conditions is too small to explain the excess of circulatory disease in ever-users. Furthermore, two-thirds of the circulatory deaths were attributed to either myocardial infarction or subarachnoid hæmorrhage, neither of which was suspected as a complication of oral-contraceptive use at the time when most deaths occurred. Nor is there any indication that a differential loss to follow-up between the ever-users and controls could explain these findings. When a woman changes her address and transfers from one general practitioner to another, she is automatically withdrawn from the study. This is responsible for the large majority of the losses to follow-up[1] and they are unlikely to be related to the patient's morbidity or contraceptive use.

An important consideration in interpreting the differences in disease patterns between ever-users and controls is that oral-contraceptive users are a selected population. They are self-selected, as they choose to take the pill, and they are medically selected, as they must obtain a prescription from a doctor. They tend to have had fewer serious past illnesses,[1,2] to use less medications,[8] but to smoke more than non-users.[1,2] Adjustment can be made for the major differences by excluding those with pre-existent disease and standardising for risk factors such as age and smoking habit. Small differences between ever-users and controls may still remain after these adjustments, but they could not explain mortality differentials of the size observed for circulatory diseases. On the other hand, they may explain small differences such as the excess of accidents, suicide, and homicide and the deficiency of cancer and other diseases in the ever-takers. These may be chance findings or they may reflect psychological and other differences between ever-users and controls.

Conclusions

The differences in death-rate from diseases of the circulatory system between ever-users of oral contraceptives and controls is 20 per 100,000 women per year, which represents an increase of 1 death per 5000 ever-users per year. This accounts for the excess total mortality in ever-users (table 1). It is substantially larger than previous estimates which considered only the risks of thromboembolism and myocardial infarction,[9] but is similar to that based on observations of recent trends in mortality among young women.[6] This rate is more than double the mortality-rate from all accidents in the study population. It is also important to note that the increased mortality associated with oral-contraceptive use is much greater than the excess mortality (1.8 per 100,000 women per year) associated with the larger number of pregnancies in the controls.

Although the death-rate from circulatory diseases was increased by 1 death per 5000 ever-users per year, this risk was concentrated in older women, in those with a long duration of oral contraceptive use, and in cigarette smokers. It can be estimated from table 5 that the excess annual death-rate was about 1 per 20,000 ever-users aged 15 to 34, but it increased to 1 per 3000 ever-users at age 35 to 44 and to 1 per 700 at age 45 to 49. Similarly, the excess annual rate was about 1 per 8000 women who had used oral contraceptives continuously for less than 5 years, but 1 per 2000 for continuous users of more than five years duration (Table 6). Also, the excess annual death-rate was 1 per 10,000 ever-users who do not smoke, but 1 per 3000 ever-users who also smoke (Table 4). These estimates are based on small numbers and are necessarily approximate. Without more data it is not possible to examine the interrelationships of age, smoking, and duration of oral-contraceptive use, nor to compare the effect of continuous oral-contraceptive use with intermittent use.

The excess mortality among oral-contraceptive users is of sufficient size to warrant a careful reassessment of pill usage by older women unless there are strong social, personal, or other reasons to use them. It must be stressed that the size of the risks described here are approximate. Moreover, they would not apply in other countries where the prevalence of circulatory disease is different. Continued observation of these and other groups of women will be required to permit a more detailed evaluation of the risks and benefits of oral-contraceptive use.

Discussion

Women who had used oral contraceptives had a mortality-rate from circulatory diseases which was 4.7 times that of women who had never used them. While these and comparable prospective data from the Oxford/Family Planning Association study[2] support the conclusions of earlier case-control studies[3-5] they also indicate that the vascular diseases associated with oral-contraceptive use are more varied than has previously been recognised. The deaths, all in oral-contraceptive users, from sub-arachnoid hæmorrhage, malignant hypertension, cardiomyopathy, and mesenteric-artery thrombosis in this study and from congenital and rheumatic heart-disease in the Oxford study illustrate the diversity. These have occurred despite a lower prevalence of vascular and other circulatory diseases in users than in non-users before recruitment into the studies.[1,2] These findings closely fit Beral's predictions, based on an analysis of mortality trends in young women from twenty-one countries.[6] She suggested that the range of vascular diseases affected by oral-contraceptive use and

the size of the risk involved were substantially greater than the combined risks of thromboembolism and myocardial infarction.

The present findings suggest that the risk of circulatory disease increases with the duration of oral-contraceptive use and may persist after the pill is discontinued. The increased mortality of the ex-takers could not be explained by a transfer of seriously ill women from the "taker" to the "ex-taker" category. The ratio of the mortality-rate from circulatory disease in ex-takers to controls is still 3.7 to 1 even after excluding the 2 deaths from malignant hypertension, where oral-contraceptive use was stopped because of the onset of hypertension. This suggests that oral contraceptives induce changes in the circulatory system which are not immediately reversible. Since only small numbers of deaths are involved and since the relationship of duration of oral contraceptive use to the risk of death from circulatory diseases could be assessed only for women who had used oral contraceptives continuously, it is premature to draw firm conclusions about the long-term and residual vascular effects of oral contraceptives; but clearly they require further study as additional data become available.

The ratio of the death-rate from circulatory diseases in ever-users to that in controls was similar for smokers and non-smokers (Table 4). This suggests that the relative increase in mortality associated with oral-contraceptive use is independent of smoking habit. In contrast, the ratio of the death-rate from circulatory diseases in ever-users to that in controls increased from 2.0 at age 25 to 34 to 4.5 at age 35 to 44 (Table 5). The increase in mortality ratio with age in part reflects the longer average duration of oral-contraceptive use by older women, but the number of deaths is at present too small to permit a detailed analysis of the inter-relationship between age, duration, of oral-contraceptive use and risk of death from circulatory disease.

It is very unlikely that any form of bias could explain these findings. The over-reporting of symptoms by women using oral contraceptives was considered to be the major source of bias in interpreting the morbidity findings in this population;[1] but this is eliminated by confining the analysis to mortality data. General practitioners should find out about all deaths, regardless of where they occur when, as part of the routine administration of the National Health Service, the deceased's name is removed from their practice list. Although the deaths would not be missed, the mortality-rate in this population is lower than that in the general population.[7] This is because, as in the Oxford study,[2] the study population tended to be healthier and of higher social class than the general population, and also because 17 deaths from causes diagnosed before recruitment were excluded from the analyses.

The cause of death used in these analyses is that recorded by the general practitioner. The validity of their recording of diagnoses for hospital admissions has already been demonstrated.[1] To uphold the important principle of confidentiality, which is basic to the conduct of the study, copies of the death certificates have not so far been collected. If the general practitioners agree to divulge the patients' names, it is hoped to examine the consistency of their recording of the cause of death with that recorded on each woman's death certificate. Examination of the source documents suggests no inconsistency between pill users and controls in the manner of recording the causes of death.

Acknowledgments

We thank the 1400 general practitioners who are contributing all the data for this survey. The study is supported by a major grant from the Medical Research Council. The costs of the pilot trials and current supplementary expenditure have been met by the Scientific Foundation Board of the Royal College of General Practitioners. The Board gratefully acknowledge the receipt of funds for research into oral contraception from Organon Laboratories Ltd, Ortho Pharmaceutical Corporation, Schering Chemicals Ltd, G. D. Searle and Co. Ltd, Syntex Pharmaceuticals Ltd, and John Wyeth and Brother Ltd.

Addendum

Since completing this report, we have seen collecting death certificates for a comparison of coding. So far 97 death certificates have been analysed out of 173 deaths among study women in England and Wales (a greater number than has yet been analysed). The coding was identical to ours in 68 (70 per cent). In 28 there were minor differences which would not have affected our analyses. In 1 case a control who had died of cerebral hæmorrhage had been included in our analyses in that category, but obesity had been coded as the underlying cause of death on the certificate. A full account of the comparison of the coding will be published elsewhere.

REFERENCES

1. Royal College of General Practitioners. Oral Contraceptives and Health. Putman: London, 1974
2. Vessey, M. P., McPherson, K., Johnson, H. Lancet, 1977, ii, 731
3. Inman, W. H. W., Vessey, M. P. Br. Med. J. 1968, ii, 193
4. Mann, J. I., Inman, W. H. W. ibid. 1975, ii, 245
5. Collaborative Group for the Study of Stroke in Young Women. JAMA 1975, 231, 718
6. Beral, V. Lancet, 1976, ii, 1047
7. Registrar General's Statistical Review of England and Wales, 1973. H. M. Stationery Office
8. Rabin, D. L., McCarthy, P. Prev. Med. 1974, 3, 268
9. Vessey, M. P., Doll, R. Proc. R. Soc. Lond. B, 1976, 195, 69

The Spectrum of Otitis Media in Family Practice*

Jack Froom, James Mold, Larry Culpepper, and Vincenza Boisseau

Individual and family factors which relate to acute purulent otitis media were investigated in a family practice population. In a practice with more than 11,000 patients, 442 persons had 527 episodes of otitis media during a one-year period. More than 20 percent of the cases occurred in patients of age 15 years and over, but the case rate per year for this group was 11 cases per 1,000 as opposed to 109.7 cases per 1,000 for patients under the age of 15 years. Twenty percent of young children had two or more episodes during the year as compared with five percent for adults. Females had more multiple episodes than did males. The incidence of multiple cases in families is greater than would be expected if cases were distributed randomly (P < 0.05). However, significantly fewer families with three or more children reported cases of otitis media as compared with smaller families (P < 0.05).

Otitis media is an important health problem because of its frequency of occurrence and possible adverse consequences. Although the pathogenesis, causative organisms, associated co-illness factors, and therapy have received careful study, several facets of the disease have been inadequately explored. These include incidence relative to defined populations, presentation in adult patients, and family factors. This communication reports data from the patient population of

Presented in part at a Meeting of the World Organization of National Colleges, Academies and Academic Associations of General Practitioners/Family Physicians (WONCA), Montreux, Switzerland, May 14-19, 1978.
*Reprinted by permission from *The Journal of Family Practice*, 10:599-605, 1980.

the Rochester Family Medicine Medical Center which relates to these several factors.

Literature Review

Acute purulent otitis media is defined by the presence of purulent fluid in the middle ear.[1] Dysfunction and/or obstruction of the eustachian tube are thought to be the principal pathogenic mechanisms. Obstruction may be extrinsic from enlarged adenoids or intrinsic from allergy or infection. Functional obstruction may occur with increased eustachian tube compliance as seen with cleft palate or from nasal obstruction with reduced nasopharyngeal volume, which can result from either allergy or infection.[2] Streptococcus pneumoniae, Haemophilus influenzae, and beta hemolytic streptococci are the organisms most frequently cultured from infected ears, although in up to 44 percent of cases, no pathogenic agent can be identified.[3] The relative frequency of pathogens is age related, with H influenzae more common in young children beyond the sixth week of life. In the first six weeks of life, Escherichia coli, Klebsiella pneumoniae, and Staphylococcus aureus are the predominant organisms.[4] Attempts to isolate viruses and mycoplasmas from middle ear fluid aspirates are largely unsuccessful.[5] Amoxicillin, ampicillin, penicillin V, and erythromycin either alone, or the latter two in combination with sulfa drugs, are effective therapeutic agents depending upon the infecting organisms.[6-8] All antibiotic regimens are more effective than placebo.[9] Myringotomy does not hasten resolution of pathology or improve clinical response, but does relieve discomfort in a small group with severe pain.[10] Chemoprophylaxis can reduce the incidence of recurrent infection.[11,12]

The clinical diagnosis of otitis media is most often made by abnormal appearance of the tympanic membrane. The diagnostic value of specific abnormalities, however, such as redness, distortion of bony landmarks, and impaired mobility, is uncertain.[1] Symptoms of ear pain and fever are confirmatory evidence but appear to vary with the pathogenic organisms. Pneumococcus is more likely to cause severe pain and high fever, whereas infections caused by H influenzae are more likely to be bilateral.[13]

Bottle feeding and feeding infants in a reclined position,[14] allergy,[15] cleft palate,[16] and prematurity[4] predispose to infection. Eskimo and other Alaskan natives, Canadian Indians, and Swedish Lapps all have unusually high incidence of purulent otitis media.[17,18] Although reasons for excessive incidence in these populations are unknown, primitive and crowded housing, poor sanitary conditions, impaired access to medical care, recently increased prevalence of bottle feeding, and racial factors are thought to play a role.[18]

Recurrent or incompletely resolved infection can lead to hearing loss. In one study of children with no preceding history of chronic otitis media or loss of hearing, 12.2 percent had audiometrically demonstrated hearing impairment six months following an acute infection.[19] Hearing loss in children has been correlated with speech problems and reduced scholastic achievement.[20]

Otitis media accounted for over ten million visits (tenth most frequent diagnosis) to United States' office-based physicians during the year May 1973 through April 1974. Twenty-five and one half percent of visits were to general practitioners/family physicians.[21]

Method

Demographic data on all persons who received one or more diagnoses of otitis media during the period July 1, 1975, through June 30, 1976, were retrieved from a computerized diagnostic index.[22] Detailed analyses of the clinical course and management were made from a random sample of medical charts stratified by patient age (94 patients under age 15 and 73 patients age 15 years and over). The 94 patients were a subset of the total cases for the study year. Appropriateness of diagnosis and therapy (for the subset) was judged using a protocol developed by a group of family physicians, pediatricians, and otolaryngologists (Appendix).[23]

Results

From a practice population of over 11,000 patients, 442 persons had 527 episodes and 849 visits for acute purulent otitis media during a one-year period. The age and sex distribution of these patients is given in Table 1. Of interest is that 21.5 percent of affected persons were aged 15 years and over. This group, however, comprises 73.1 percent of the patient population and the case rate difference between the two age groups (under 15 years vs 15 years and over) is considerable (109.7 vs 11.0 cases per 1000 per year).

Table 2 details recurrences during a one-year period. Approximately 20 percent of young children had two or more

Table 1. *Age/Sex Distribution of Patients with Otitis Media: 1975–1976 (in Percent of Total Cases)**

Age Group (Years)	Male N = 221	Female N = 221	Total N = 442
<1	3.6	2.9	6.5
1–4	21.0	18.5	39.5
5–14	16.7	15.6	32.3
15–24	2.7	5.4	8.1
25–44	4.8	6.6	11.3
>44	1.1	0.9	2.0

*Case rates: <15 years = 109.6/1,000 patients/yr; >15 years = 11.0/1,000 patients/yr; All patients = 37.6/1,000 patients/yr.

Table 2. *Percent of Multiple Episodes of Otitis Media by Age/Sex Groups (527 Episodes)*

Age Group	Number of Episodes		
	1	2	3 or More
	Percent of Patients		
<15 Years			
Male	82.3	15.1	2.7
Female	79.4	18.8	1.9
≥15 Years			
Male	97.5	2.5	—
Female	94.9	5.1	—

episodes during the year, but less than 5 percent of adults had recurrent attacks in the same period. Females had more multiple episodes than did males. In the study population there were 1.61 visits per episode. The socioeconomic distribution of otitis media patients in the population served by the Rochester Center as compared with that of Monroe County indicates only a slight trend toward increased incidence in patients living in census tracts designated as low in socioeconomic status (Table 3).

The relationship of family size to the incidence of otitis media is given in Table 4. Significantly fewer families with three or more children reported cases of otitis media ($P < 0.05$). The percentage of families with two or more affected children

Table 3. *Socioeconomic Distribution of Otitis Media Cases: Percentage Comparison of Monroe County and Family Practice Populations*

SES*	Monroe County (N = 711,917)	Family Practice (N = 11,765)	Otitis Media (N = 442)
I	14	12	10
II	33	24	19
III	37	45	48
IV	10	15	19
V	5	3	4

*SES = Socioeconomic status, SES I is highest.

Table 4. *Relationship of Family Size to Distribution of Otitis Media*

Number of Children in Family	Percent of Families with One or More Cases
1	32.6
2	31.1
3 or more	25.4*

*$P < 0.05$.

is given in Table 5. The incidence of multiple cases in families is greater than would be expected if cases were distributed randomly ($P < 0.05$).

A comparison of symptoms recorded for patients in three age groups (less than 1 year, 1 to 14 years, and 15 years and over) is presented in Table 6. Fever and gastrointestinal symptoms which are more evident objectively predominate in patients less than one year of age. The subjective symptoms of pain and diminished hearing are more frequent in the older groups. Table 7 contains a similar comparison for objective findings. No marked differences are noted except for fever which is more common in the less than one year group and external canal inflammation, noted more frequently in adults.

Of 206 episodes examined by chart review using a protocol (Appendix), 83 percent had sufficient documentation to satisfy the diagnostic criteria in the protocol.

Table 5. *Multiple Cases of Otitis Media in Families (Total Cases, July 1975–June 1976)*

	Percent of Families (N = 382)	Percent of Patients (N = 442)
1 Case Families	86.1	74.4
2 Case Families	12.2	21.3
3 Case Families	1.3	3.4
4 Case Families	0.2	0.9

Note: Expected incidence 2.76% (2 or more cases in family); observed incidence 6.38% (2 or more cases in family).
*$P < 0.05$.

Table 6. *Symptoms of Otitis Media in 204 Episodes*

Symptom	All Episodes		Age Groups in Percent		
	N	%	<1 yr	1-14 yr	15+ yr
Pain	98	48	0	47	69
Fever	97	48	94	61	21
Rhinitis	48	24	18	25	23
Sore throat	37	18	0	14	31
Ear fullness	29	14	0	2	35
Vomiting	22	11	21	11	7
Diarrhea	17	8	18	8	4
Decreased hearing	13	6	0	4	12

Ninety-one percent of these episodes were treated with appropriate antibiotics. Decongestants were prescribed in 56 percent of cases.

Discussion

The incidence of acute purulent otitis media in North Americans has not been reported with precision because few health service groups can accurately define the patient populations served. A report of 28 physicians in 13 United Kingdom practices with more than 47,500 patients gives an annual incidence of 85.8 cases/1,000 for patients under age 15 years, and 5.3 cases/1,000 for those 15 years and older.[24] These rates are less than those in the Rochester Center patient population. The differences could be due to the different diagnostic criteria utilized by the two groups. The United Kingdom physicians did not follow any standard criteria, while the center physicians generally used the protocol guidelines (Appendix). Differences in climate, patient health-care-seeking behavior, and the ability to define the population at risk are additional possible explanations for the different rates. The English physicians also reported a somewhat lower incidence of multiple episodes during a one-year period than the present authors did: 12.7 percent vs 19.2 percent for children under the age 15 years, and 2 percent vs 3.8 percent for those 15 years and over.

Although a predominance of severe cases of chronic otitis media has been reported in socially deprived families,[25] this study showed little effect of socioeconomic status (SES) on incidence. The low SES patients generally have free access to medical care which may explain the small effect of SES on infection rates.

Table 7. *Objective Findings in Otitis Media in 204 Episodes*

Objective Findings	All Episodes		Age Groups in Percent		
	N	%	<1 yr	1-14 yr	15+ yr
Redness of TM	153	75	74	82	65
Difference between TMs	90	44	41	41	48
Loss of landmarks	79	39	35	33	47
Abnormal mobility	64	31	35	32	29
Bulging TM	58	28	27	30	27
Dullness of TM	45	22	27	22	20
Fever	43	21	29	14	13
Toxic appearance	22	11	9	13	9
Inflammation of external canal	18	9	—	4	18
Drainage from middle ear	13	6	—	7	8
Rupture of TM	7	3	—	2	7

TM = tympanic membrane.

The decreased incidence in families with three or more children is surprising. Although otitis media is probably not a contagious disease, attacks are often preceded by upper respiratory tract infections which are apt to be more frequent in larger households. The greater tendency for multiple cases in selected families, however, may imply a genetic component in the pathogenesis.

The finding of this study related to family factors and incidence must be interpreted with caution. It is difficult to accurately define patient populations in North American practices. Emergency Room visits for acute otitis media are frequent and the recorded incidence of otitis media for some study patients and families may, therefore, be incorrect. In addition, estimates of total patient population are subject to error.[26]

The incidence of otitis media in patients 15 years and over has generally not been appreciated because most reports concern the manifestations in children. Although the age adjusted case rate is lower for adults than for children, the age distribution of most family practice populations is such that many adult patients with otitis media will be treated by family physicians. Adults present somewhat different symptoms than do children. They are less likely to experience fever but more apt to complain of pain, ear fullness, and decreased hearing. Young children frequently have gastrointestinal symptoms and are less able to complain of symptoms described by adults. The tympanic membrane abnormalities appear similar in all age groups. The increase in external ear canal inflammation seen in adults is of interest but unexplained.

The diagnostic and therapeutic dilemmas facing primary care physicians who treat otitis media have recently been described.[27] Although the usual diagnostic criteria utilized by physicians are of uncertain value, it is nevertheless necessary to establish a diagnosis and to employ rational therapeutic measures. Until more accurate diagnostic tools become available, a protocol for diagnosis and management which represents the best judgment of a group of physicians can be a useful device for family physicians.

Appendix
Protocol for the Diagnosis
and Management of Otitis Media

This protocol was developed by Team B with advice from other members of the faculty and resident staff and community pediatricians and otolaryngologists. We believe this is a practical plan for the diagnosis and management of otitis media as seen in the family practice office setting. We recognize that alternative and suitable protocols are possible and do not suggest that providers must adhere rigidly to this protocol. Instead, it is offered as one rational plan for the diagnosis and management of a common condition.

I. Acute Otitis Media

A. Minimal diagnostic criteria—one or more of the following:
    1. Redness and bulging of tympanic membrane (in the absence of bullous myringitis)
    2. Redness and abnormal mobility and the tympanic membrane
    3. A difference between the two tympanic membranes in redness or mobility

    4. Redness of the tympanic membrane plus one or more of the following: Pain, fever, loss of landmarks

B. Laboratory work
    1. If patient with fever is less than six weeks of age, do the following: Hospitalize and perform lumbar puncture, blood culture, chest x-ray, tympano-centesis (optional), urine culture

Appendix (continued)

2. If patient with fever is six weeks to three months of age: Hospitalization is optional, but patient requires lumbar puncture, blood culture, and chest x-ray (particularly if child appears toxic)

3. If patient is three months of age: No laboratory work is required

C. Treatment
   1. Antibiotics
      a. If patient is less than six weeks of age, hospitalize. Antibiotics will depend upon susceptibility of Gram-negative organisms.
      b. If patient is six weeks to three months of age, the following antibiotics are appropriate:
         i. amoxicillin 30 mg/kg per day
         ii. ampicillin 50–75 mg/kg per day
         iii. if patient is vomiting, use 600,000 units of CR Bicillin plus oral Gantrisin (if patient is more than two months of age, use 150 mg/kg per day in divided doses or IM ampicillin 125–250 mg). Then use either oral amoxicillin or ampicillin
      c. If patient is over three months of age, use any of the following:
         i. 1,200,000 units CR Bicillin if patient is greater than 30 kg; 600,000 CR Bicillin if less than 30 kg
         ii. amoxicillin 30 mg/kg per day; amipicillin 50–75 mg/day
         iii. oral penicillin ½ gm/day if patient is less than 30 kg; 1 gm/day if greater than 30 kg
         iv. erythromycin and Gantrisin in combination are particularly useful in the penicillin allergic patient
   2. Decongestants and/or antihistamines
   Perhaps useful if the child is allergic. There is no evidence of their value in the treatment of otitis media
   3. Follow-up
   Two weeks. Check movement and morphology of tympanic membrane. Ask about and/or check hearing. If hearing is impaired at this visit reschedule visits monthly until hearing returns to normal

II. Recurrent Otitis Media

A. Definition: Three or more infections in one year

B. Treatment: Oral Gantrisin 500 mg twice a day (only "proven" benefit is in males under six years old)

III. Prevention of Acute or Recurrent Otitis Media

A. Education of mother to feed baby in upright position

B. All children with cleft palate need polyethylene (PE) tubes as soon as feasible (usually about three to five months of age)

IV. When to Refer Cases of Acute or Recurrent Otitis Media

A. In cases of incomplete resolution of acute otitis media with appropriate therapy manifested by
   1. Persistent decreased (> 25 db) hearing at three months after onset of infection; or severe hearing loss at one month
   2. Persistence of middle ear fluid at three months or hemotympanum at any time
   3. Atelectatic tympanic membrane

B. Recurrent otitis media which may benefit by the placement of PE tubes

C. At parents' request

D. For allergic work-up if this appears to be a prominent feature of the illness

V. Tonsillectomy and/or Adenoidectomy

Need: Probably none. Occasionally, adenoidectomy is useful at the time of PE tube insertion

VI. Myringotomy

Need: Rare. Only proven benefit is for acute relief of pain

REFERENCES

1. Rowe DS: Acute suppurative otitis media. Pediatrics 56:285, 1975
2. Bluestone CD, Shurin PA: Middle ear disease in children: Pathogenesis, diagnosis and management. Pediatr Clin North Am 21:379, 1974
3. Feingold M, Klein JO, Haslam GE, et al: Acute otitis media in children: Bacteriological findings in middle ear fluid obtained by needle aspiration. Am J Dis Child 111:361, 1966
4. Bland RD: Otitis media in the first six weeks of life: Diagnosis, bacteriology and management. Pediatrics 49:187, 1972
5. Tilles JG, Klein JO, Jao RL: Acute otitis media in children: Serologic studies and attempts to isolate viruses and mycoplasmas from aspirated middle ear fluids. N Engl J Med 277:613, 1967
6. Howard JE, Nelson JD, Clahsen J, et al: Otitis media of infancy and early childhood: A double-blind study of four treatment regimens. Am J Dis Child 130:965, 1976
7. Nilson BW, Poland RL, Thompson RS: Acute otitis media: Treatment results in relationship to bacterial etiology. Pediatrics 43:351, 1969
8. Bass JW, Frostad AL, Schooler RA: Antimicrobials in the treatment of acute otitis media: A second clinical trial. Am J Dis Child 125:397, 1973
9. Howie VM, Ploussard JH: Efficacy of fixed combination antibiotics versus separate components in otitis media: Effectiveness of erythromycin estolate, triple sulfonamide, ampicillin, erythromycin estolate and triple sulfonamide, and placebo in 280 patients with acute otitis media under two and one-half years of age. Clin Pediatr 11:205, 1972
10. Roddey OF, Earle R, Haggerty R: Myringotomy in acute otitis media: A controlled study. JAMA 197:849, 1966
11. Maynard JE, Fleshman JK, Tschopp CF: Otitis media in Alaskan Eskimo children. JAMA 219:597, 1972
12. Perrin JM, Charney E, MacWhinney JB et al: Sulfisoxazole as chemoprophylaxis for recurrent otitis media: A double-blind crossover study in pediatric practice. N Engl J Med 291:664, 1974
13. Howie VM, Ploussard JH, Lester RL: Acute otitis media: A clinical and bacteriological correlation. Pediatrics 45:29, 1970
14. Beauregard WG: Positional otitis media. J Pediatr 79:294, 1971
15. Dees SC, Lefkowitz D: Secretory otitis media in allergic children. Am J Dis Child 124:364, 1972
16. Paradise JL, Bluestone CD, Felder H: The universality of otitis media in 50 infants with cleft palate. Pediatrics 44:35, 1969
17. Kaplan GJ, Fleshman JK, Bender TR, et al: Long-term effects of otitis media: A ten-year cohort study of Alaskan Eskimo children. Pediatrics 52:577, 1973
18. Schaefer O: Otitis media and bottle feeding: An epidemiological study of infant feeding habits and incidence of recurrent and chronic middle ear disease in Canadian Eskimos. Can J Public Health 62:478, 1971
19. Omstead RW, Alvarez MC, Moroney JD, et al: The pattern of hearing following acute otitis media. J Pediatr 65:252, 1964
20. Holm VA, Kunze LH: Effect of chronic otitis media on language and speech development. Pediatrics 43:833, 1969
21. National Ambulatory Medical Care Survey: 1973 summary: United States, May 1973–April 1974. In National Center for Health Statistics (Rockville, Md): Vital and Health Statistics, series 13, No. 21. DHEW publication No. (HRA) 76-1772. Government Printing Office, 1975
22. Froom J, Culpepper L, Boisseau V: An integrated medical record and data system for primary care: Part 3: The diagnostic index: Manual and computer methods and applications. J Fam Pract 5:113, 1977
23. Froom J, Culpepper L, Becker L, et al: Research design in family medicine. J Fam Pract 7:75, 1978
24. Medical Research Council: Acute otitis media in general practice. Lancet 2:510, 1957
25. Miller FJW, Court SDM, Watten WS, et al: Growing up in Newcastle-upon-Tyne. London, Oxford University Press, 1960
26. Froom J: An integrated medical record and data system for primary care: Part 1: The age-sex register: Definition of the patient population. J Fam Pract 4:951, 1977
27. Bain DJG: Acute otitis media in children: Diagnostic and therapeutic dilemmas. J Fam Pract 6:259, 1978

Symptomatic Urinary Infection in Childhood:
Presentation During a Four-Year Study in General Practice and Significance and Outcome at Seven Years*

D. Brooks, I. B. Houston

Thirty-eight children (12 boys and 26 girls) with symptomatic urinary infection have been studied in general practice. Patients were collected over a four-year period and we report an incidence of urinary infection according to Kass's criterion of 7.7 per 1,000 girls at risk per year and 3.8 per 1,000 boys at risk per year. Eighty-four per cent of the children had symptoms which suggested an origin in the genitourinary tract. *Proteus* infection was found in five of the boys and only one of the girls. At the end of the four-year study period follow-up had taken place over a mean period of 25 months and recurrent infection had been demonstrated in four boys and 12 girls. All the children had an excretion urogram and two children, both girls, were found to have pyelonephritic scarring. Twelve children with recurrent infection were investigated for vesicoureteric reflux, which was found only in the two children with scarring. At seven years 31 of the children remained in the practice and, with a mean follow-up of 42 months, no significant alteration in the figures for recurrent infection was demonstrated. Guidelines are suggested for the management of childhood urinary infection in general practice.

Introduction

A relationship between recurrent urinary infection and radiological evidence of pyelonephritic scarring has been observed

*Reprinted by permission from *Journal of the Royal College of General Practitioners*, 27:678–683, 1977.

only in children (Hodson and Wilson, 1965). Hospital studies on the presentation and significance of symptomatic childhood infection have been reported (Smellie *et al.*, 1964; Smallpiece, 1966; Bergstrom, 1972) but they have inevitably been carried out on selected populations. Screening studies of bacteriuria in schoolgirls (Kunin, 1970; Savage *et al.*, 1973), and schoolgirls and schoolboys (Cohen and Eirew, 1973) have also been reported, but unselected studies of symptomatic infection by definition need to be carried out in primary medical practice unless it can be said that accurate diagnosis and hospital referral are for all practical purposes invariable. Although many studies of urinary infection in adults have appeared from domiciliary practice (Fry *et al.*, 1962; Loudon and Greenhalgh, 1962; Brooks and Mandar, 1972), with the exception of one study into asymptomatic bacteriuria (Mond *et al.*, 1970) and one public health laboratory study of general-practitioner referrals (Hallett *et al.*, 1976) childhood infection has been neglected.

Method

The Practice

The practice is situated in an urban area at the northern edge of the Manchester city boundary. The practice population is unbiased in that it accurately reflects the Registrar General's figures for age and social class for the population of south-east Lancashire as a whole. On 1 July 1969 the prac-

81

tice consisted of 3,908 females and 3,482 males; 838 girls and 794 boys were aged 14 or under, and the total number of patients was the medical responsibility of three principals and one trainee general practitioner.

Criteria

From 1 August 1970 until 31 July 1974 all children under 15 years of age presenting with symptoms that could conceivably be caused by urinary infection, and many other children with vague symptoms in whom a definite diagnosis could not be made, had an "Oxoid" dip-slide culture of a clean-catch specimen of urine. This was incubated at 37°C on the practice premises for 24 hours. The presence of an organism count $> 10^5$ per ml was considered to indicate a urinary infection, this being the sole criterion of infection. A few children provided a second specimen of urine, which in no case altered the diagnosis. The positive dip slides were then taken to a local hospital pathology laboratory where the organisms were subcultured and identified by conventional biochemical tests.

Management

All children with proven urinary infection were seen by one of us (D.B.) and a careful history and general physical examination followed. The medical records were studied and relevant information was collected, in particular details of past illnesses which, with the benefit of hindsight, might have been caused by urinary infection.

All patients received appropriate therapy (usually cotrimoxazole) for ten days, after which a follow-up urine specimen was obtained. Regular follow-up appointments for a period of up to four years were then made. At first these were arranged monthly, but in those patients in whom a low recurrence rate had been demon-

strated, a longer interval was allowed. On these occasions details of intercurrent illnesses were obtained and a urine specimen (handled as before) was taken.

In addition, all patients were referred to a paediatric hospital renal outpatient department, where they were seen by one of us (I.B.H.) for clinical and bacteriological assessment. All patients had excretion urograms, and micturating cystograms were carried out if recurrent infection was demonstrated.

A few patients (four in all) had their urinary infections diagnosed primarily in hospital, having been referred and followed up for reasons usually unconnected with the genitourinary tract.

Three years after the end of the study period the records of the children who remained in the practice were studied and relevant details were extracted.

Results

Incidence of Infection

Over the four-year study period 38 children in the practice were found to have bacteriologically confirmed urinary infection. We are aware of the diagnosis being suspected on clinical grounds in a further four children, but bacteriological confirmation was not obtained when their urines were examined. Four of the 38 children with infection were diagnosed in hospital rather than in the practice. Of the total of 38 children with infection, 12 were boys and 26 were girls, giving a total incidence of infection in childhood of 5.8 per 1000 children at risk per year with a girl:boy ratio of 7.7 per 1000 to 3.8 per 1000; that is, 2:1.

Age on Entry to the Study

The age on entry to the study is presented in Figure 1 as an age-specific incidence rate (i.e. per 1000 children at risk per year). No

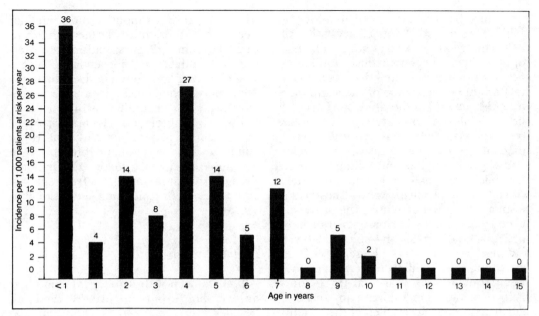

Fig. 1. Age-specific incidence rates (per 1,000 children at risk per year) for 38 children with symptomatic urinary tract infection in general practice.

children presented between the ages of 11 and 15 and most children were aged seven years or under. With the exception of one boy, aged two, whose acute dysuria and frequency resulted in his mother ringing for an ambulance (the practice doctors were all on their morning visits), all four hospital-diagnosed infections occurred in infants under the age of one year.

Organisms Isolated

Thirty-one (82 percent) of the 38 children had a pure growth of *Escherichia coli* in their urines. Six children (five were boys) had *Proteus* infections. One girl had a mixed infection with *Escherichia coli* and *Streptococcus faecalis*. Thus, 42 percent of infections in boys were caused by *Proteus* species compared with only four percent in girls. The girl in question (C.M.) was subsequently found to have an abnormal genitourinary tract.

Presenting Features in the Children With Proven Infection

Dysuria, usually associated with frequency of micturition, was present in 27 (71 percent) of the children, loin pain in three, loin tenderness in two, and vague abdominal pain in 12. Fever was found at the time of the examination or suggested by the history in only eight children. Seven children, according to their mothers, had offensive urine. Nine children had enuresis (defined as bed wetting in children who were normally dry at night) and two children had daytime incontinence; in all cases this was unusual. Haematuria was an unusual symptom, being present in only one girl. One girl had a rigor. None of the children had a raised blood pressure or palpable kidneys.

All these symptoms were, as a rule, of short duration. Only one child had a history of acute symptoms for longer than three days. Only three of the children looked ill and seemed to be seriously upset by their symptoms, but the parents of nine of the children requested a domiciliary visit. All the ill children were seen at home. The history (as obtained spontaneously and by direct questioning) indicated that the urinary tract might be the source of the symptoms in 32 (84 percent) of the children. Three of the six children with atypical symptoms were infants under the age of one year. One infection was diagnosed in a premature infant who was irritable and failing to thrive in a special care baby unit, and one other, with a feeding problem, was diagnosed at a hospital infant welfare clinic; the third was taken to hospital by her parents after having had a mild convulsion—she had a fever and there was a history of loose stools. The remaining three children were aged between four and six years; all three complained of vague abdominal pain and one had an associated fever. Ten of the 38 children had suffered previous episodes of symptoms which could have been due to urinary infection, although this is not certain as these symptoms were only characteristic in two and bacteriological examination of a urine specimen had not been carried out. The rest were apparent first attacks.

Associated Observations

Five of the 38 children had an associated upper respiratory infection either at the time they presented with the acute urinary infection or within the preceding seven days. Three of the children had chronic constipation and encopresis. Two boys had chronic recurrent balanitis and two girls had recurrent vulvitis. The 38 children with infection included one pair of siblings, and one child had an allergic diathesis.

Recurrent Infection

At the end of the study period all children had been followed up for a period of up to four years. The shortest follow-up period was two months and the longest 48 months,

with a mean of 25 months and a median period of 18 months. Fifteen children, three boys and 12 girls, had experienced recurrent infection. Nine children had a single recurrence, four children had two recurrences, and two children had four recurrences. Ten of the 25 recurrent infections were symptomatic. The majority were diagnosed in general practice but three children with asymptomatic infection were diagnosed on hospital follow-up. One boy, though asymptomatic, gave frequent low count specimens containing species of *Proteus*.

Further Investigation

All 38 children with urinary infection had an excretion urogram; three of these, all females, were reported as abnormal: patients C.M., aged four, S.L.B., aged two, and K.S., aged seven. Patient C.M. had a poorly functioning shrunken left kidney with what appeared to be clubbed calyces probably due to pyelonephritic scarring, although a congenital anomaly could not be excluded. The right kidney was more reasonable in size and functioned better, though one or two calyces looked clubbed and the right ureter was dilated. Patient S.L.B. was found to have a bifid left ureter of which the upper radical was relatively poorly defined and the joint of junction was not apparent. There was a full calyceal pattern on the right. The bladder appeared normal. Further investigation of the renal system appeared to be warranted. Patient K.S. did not demonstrate hydronephrosis or hydroureter but there was a straightened right lower pole calyx and inadequate filling of the upper and middle pole calyces on the right side. While the radiologist thought it was probably normal, he considered that a right retrograde pyelogram would be advisable.

Patient C.M. was admitted for cystogram and cystoscopy. She was found to have gross bilateral vesicoureteric reflux and patulous ureteric orifices. Bilateral ureteric reimplants were performed.

Patient S.L.B. was also admitted for further investigation. Cystoscopy revealed a left-sided ureterocele with an incompetent ureteric orifice above it. Right retrograde catheterisation showed a normal single system with a bifid pelvis. Left-sided catheterisation was not possible. The ureterocele was excised and its ureter brought onto the surface as a separate opening. A second ureter on the left side was incompetent and was freed, mobilized, and then reimplanted. At a second operation three weeks later, in view of the fact that the urine from the upper pole ureter opening onto the surface was not draining, a left heminephroureterectomy was performed. Histology revealed a tortuous ureter reaching 2 cm in diameter in its middle third. The kidney showed pyelonephritis with scarring.

Patient K.S. was admitted for cystoscopy, which revealed some infection over the trigone area. The ureteric orifices were normal and competent. Retrograde pyelography on the right side revealed slightly irregular calyces but the findings were not considered pathological.

Twelve children (32 percent) had a cystogram but only two of them (C.M. and S.L.B.) were abnormal.

Subsequent Progress 1974 to 1977

Although the study period ended in 1974, the records of 31 children involved in the study who remained patients of the practice were examined three years later and details of subsequent urine examinations and other relevant information were extracted. Taking the last recorded urine examination as the end of follow-up the total follow-up period was thereby extended up to a maximum of 58 months and a minimum period of eight months (mean 42 months; median period 33 months). The informa-

tion resulting from this exercise did not significantly alter the results already reported. With one exception, all the children who originally had recurrent infection remained on the list including the two children with renal scarring, one of whom went on to have three asymptomatic infections during this period. Two of these children with recurrent infections who had already had normal cystograms went on to further episodes of infection. In one girl infection was always symptomatic and occurred on three occasions between 1974 and 1977, the last episode being two years ago, three years after the original infection. One girl originally placed in the non-recurrent group developed an asymptomatic recurrence within two years of the original infection and she was referred for a cystogram which proved to be normal.

Patient S.L.B. This girl was readmitted 12 months after surgery and a cystogram showed a normal bladder, bladder neck, and urethra, and no reflux. Clinically her progress was very satisfactory with no symptomatic infections and only three asymptomatic infections.

Patient C.M. This girl was also readmitted 12 months after surgery; a cystogram showed a normal bladder with no reflux. Excretion urogram showed quite marked improvement on the right side but there was still a very small scarred kidney on the left, which will probably need to be removed. The dilated right ureter in the original film had disappeared.

Discussion

Little information is available about the incidence of symptomatic childhood urinary infection in general practice. Loudon and Greenhalgh (1962) in a study primarily involving adults identified 16 children over a two-year period, diagnosis being confirmed by a "positive culture at a local laboratory." Incidence rates were reported as 11.3 per 1000 girls at risk per year and 2.6 per 1000 boys at risk per year, giving a girl:boy ratio of 4:1 under the age of 15. Fry and his colleagues (1962), studying 13 children and 159 adults identified in 1955, 1956, and 1957, gave a rate of 21.0 per 1000 girls at risk per year and 7.0 per 1000 boys at risk per year under the age of ten years, giving a total girl:boy ratio of 3:1. Our risks of 7.7 per 1000 girls and 3.8 per 1000 boys at risk per year, giving a sex ratio of 2:1, can be directly compared with the figures reported by Loudon and Greenhalgh, as similar populations (under the age of 15) were reported. We found a slightly lower incidence in girls and a slightly higher incidence in boys, possibly explained in part by different diagnostic criteria. Sex ratios for symptomatic infection in hospital series have been reported as 2.8:1 (Smellie et al., 1964) and 3.3:1 for screening studies (Cohen and Eirew, 1973). We identified only one child with infection between the ages of ten and 15 years, who later developed infection at the age of 14. Excluding four infants under one year of age, of whom three were diagnosed in hospital without suprapubic aspiration, most children presented between the ages of two and seven with a peak at four years. The commonest organism isolated was *Escherichia coli,* which was found in 82 percent of children. Yet out of six children with infection due to *Proteus* species, five were boys; this sex difference failed to reach statistical significance with the numbers involved in this study. However, an increased likelihood of *Proteus* infection in boys has been reported elsewhere (Bergstrom, 1972; Hallett et al., 1976). Bergstrom stated that two thirds of male infections were caused by organisms other than *Escherichia coli.*

Eighty-four percent of the children had symptoms which suggested an origin in the genitourinary tract, although on occasions these had to be elicited by direct questioning. A similar proportion of typical symptoms was found in a study of urine specimens from boys sent by general practitioners to a public health laboratory (Hallett

et al., 1976). The commonest symptoms were dysuria and frequency, vague abdominal pain, nocturnal enuresis, and offensive urine. Three out of four infants under the age of one year had the vague symptoms described by Smellie and her colleagues (1964). Three older children, however, complained only of vague abdominal pain. Enuresis was an interesting symptom in that although present in nine children, it was rarely the presenting symptom and never a solitary symptom. It was, in fact, often obscured by other symptoms such as fever, dysuria, and frequency and was usually elicited only by direct questioning. Smellie and her colleagues (1964) found that 45 percent of children in their hospital series had symptoms beginning in the first year of life. Only ten of the children in our group had previous symptoms that might have been due to infection, and these rarely went back quite so far. They found that only 22 percent of their patients had dysuria and frequency compared with our figures of 71 percent, and only 30 percent of their children were referred with the correct diagnosis. Covert symptoms in screening studies were often more characteristic (Savage et al., 1973), but although frequency and urgency and nocturnal enuresis were not uncommon, dysuria was found in only 13 percent.

Urinary infection in childhood in hospital series often points to underlying renal tract abnormalities. Smellie and her team (1964) found that 13 percent of children with symptomatic infection had pyelonephritic scarring, and 34 percent had reflux; these figures were higher when children with recurrent infection were considered separately. However, more recently, Welch and his colleagues (1976) pointed out that infection associated with typical symptoms and minimal reflux can have a good prognosis in terms of renal damage, even when attacks recur frequently.

In our series only two children had pyelonephritic scarring, and of 12 children investigated for reflux only two had this defect. There is evidence, however, that our group differed from the group reported by Smellie and her colleagues in that, as mentioned above, children in the hospital series tended to be younger and have atypical symptoms in a higher proportion of cases; in addition, symptoms could more often be traced back to the first year of life. The relatively low incidence of children aged one, two, and three in our series may reflect the greater difficulty in recognizing illness of any sort in babies, and urinary symptoms in particular; indeed three of four practice children whose infections were diagnosed in hospital were less than 12 months old. It is possible that hospital series tend to contain a higher proportion of clinically atypical infections occurring in a younger population, whereas this general-practice study contained a higher proportion of clinically typical infections, with a lower recurrence rate, limited to the lower urinary tract: children with these infections are probably only rarely referred to hospital. These observations, plus the likelihood that infection and reflux are a greater hazard in the younger child, suggest that our figures for the incidence of scarring and reflux are not incompatible with hospital series and that large-scale general-practice studies are needed.

When screening studies in the community are considered Savage and his colleagues (1974) found that 35 percent of primary schoolgirls with urinary infection had reflux and 23 percent had radiological evidence of pyelonephritis. In general practice Mond and others (1970) investigated eight children with significant bacteriuria, and five had radiological abnormalities. However, screening studies can be expected to be more likely to pick up children with persistent or frequently recurring bacteriuria.

In our series 54 percent of the girls and 75 percent of the boys had no recurrence over a mean follow-up period of 25 months, and only one child had a history of acute symptoms lasting longer than three days; only two children had a past history of symptoms actually suggesting urinary infection. In the series published by Savage and his colleagues, however, 70 percent of the girls had a history of covert symptoms such as frequency, urgency, and nocturnal enuresis.

This study has enabled us to suggest some guidelines for the management of childhood urinary infection in general practice. The significance of the condition has been demonstrated by the discovery of two girls with treatable renal tract lesions: they did not have any particular distinguishing features other than a *Proteus* infection in one case and rapid recurrence of infection in both cases. It seems that all children with urinary tract symptoms and many children with vague symptoms require bacteriological assessment in general practice if those with treatable renal tract lesions are to be identified. The study has demonstrated the feasibility of shared care. Traditional attitudes towards further investigation of children with urinary infection have differentiated between boys and girls in that girls have often been allowed to have more than one infection before undergoing radiological investigation. Since both children with abnormalities in our series were girls we feel that our policy of an excretion urogram in all children after a first attack has been justified. As the children received careful follow-up in general practice as well as at hospital, micturating cystograms and more involved investigations could be delayed, to be carried out in the presence of a pyelographic abnormality or recurrent infection. Since nearly all recurrent infections occurred in the first two years after the original attack, children with infection should be followed up routinely for this period unless reflux has been discovered, when careful follow-up until adolescence is indicated. Much of this follow-up work should take place in general practice and we feel that this study lends further weight to the argument that dip slides and small incubators should be available in all practices.

Acknowledgments

We thank Dr. A. D. Clift and Dr. J. A. Maudar for helpful criticism and for referring patients for inclusion in the study. We are grateful to Mr. S. J. Cohen for the surgical management of some of the children and Dr. R. Postlethwaite for some of the outpatient management in the renal clinic. The Radiology Department at Booth Hall Hospital and the Bacteriology Departments at Booth Hall and Oldham and District General Hospital actively co-operated in the investigation of the patients and we are grateful for this assistance.

Addendum

Since the submission of this paper for publication we have become aware of a large-scale general-practice survey carried out by the Victoria Faculty of the Royal Australian College of General Practitioners involving 135 practitioners (Williams, C. M. (1976) Australian Family Physician, 5, 340). Dr. Williams reports that urinary infection was found in 24 percent of children who admitted to symptoms of frequency and dysuria, and of 116 children with proven infection investigated radiologically 36 had an abnormality of some sort, most commonly reflux. Three children were found to have serious bilateral renal disease.

REFERENCES

Bergstrom, T. (1972). Archives of Diseases in Childhood, 47, 227–232

Brooks, D. & Mandar, A. (1972). Lancet, ii, 893–898

Cohen, S. J. & Eirew, R. C. (1973). In Urinary Tract Infection, eds. Brumfitt, W. & Asscher, A. W. London: Oxford University Press

Fry, J., Dillane, J. B., Joiner, C. L. & Williams, J. D. (1962). Lancet, i, 1318–1321

Hallett, R. J., Pead, L. & Maskell, R. (1976). Lancet, ii, 1107–1110

Hodson, C. J. & Wilson, S. (1965). British Medical Journal, 2, 191–194

Kunin, C. M. (1970). Journal of Infectious Diseases, 122, 382–393

Loudon, I. S. L. & Greenhalgh, G. P. (1962). Lancet, ii, 1246–1248

Mond, N. C., Gruneberg, R. N. & Smellie, J. M. (1970). British Medical Journal, 1, 602–605

Savage, D. C., Wilson, M. I., McHardy, M., Dewar, D. A. E. & Fee, W. M. (1973). Archives of Disease in Childhood, 48, 8–20

Smallpiece, V. (1966). Lancet, ii, 1019–1021

Smellie, J. M., Hodson, C. M., Edwards, D. & Normand, I. C. S. (1964). British Medical Journal, 2, 1222–1226

Welch, T. R., Forbes, P. A., Drummond, K. N. & Nogrady, M. S. (1976). Archives of Disease in Childhood, 51, 114–119

Depression in Family Practice:
Long-Term Prognosis and Somatic Complaints*

Remi J. Cadoret, Reuben B. Widmer, and Carol North

Somatic pain, functional, and anxiety complaints of 154 depressed patients were followed during the course of their initial depression and were found to parallel the depression: these complaints increased in number just prior to diagnosis of depression and decreased to normal levels after one year's treatment of the depression. Persistence of these types of somatic symptoms after one year's treatment predicted eventual chronicity of the depression. Older patients were also more likely to develop chronic depressions, and there was some indication that those individuals who had an initial remission of a depression followed by a second depression which then became chronic had longer first depressions.

In a previous paper,[1] patients were found to increase their number of visits to a family physician prior to being diagnosed as depressed. At the same time somatic complaints consistent with anxiety and with varied "functional" disorders increased significantly. This presented a picture of a developing depression characterized by multiple somatic complaints.

In a remitting but recurrent condition such as depression, prognosis of the course of the illness is important for primary care. Since these same patients were followed over a number of years, one of the purposes of this paper is to detail the changes in complaints as the depression was treated. One of the features of depression is the tendency in a certain number of individuals to run a chronic course in contrast to the more usual remitting one. In samples of hospitalized depressed patients, older females

*Reprinted by permission from *The Journal of Family Practice*, 10 (4):625–629, 1980.

have been described as having increased chances for developing a chronic depression. Other factors associated with longer episodes and chronicity are age of onset of depression and pre-existing deviant personality features. These studies, however, are based on individuals with more serious or severe depressions as evidenced by the need for hospitalization. In family practice, depressed patients represent on the average a less seriously ill group and accordingly most are treated successfully as outpatients. Prediction of chronicity or of a protracted course in such a different group is necessary in primary care. Accordingly, a further purpose of this paper is to determine whether somatic complaints might be of prognostic value in predicting the course of depression.

Methods

Sample selection was described in a previous paper.[1] One hundred fifty-four depressed patients were studied who were treated over a 24-year period in a solo family practice. Depressions included both exogenous and endogenous types. Diagnosis was usually made on the basis of a low or depressed mood associated with other symptoms of depression such as low energy and insomnia. Functional, pain, and anxiety complaints did not alone suffice for a diagnosis of depression.

In order to characterize changes in symptoms over time, 4 seven-month periods were sampled as shown graphically in Figure 1:

Period 1—starting 19 months prior to date of diagnosis
Period 2a—starting 7 months prior to date of diagnosis

Depressed Patients

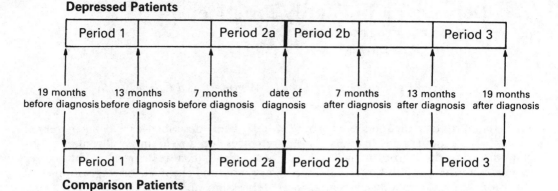

Comparison Patients

Fig. 1. Sampling scheme for complaints and visits of depressed and comparison patients.

Period 2b—starting at date of diagnosis of depression

Period 3—starting 1 year after date of diagnosis of depression.

Number of office visits and number and type of patient complaints were recorded for each of these periods.

Patient complaints for each of these periods were divided into categories described in reference 1 as: definite diagnoses, infections, (functional) pain complaints, other functional somatic complaints, and anxiety complaints.

Comparisons of incidences of factors between depressed and control groups were analyzed by chi-square test and reported (two-tailed) as significant if the five percent level was achieved. Contrasts within the depressed group involving changes in reported symptoms from one period to the other were analyzed by the sign test and these are reported significant if the two-tailed probability reached at least the five percent level.

Results

Course of Complaints During Depression

Figure 2 shows the percentage of depressed patients with definite diagnoses, infections, pain complaints, functional complaints, and anxiety complaints during the seven-month period immediately following diagnosis of depression (period 2b) and the seven-month period starting one year after the diagnosis of depression (period 3). For comparison, the same type of data for periods 1 (the seven-month period starting 19 months previous to diagnosis) and 2a (the seven-month period starting seven months prior to diagnosis) are included in the table. Because age and sex breakdown of these data showed no statistically significant differences, results for the total depressed sample are presented.

Number of pain, functional, and anxiety complaints peak in the periods just before the diagnosis of depression is made (period 2a), and decline thereafter during the period of active treatment (period 2b). One year later (period 3) they appear at approximately the levels shown by individuals one year before their diagnosis of depression (period 1). That these particular complaints parallel the course of the episode of depression is further borne out by the following finding: at one year's time (period 3), 16 of the original 154 patients were described in the clinical record as still depressed. Fifteen of these 16 (94 percent) had at least one symptom in the pain, functional, and anxiety complaint categories. In contrast to this, when depression was not mentioned during period 3, only 42 of the remaining 135 patients (31 percent) had a symptom in

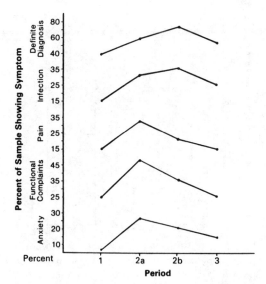

Fig. 2. Complaints in depressed patients by period.

the pain, functional, or anxiety category (χ^2 difference = 21.29, df = 1, P < .001). When the pain, anxiety, and functional complaints of these 16 depressed patients in period 3 are subtracted from those of the nondepressed patients, the incidence of all three types of complaints for the entire sample is lowered to that shown one year previously.

Definite diagnoses show a significant increase in number in period 2b compared to period 2a as determined by the sign test, but this is due almost entirely to individuals who returned for check-ups while on antidepressant medication. Otherwise the quality of definite diagnoses did not materially change from period 2a to period 2b. The dip shown in the definite diagnosis line (Figure 2, line 1) from period 2b to period 3 reflects mainly the decrease in visits for antidepressant medication check-ups and is not statistically significant.

Infection diagnoses (Figure 2, line 2 from top) show slight but insignificant changes from period 2a to period 2b, and from period 2b to period 3. The increase shown from period 1 to period 2b, however, is statistically significant. The increase in

number of infection diagnoses is not due to a qualitative change in the diagnosis, since during *each* of the four time periods about 50 percent of the infection diagnoses involved the respiratory tract: bronchitis, sinusitis, upper respiratory tract infection, or pharyngitis.

Individuals who had a larger number of functional complaints during periods 2a and 2b tended to have larger number of pain complaints during these same periods. Although these correlations as tested by a 2 × 2 × 2 contingency table were substantial, the majority of patients during both periods had no pain or functional complaints. However, if an individual had a functional complaint during period 2a, he was more likely to have a functional complaint during period 2b as well, but the quality of the complaint was often different from one period to the next so that the clinical picture was one rather of shifting functional complaints than persistence of one type of complaint throughout both periods.

In summary, the course of pain, functional, and anxiety complaints appears to parallel the course of depression. The quality of functional complaints during period 2b when almost all patients were receiving tricyclic antidepressants does not suggest they are medication side effects since overall they are similar to the quality of complaints seen during period 2a when no antidepressant medication had been prescribed.

Chronic Depression

Of the 154 index depressed patients, a substantial number remained on the antidepressant medication (almost invariably a tricyclic antidepressant) over an extended period of time during the 24 years covered by this study. The physician (RBW) generally tried to taper the medication during the 6- to 12-month period following initiation of antidepressants, but often found that symptoms recurred, requiring an increase in antidepressant dosage. The latter maneuver was almost always effective in causing symptoms of depression to remit.

Of the 154 depressed patients, 61 (39 percent) were on antidepressant medication for one or more years. For analytical purposes these patients were dichotomized into a "short chronic" group composed of individuals who took antidepressants for one year to three years and eleven months (N = 33) and a "long chronic" group composed of individuals taking antidepressants for four years or longer (N = 28).

Approximately two thirds of the individuals comprising these two chronic groups were female. This sex ratio is indistinguishable from that found in the remaining 93 nonchronic depressed patients. In contrast, age of onset of index depression proved to be a significant factor associated

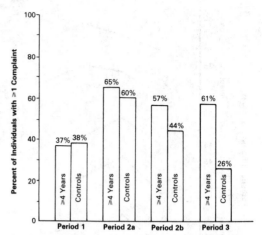

Fig. 4. Total number of individuals with either pain, functional, or anxiety complains in each period for chronic depressive patients of 4 years vs control patients.

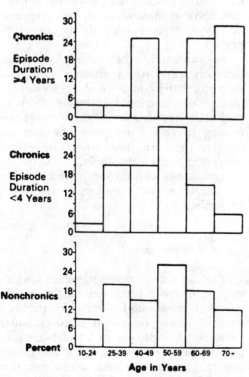

Fig. 3. Age of onset of depression in chronic and nonchronic patients.

with chronicity. Figure 3 shows histograms of age of onset of index depression for "long chronic," "short chronic," and nonchronic depressed groups. The "long chronics" had a significantly older age of onset of index depression as determined by testing the difference between age distributions shown in Figure 3 by χ^2. Average age of onset for "long chronics" of 63.4 years contrasted with 52.3 years for "short chronics."

One other condition was found to be predictive of chronicity: if an individual had either a pain, functional, or anxiety complaint one year after the time of index diagnosis of depression that person was more likely to fall into the "long chronic" group. This is shown in Figure 4 in which number of pain, functional, and anxiety complaints of "long chronics" are contrasted with those made by an age- and sex-matched comparison group from the nonchronic depressed patients. It is apparent that both groups have similar incidences of these complaints just prior to diagnosis of depression (periods 1 and 2a) and immediately after diagnosis of depression (period 2b), but diverge significantly at one year (period 3). The difference shown by chi-square test between 61 percent and the comparison group's 26 percent is significant at the five percent level. For this last period the comparison group returned to the one-year predepression level (period 1) but the "long chronic" group remained elevated. The "short chronic" group, on the other hand, was indistinguishable from an age- and sex-matched comparison group from the nonchronic depressed patients. This evidence for somatic symptoms persisting for one year suggests that these individuals may have longer depressions. To check this the authors looked at the length of depression in the nine "long chronics" patients who had one episode of depression with a remission prior to the onset of their chronic depressions. Comparing these nine "long chronics" with nine age- and sex-matched controls from the nonchronic group, it was found that seven of the nine "long chronics" had longer depressions than their controls, with a mean length of 2.2 years for "long chronics" vs 0.3 years for the nonchronic controls. This difference is not statistically significant when tested by both the sign test and the median test. Further, at one year's time after diagnosis of their first depression which remitted (period 3), eight of these nine "long chronics" (89 percent) had at least one pain, functional, or anxiety complaint. Thus, there is only suggestive evidence that length of first depression (in those who have more than one episode) might predict chronicity, and that somatic symptoms (pain, functional, or anxiety complaints) present as late as one year after diagnosis of depression predict eventual chronicity.

Discussion

This study has found a correlation of the incidence of varied somatic complaints with the course of depression. Although many individuals with depression do not complain of somatic symptoms, when they do so they are more likely to report other somatic complaints as well while depressed. With remission of depression the number of somatic complaints decreases. Even during treatment for depression, however, new somatic complaints are likely to develop which do not necessarily represent medication side effects, nor do they correlate with type of somatic symptoms present earlier in the course of the depression.

The shifts of somatic symptoms observed in the longitudinal course of some of these depressed patients suggest that appearance of somatic symptoms during a depression need not elicit a flurry of diagnostic tests on the part of the primary care physician. Rather, a careful history would reveal that the complaints might better be ascribed to the depression (if not a side effect of medication) and treated as such. The complaints in the pain, functional, and anxiety categories found in this study did not suggest a diagnosis which had to be immediately and extensively pursued with an elaborate work-up. This finding suggests that the physician should temporize in dealing with these complaints in a depressed patient. Time is a powerful tool which can work to the advantage of both the family physician and his/her patients. If the somatic complaints do not clear with amelioration of the depression, then further diagnostic maneuvers are indicated. Obviously one cannot temporize with complaints which suggest serious medical emergencies, such as symptoms of acute appendicitis.

The presence of somatic symptoms 12 to 19 months after the diagnosis of depression appears to predict a more chronic course. The somatic symptoms in some individuals appear to be associated with a longer episode of depression when remission does occur, and length of first depression does predict a "long chronic" course.

The finding that greater age of onset of depression is associated with chronicity is consistent with findings reported by Winokur et al,[2] in a sample of hospitalized patients from the state of Iowa, where age at onset of last depression was predictive of chronicity in the female patients. Thus, age of onset could be a valid predictor of eventual chronicity of depression; however, more studies of outpatient samples to confirm the present findings in one family practice are in order.

REFERENCES

1. Widmer RB, Cadoret RJ: Depression in primary care: Changes in patterns of patient visits and complaints during a developing depression. J Fam Pract 7:293, 1978
2. Winokur G: Genetic and clinical factors associated with course in depression. Pharmakopsychiatr Neuropsychopharmakol 7:122, 1974

An Epidemic of Gastro-Enteritis in West Lothian*

E. M. Melville

This article describes an epidemic of gastro-enteritis due to *Salmonella typhimurium* in a semi-rural practice. Methods of investigation and control of the outbreak are outlined, clinical features are described, and management of 97 patients discussed. Attention is drawn to the prolonged carrier state which may occur, and to the possible hazards of antibiotic therapy.

Introduction

The practice has three full-time partners, providing a 24-hour service for a list of approximately 7600 patients. This is virtually the entire population of five small villages situated along a five-mile stretch of trunk road, and the immediate hinterland. The compact and self-contained nature of the practice aids the investigation and control of such an epidemic.

Outbreak

On Sunday, 24 September 1978, calls were received from five patients suffering from colicky mid-abdominal pains, vomiting, and diarrhoea. Later in the week it became clear that there was an explosive outbreak of gastro-enteritis in the practice, judging from the number of calls and enquiries received from patients with enteric symptoms. Stools from the five initial patients were sent to the laboratory at Bangour Hospital, and by 28 September *Salmonella typhimurium* had been isolated from all five.

*Reprinted by permission from *Journal of the Royal College of General Practitioners*, 30:293–296, 1980.

Cases were notified to the Community Medicine Specialist, by the practice and the laboratory. Investigative and control measures were instituted by the Community Medicine Specialist in collaboration with environmental health officers of the West Lothian District Council. Through their courtesy the full data on the epidemic were obtained.

Figure 1 shows the course of the epidemic by dates of notification. The largest number of cases (21) was recorded on 9 October 1978. The last new case detected was on 6 November.

Figure 2 shows the cumulative total of cases, 97 in all.

Early in the epidemic, guidelines were issued by the Community Medicine Specialist on "Procedures to be adopted in the control of salmonellosis". A high-risk group of bacteriologically positive patients was identified. This included food handlers, nurses, dentists, teachers, and play-group supervisors. These people stayed away from work until six negative stools at intervals of not less than two days had been obtained. Absence from work or school was less stringently imposed on other workers, children, and contacts, one to three negative stools being required before return.

It was valuable to have a uniform policy from the outset, because we found that patients requested information not only from ourselves and our staff, but from the environmental health officers, district nurses, and the Community Medicine Specialist's office.

Each household with a bacteriologically proven case of salmonellosis was visited by the environmental health officers, who compiled a list of where each family obtained food and milk, and had meals away

95

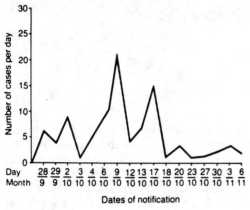

Fig. 1. Number of cases notified during the epidemic.

from home. From the enquiries the one common factor that emerged was that 53 out of 56 households obtained their milk from one particular dairy farm.

Clinical Features

The more severely affected patients were seen in the early stages of the epidemic. Of the five patients seen on the first day, all

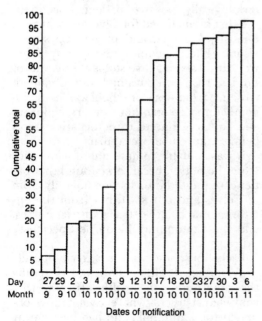

Fig. 2. Cumulative total of cases.

were febrile: one youth had high fever with rigors. All had colicky abdominal pain and profuse diarrhoea, three with fresh blood in the stool. Four had vomited several times. Three adults reported headache, dizziness, and generalized aches and pains. This pattern of symptoms continued in varying degrees throughout the epidemic. Symptomless carriers were also detected. All age groups in the community were affected, from babies to the very old. No deaths attributable to salmonellosis occurred during the epidemic, but there was a considerable toll in ill health and time lost from work and school.

Three patients became seriously ill and required admission to hospital:

Patient 1

A 62-year old man who regularly drank milk as well as whisky had persistent vomiting and diarrhoea, and became dehydrated. On the third day of the illness he developed delirium tremens. In hospital he became comatose and developed pneumonia. He required intensive intravenous therapy and antibiotics before making a complete recovery.

Patient 2

A 36-year-old man from whose stool *Salmonella typhimurium* had been isolated developed persistent rectal bleeding. A diagnosis of ulcerative proctitis was made after sigmoidoscopy.

Patient 3

Two weeks after a mild attack of diarrhoea and vomiting lasting for two or three days, a 38-year old woman developed joint pains affecting both knees, left ankle, and right hip. *Salmonella typhimurium* was isolated from her stool for the first time when the joint pains occurred. A large effusion developed in the left knee, and she became constitutionally ill. The effusion was aspirated later in hospital, but no pathogen was isolated. The patient was incapacitated by joint pains for six weeks but had fully recovered by 12 weeks.

A further case of joint effusion affecting the left knee occurred in a bacteriologically positive boy of 15 years, three weeks after the onset of diarrhoea and vomiting. The effusion persisted for three weeks after which complete recovery took place. Hospital admission was not required. The boy continued to complain of pain and occasional swelling of the knee during the subsequent year.

Management

Three severely ill patients were admitted to hospital. The remaining 94 were treated at home on a régime of bed-rest, 'fluids only' for 24 to 48 hours until the vomiting ceased, and symptomatic remedies such as chalk and opium mixture BP and diphenoxylate hydrochloride with atropine sulphate (Lomotil). Symptoms usually subsided in two to three days although in four patients moderate diarrhoea persisted for 10 to 14 days. In these patients dehydration was not a problem.

Stool cultures were repeated at intervals of two to three days until negative cultures were obtained. Within four weeks the majority of stool cultures were reported negative. Five patients continued to excrete *Salmonella typhimurium* at eight weeks—two adults and three infants. At 13 weeks, one adult and three infants continued to excrete the organism, and two infants and one adult were still doing so at 26 weeks (Table 1).

Of the five patients remaining at home who continued to excrete *Salmonella typhimurium* for eight weeks or longer, four had been treated with antibiotics, without apparent effect on the carrier state. Patients 1 and 3, who were admitted to hospital, were treated intensively with ampicillin and chloramphenicol respectively, in a dosage of 1–2 g daily for two to four weeks after which their stools became negative on six occasions. The remaining 90 patients were not treated initially with antibiotics for their salmonella infection.

Discussion

In the majority of patients, the illness was confined to symptoms of gastro-enteritis, but in two patients out of 97, joint symptoms occurred, an incidence of just over 2 percent. After dysenteric infections of all types—salmonella, shigella, *Yersinia enterocolitica,* and possibly enterovirus, typical Reiter's syndrome with conjunctivitis, urethritis, and arthritis, with or without fever, can occur. At times arthritis only occurs, often tending to flit initially and then settling in a few joints. This is described as 'reactive' or 'incomplete' Reiter's syndrome. Other inflammatory bowel disease, such as ulcerative colitis and regional enteritis may

Table 1. *Treatment of Five Patients Continuing to Excrete Salmonella typhimurium Up to 26 Weeks*

Patient	Sex	Date of Birth	First Positive Stool Culture	$\frac{8}{52}$	$\frac{13}{52}$	$\frac{26}{52}$	Antibiotic Therapy
1.	M	3.2.78	24.9.78	+	+	+	Neomycin for 7 days from 24.9.78 "Ceporex" for 7 days from 20.12.78
2.	F	24.2.78	29.9.78	+	+	+	Pivmecillinam for 10 days from 18.11.78 Neomycin for 7 days from 21.12.78
3.	M	4.1.78	29.9.78	+	+	−	Ampicillin for 7 days from 27.12.78
4.	F	23.11.40	6.10.78	+	+	+	Pivmecillinam 1.2 g daily for 10 days from 15.11.78
5.	M	28.6.43	27.9.78	+	−	−	No antibiotic

be preceded or accompanied by recurrent transient synovitis (Ansell, 1978; British Medical Journal, 1979).

Joint symptoms are becoming increasingly recognized as a complication of salmonellosis: commonly the effusion is sterile suggesting a hypersensitivity reaction but septic arthritis following bacteraemia may also occur.

Proctitis is another well known complication of salmonellosis. It is thought that an acute enteric infection such as salmonellosis may 'unmask' an ulcerative colitis (Dickinson et al., 1979).

Of the five prolonged excretors of salmonella, three were infants aged seven to eight months at the onset of symptoms. One infant had been breast fed for six and a half months, and the other two had been bottle fed, but all were receiving cows' milk when they became infected. Two infants continued to excrete salmonella after seven months. One adult remained positive after six months. This woman had a course of pivmecillinam 1.2 g daily for 10 days in November 1978. It therefore seems that antibiotics are of little value in treatment of the disease, and eradication of the carrier state requires intensive and prolonged antibiotic therapy.

Infants appear particularly liable to become prolonged carriers, perhaps owing to their immature immune system.

The Salmonella typhimurium RDNC I isolated in this epidemic was originally sensitive to all commonly used antibiotics: tetracycline, co-trimoxazole, ampicillin, nalidixic acid, cephaloridine, nitrofurantoin and neomycin. Sensitivity patterns were not performed routinely during the epidemic, but the sensitivity pattern in the two persistent excretors of salmonellae has remained unchanged. One of the dangers of indiscriminate use of antibiotics in enteric infections is the development of resistant strains of organisms. Salmonella and E. Coli in particular can develop multiple antibiotic resistance via transmissible R-factors. The hazards of spread of such organisms are obvious. Should severe disease occur, the choice of antibiotic available to the clinician would be very limited (Threlfall et al., 1978).

Salmonellae were not cultured from the specimens of milk submitted for examination. The evidence incriminating the milk was therefore circumstantial but very convincing:

1. In the week before the epidemic in our practice, an outbreak of salmonellosis had been reported amongst cattle at the dairy farm. The salmonella isolated from the cows was of the same phage type RDNC I as that isolated from our patients. The farmer himself and two of the milk delivery boys were found to be carrying the same organism in their stools.
2. Of the 97 patients with salmonellosis, 94 got their milk supply from the farm.
3. The initial patients with severe gastroenteritis all habitually drank raw milk.
4. The explosive nature of the outbreak was compatible with a milk-borne epidemic. The milk in this outbreak was unpasteurized, although the cattle were tuberculin tested and brucellosis accredited.

Possible sources of infection for the cattle came under investigation by the health authorities. Enquiry revealed that in April/May 1978 slurry from the local sewage works, mixed with washings from a poultry processing plant, had been spread on fields in the area, including those belonging to the dairy farm concerned. The slurry had not been ploughed in and cattle had been allowed to graze on the fields seven to eight weeks later. Salmonella typhimurium may remain viable in water, faeces, and pasture for as long as 28 weeks (Cruickshank and Gillies, 1975). Swabs from the local sewage works grew pathogenic salmonellae for example, Salmonella Newport, Salmonella Virchow. Washings from the poultry plant contained Salmonella typhimurium RDNC I. Methods in common use for treating sewage greatly reduce the content of pathogenic organisms such as salmonellae, tuberculosis, brucellae, and viruses, but should there be short-circuiting, for example, for reasons of expense, hazards could arise for human and animal health, where sewage is spread on agricultural land.

Animal feeding stuffs are a potential source of salmonella infection. It is modern practice in the poultry industry to recycle waste products such as excreta and bones, after sterilization, into feeding stuffs. Few would deny the value of recycling waste products, which provide valuable fertilizer and nutrients, but safeguards must be comprehensive and rigidly enforced to prevent hazards from infection.

Pasteurization of milk for human consumption constitutes a second line of defence against epidemics of similar origin. The fact that the farmer concerned promptly agreed to pasteurize the milk and the early control measures instituted by the health authorities undoubtedly helped to cut short this epidemic of salmonellosis in West Lothian.

Acknowledgments

My thanks are due to my partners Dr. F. McRae and Dr. D. J. Kerr, Dr. R. Burnett, Community Medicine Specialist, the environmental health officers of West Lothian District Council, Dr. R. Wiseman, Consultant Bacteriologist, and the staff of the Bacteriology Laboratory, Bangour General Hospital, to our office staff for their untiring help, and to our patients for their goodwill and co-operation.

REFERENCES

Ansell, B. M. (1978). Early diagnosis of rheumatic diseases in children. Practitioner, 220, 42–48

British Medical Journal (1979). Rheumatoid arthritis and the gut. Editorial, 1, 1104

Cruickshank, R. & Gillies, R. R. (Eds.) (1975). A Guide to Laboratory Diagnosis and Control of Infection. Vol. 2. Practice of Medical Microbiology. 12th edn. Edinburgh: Churchill Livingstone

Dickinson, R. J., Gilmour, H. M. & McClelland, D. B. (1979). Rectal biopsy in patients presenting to an infectious disease unit with diarrhoeal disease. Gut, 20, 141–148

Threlfall, E. J., Ward, I. R. & Rowe, B. (1978). Spread of multiresistant strains of salmonella typhimurium phage types 204 and 193 in Britain. British Medical Journal, 2, 997

Prognostic Indicators in Low Back Pain*

P. A. Pedersen

Nearly 4 percent of the population over the age of 15 years in a Danish general practice reported episodes of low back pain at least once a year. A one-year follow-up of 72 patients provided data regarding symptoms, length of absence from work, use of analgesics and bed rest. An indication of the prognosis was reached by relating these data to the history (including occupation), symptoms, and signs noted at the initial interview. The following factors indicated a long or relapsing course: (1) More than three previous episodes of low back pain; (2) gradual onset of symptoms; (3) pain referred distal to the femur; and (4) more than four weeks' delay in reporting symptoms. Other factors of prognostic significance were difficulty in moving, onset in relation to work, absence from work, positive straight leg raising test and unilateral pain in the loin.

Introduction

Management of low back pain in general practice involves determining the prognosis early on in episodes of the condition. Previous studies of the prognosis of low back pain in general practice have selected patients by certain kinds of work (Bergquist-Ullman and Larsson, 1977), by method of investigation (Sims-Williams *et al.*, 1978), or by certain types of pain (Dillane *et al.*, 1966). Dillane and colleagues found that, among patients suffering from acute low back pain severe enough to seek medical advice, positive signs of nerve root pressure indicated a duration of two weeks or more. Duration was measured by the

*Reprinted by permission from *Journal of the Royal College of General Practitioners*, 31:209–216, 1981.

time from first contact to last consultation (though the last consultation is no valid indication of the end of symptoms). Sims-Williams and colleagues found that recovery was more frequent if the pain had lasted less than one month. No other prognostic indicators were found. The patients in the latter study were those referred for x-ray examination. However, only a minority of general practice cases are referred for x-ray.

Aims

The aim of this study was to investigate, by clinical means alone, prognostic indicators in unselected patients reporting new episodes of low back pain by relating clinical features at the initial contact to the subsequent course in the following year. If this could be done, then more refined procedures might be superfluous.

Method

I defined low back pain as pain located within an area limited by a horizontal line through the third lumbar spine, the lateral edges of the quadrati lumborum, the iliac crests and the upper edge of the sacrum. Diseases of the skin, the subcutaneous tissues or abdomen were excluded.

All patients aged 16 or over who reported a new episode of low back pain were included in the study (Table 1). I made a standardized initial assessment; follow-up was performed by questionnaires after one, three and six months, and by interview after 12 months.

The study practice is single-handed, suburban and located 10 kilometres outside

Table 1. *Patients Reporting New Episodes of Low Back Pain at Least Once in One Year*

Age	Men		Women		Total	
	Number	*Percentage of Practice*	*Number*	*Percentage of Practice*	*Number*	*Percentage of Practice*
16–24	10	*4.1*	4	*1.6*	14	*2.8*
25–34	11	*4.9*	11	*3.4*	22	*4.0*
35–44	18	*4.9*	12	*3.5*	30	*4.2*
45–54	7	*4.4*	4	*3.4*	11	*4.0*
55–64	1	*2.0*	1	*1.9*	2	*1.9*
65–74	1	*4.2*	3	*16.7*	4	*9.5*
Total	48	*4.5*	35	*3.1*	83	*3.8*
		*(3.3–5.9)**		*(2.2–4.3)**		*(3.1–4.7)**

*95 percent confidence limits.

Copenhagen. The practice population comprises more skilled and unskilled workers than the standard Danish population.

On 1 October 1976, there were 2188 people aged 16 or more in the practice (males 1070, females 1118). Of these, 83 reported low back pain at least once during the year starting 8 September 1976. Five patients were excluded since follow-up would not have been possible (two were non-nationals, two were leaving the practice and one was suffering from a psychiatric disorder). This left 78 patients who were admitted to the study. One observer (P.A.P.) collected information on a standard questionnaire about the previous history of the patients and their symptoms, signs and work conditions. This questionnaire covered location, radiation, onset, constancy and previous history of back pain, the relation of pain to work, time off work, and a number of signs including mobility, scoliosis, unequal leg length, tenderness of loin muscles, muscular weakness, ankle jerk and straight leg raising. These parameters were defined prior to onset of the survey. In order not to increase the workload excessively the questionnaire was completed within about 10 minutes at the initial consultation.

The follow-up covered the total number of days with:

1. Symptoms present.
2. Absence from work.
3. Rest in bed part of or all day.
4. Use of analgesics.

Ninety-five percent of the patients were followed for six months, 92 percent for one year.

Results

Initial Clinical Information

The clinical data obtained at first attendance are presented in Table 2. Twenty-one percent (16) of the patients had had no previous attack. This gave an annual incidence of 7 per thousand (95 percent confidence limits: 4 to 12).

Follow-Up Data

Figures 1 to 4 show follow-up data about the duration of symptoms, time off work, use of analgesics and number of days' bed rest.

As the aim of this study was to elicit long-term prognostic indicators, data from the initial assessment and from the follow-up period are not commented on here.

Table 2. *Clinical Information* at Initial Contact (N = 78)*

Item	Number (Percentage)
Previous low back pain	
No episodes	16 (*21*)
More than three episodes	40 (*53*)
Onset	
Sudden	34 (*44*)
Gradual	43 (*55*)
Duration prior to contact	
Less than one week	42 (*54*)
More than four weeks	20 (*26*)
Pain constant	33 (*42*)
Radiation from loin	38 (*49*)
Straight leg raising test positive	10 (*13*)
Scoliosis caused by muscular spasm	26 (*33*)
Tenderness	61 (*78*)
Bilateral/unilateral	56/21 (*72/27*)
Difficulty in moving	40 (*51*)
Unequal leg length	8 (*10*)
Fit for work	50 (*64*)
Previous absence from work caused by low back pain	29 (*37*)
Onset related to work	22 (*28*)
Hard work	25 (*32*)
Previous operation	2 (*3*)
Muscular weakness	1 (*1*)
Achilles tendon reflex diminished	2 (*3*)

*Definitions of these items of clinical information are available from the author.

Comparison of Initial and Follow-Up Data

The prognostic value of the initial clinical data was analyzed as follows. The patients were divided into groups according to the severity of disability during the observation year. For instance, patients whose symptoms continued only during the first month of the follow-up year comprised one group, and patients with relapsing symptoms throughout the follow-up year comprised a second. A comparison between the two groups was then made by testing to see whether some item of initial information had occurred more often in one group than in the other. The patients were regrouped

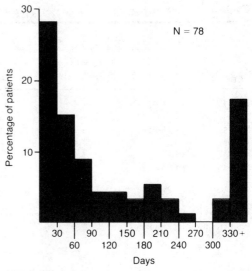

Fig. 1. Total number of days with symptoms during follow-up year. N = 78.

for each of the four items of follow-up data. In the case of continuing symptoms, the first group consisted of 12 people and the second group of 25. In the first group, only one person had had more than three previous cases of low back pain, but this had occurred in 16 of the second group. This dif-

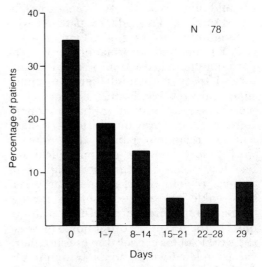

Fig. 2. Total number of days' unfitness for work during follow-up year. N = 78.

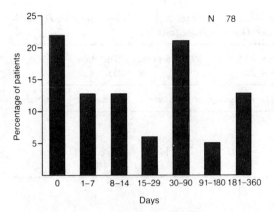

Fig. 3. Total number of days using analgesics during follow-up year. N = 78.

ference was significant by Mann-Whitney's test, p < 0.01. It follows that a history of more than three previous episodes pointed to a long or relapsing course.

Tables 3 to 6 present further comparisons made by this method. Gradual onset, more than four weeks' delay in reporting and radiation distal to the femur pointed to a long or relapsing course (Table 3). Most of the severe cases had initially had difficulty in movement (Table 4). Where patients subsequently had more than one week off

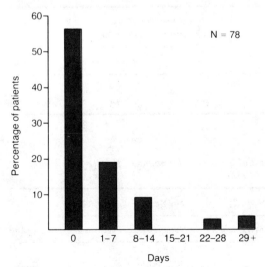

Fig. 4. Total number of days bed rest during follow-up year. N = 78.

work, this was related to the pain starting at work (Table 5). Having to stay in bed for one day or more during the follow-up year occurred more often in the group of patients who were absent from work at first contact, who had a positive straight leg raising test or whose pain was unilateral (Table 6).

Statistical tests were performed as Fisher's exact test or the chi-square test, depending upon number of observations.

Discussion

This study has shown that the clinical features presented to the general practitioner at the initial contact with patients with low back pain contain important prognostic information. Such prognostic indicators are important because they assist in the management of individual cases, enable the doctor to describe the likely course of the disability to the patient and may have a bearing on prophylactic measures for future patients.

The clinical examination of patients who entered this study did not exceed what may be considered an ordinary, fairly short practice procedure. As rather more refined techniques of medical assessment could easily be adopted, it seems feasible to elicit more prognostic information than that presented in this study.

In this study the duration of ill-effects was arrived at by totalling the number of days these were experienced in the observation year, rather than by recording only the initial period. This method takes into account courses characterized by relapses during the follow-up period as well as courses of a single period. Treatment has not been described; however, conservative treatment was applied to all patients except one. This patient was operated upon and recovered soon afterwards.

In this study it was not possible to test whether occupation was of any prognostic significance.

Table 3. *Duration of Symptoms in Follow-Up Year in Relation to Initial Information—Radiation Distal to Femur, Gradual Onset, More than Four Weeks' Delay in Reporting*

	Symptoms < 30 days (N = 22)		Symptoms > 180 days (N = 21)		
	Number	Percentage	Number	Percentage	p-value
Initial information					
Radiation distal to the femur	1	5	8	38	<0.05
Gradual onset	9	41	17	81	<0.01
More than four weeks' delay in reporting	0	0	8	38	<0.01

Table 4. *Severity of Course in Follow-Up Year in Relation to Initial Clinical Information—Difficulty in Movement*

	Mild Course (N = 8)		Severe Course* (N = 13)		
	Number	Percentage	Number	Percentage	p-value
Initial information					
Difficulty in movement	1	13	10	77	<0.02

*Severe defined as unfitness for work for more than 30 days, or use of analgesics for more than 90 days, or bed rest for more than 10 days.

Table 5. *Unfitness for Work in Follow-Up Year in Relation to Initial Clinical Information—Onset at Work*

	No Unfitness (N = 27)		Unfitness for More Than One Week (N = 28)		
	Number	Percentage	Number	Percentage	p-value
Initial information					
Onset at work	3	11	11	39	<0.05

Table 6. *Bed-Rest in Follow-Up Year in Relation to Initial Clinical Information—Absence from Work, Positive Straight Leg Raising Test, Unilateral Pain*

	Best Rest (N = 27)		No Bed Rest (N = 44)		
	Number	Percentage	Number	Percentage	p-value
Initial information					
Absent from work at first contact	20	74	7	16	<0.001
Positive straight leg raising test	8	30	1	2	<0.001
Unilateral pain	13	48	7	16	<0.01

REFERENCES

Bergquist-Ullman, M. & Larsson, U. (1977). Acute low back pain in industry: a controlled prospective study with special reference to therapy and confounding factors. Acta Orthopaedica Scandinavica, supplementum no. 170 Copenhagen: Munksgaard

Dillane, J. B., Fry, J. & Kalton, G. (1966). Acute back syndrome—a study from general practice. British Medical Journal, 2, 82–84

Sims-Williams, H., Jayson, M. I. V., Young, S. M. S., Baddeley, H. & Collins, E. (1978). Controlled trial of mobilization and manipulation for patients with low back pain in general practice. British Medical Journal, 2, 1338–1340

A Study in General Practice of the Symptoms and Delay Patterns in the Diagnosis of Gastrointestinal Cancer*

D. B. MacAdam

Gastrointestinal cancer was classified into four groups according to the site: stomach, caecum and ascending and transverse colon, sigmoid colon and rectum. The incidence of these cancers in general practice is as rare as three per 10,000 consultations. I report on a study in general practice of the symptoms and delays in diagnosis in 150 patients with gastrointestinal cancer. There was an interval of many weeks between the onset of symptoms and diagnosis in the majority of cases. In approximately 50 percent of cases there was an interval of weeks between the patient consulting the general practitioner and being referred for hospital investigation. No association was demonstrated between delay and social class, age, physical isolation, or the regular consulting rate of the patient. There was evidence that the consulting rate of some patients with gastrointestinal cancer increased in the 12 months before diagnosis because of the presence of symptoms not specific to the gastrointestinal tract.

Much more knowledge of the early symptoms of these cancers is required if the general practitioner is to be able to identify those patients with a high probability of early cancer from others who have symptoms which are common both to non life-threatening conditions and to cancer lesions.

Introduction

The five-year survival rates for patients with gastrointestinal cancer have not improved significantly over the past 20 years

despite advances in diagnostic and surgical techniques (Holland and Frei, 1973; Waterhouse, 1974). It is not known whether the survival rate could be improved if early symptoms were investigated more intensively, as little is known of the symptomatology of early gastrointestinal cancer (Lim et al., 1974). In Japan, mucosal and sub-mucosal gastric cancers have been detected in asymptomatic patients using contrast methods, cytological and endoscopy screening techniques. A significant improvement in survival rate has been achieved in such cases (Rubin, 1974). These findings have been confirmed by Elster and colleagues (1975) in West Germany. If the survival rate in Great Britain is to be improved it is important to know if mucosal and sub-mucosal gastrointestinal cancers commonly produce symptoms, and which symptom clusters are significant. It is also important to know where delay in diagnosis occurs (Hodgkin, 1973).

Aims

This study examines:

1. The symptoms which were presented to the general practitioner in patients with cancer of the stomach, caecum and ascending and transverse colon, sigmoid colon, and rectum.
2. The time elapsing before a diagnosis of gastrointestinal cancer was made was divided into:
   a. The time between the patient's realization that something was wrong and reporting it to the general practitioner.

*Reprinted by permission from Journal of the Royal College of General Practitioners, 29:723–729, 1979.

b. The time between the patient consulting the general practitioner and being referred to hospital.

c. The time between contact with the hospital (that is, date of referral) and a definite diagnosis being made.

Method

Eight general surgeons working in three hospitals in Leeds gave permission for any patient admitted under their care with gastrointestinal cancer to be invited to take part in the study. An interviewer visited the patients on the ward as soon after admission as possible, when nursing staff considered the patient well enough to be approached. The patients were invited to consent to be asked simple questions about their illness, and for their general practitioner and hospital doctor to give the interviewer details of the illness.

Questionnaire and Type of Information

The age, sex, marital status, occupation of patient or spouse, and whether or not the patient lived alone were recorded. The patient was asked about the frequency of consultation with his or her general practitioner during the five years before the present illness, and in particular about the frequency of consultation for any reason in the 12 months before the present illness began.

The patients were asked about the following symptoms: loss of energy or unusual tiredness, loss of appetite or nausea, vomiting, vomiting blood, abdominal pain or discomfort, changes in bowel habit, blood in motions, loss of weight, and other symptoms. The interviewer enquired how long each symptom had been present. As this was a retrospective study, the patient was asked for the earliest possible time it was thought the symptoms had occurred and the latest time of onset, the mean of these two recollections being recorded.

After the patient had been interviewed,

the hospital records were examined and the general practitioner seen by appointment. The following information was obtained from each source:

1. The date of referral to hospital by the general practitioner.
2. The symptoms which were recorded in the notes at hospital and by the general practitioner.
3. The date of definite diagnosis by microscopy.
4. Histology findings, either from biopsy or after surgical removal of the cancer. Only patients with cancer proven by histology were accepted into this series.

When the general practitioner was interviewed, he was asked how often the patient had consulted him in the 12 months before the onset of the symptoms thought to be due to the gastrointestinal cancer. He was asked to compare this consulting rate with the average consulting rate per year by that patient during the previous five years. At no time did the interviewer have direct access to the general practitioner records.

Co-operation Achieved During the Study

Of 154 patients who were approached to take part in the study, 150 consented. These patients were in the care of 109 practitioners, of whom one refused to be interviewed and three others were unable to help when interviewed. Not all patients had general practitioners, and of those who had, a few had never consulted them or could not answer questions about how often they consulted their doctor.

Of the 150 patients in the study there was inadequate information from general practitioners in 17 cases, inadequate information from the patient in five cases, and no general practitioner records in four cases. Information about consulting rates was available from general practitioner records for the five years before gastrointestinal cancer symptoms developed in 124 cases.

Use of Information Obtained

From the three sources of information the time of onset of each symptom was obtained, and the time recorded in weeks:

1. Before those symptoms were reported to the general practitioner.
2. Between the first report to the general practitioner and referral to hospital.
3. Between initial referral by the general practitioner and definite diagnosis by microscopy (a period which includes any waiting period for a hospital appointment as well as the consultations and investigations carried out at hospital).

Where there was a difference in the date given by the patient, general practitioner, and hospital records, the earliest date was taken either from the patient's recall of events or the general practitioner record. Such differences were not common and if the later date had been selected the findings in this study would not have been significantly different. (Details are available.)

Symptoms

Patients were grouped according to the site of the neoplasm:

1. Stomach.
2. Caecum, ascending colon, transverse colon.
3. Sigmoid colon.
4. Rectum.

The symptoms occurring in the four groups of patients with malignancies at the different sites of the gastrointestinal tract were separated into:

1. Those symptoms which were reported to the general practitioner before he decided to refer to hospital.
2. Those symptoms which were first recorded by the general practitioner on the day when he decided referral to hospital was indicated.

Results

The time elapsing before diagnosis was made histologically in all types of gastrointestinal cancer in this study is shown in Table 1.

The symptoms discussed here are those which the general practitioner selected to record. The absence of a symptom does not mean that it was not reported by the patient, but only that it was not recorded, and it is probable that in recording the general practitioner selected symptoms which seemed dominant or important rather than being comprehensively descriptive of all that the patient said. In Figures 1 to 4 the recorded symptoms arising from the different sites of carcinoma are shown, and the hatched areas indicate when that symptom was associated with the general practitioner making an immediate referral to hospital. In this study it was found that in only one instance did the general practitioner arrange for radiological investigation before

Table 1. *Time Elapsing Between Onset of Symptoms and Diagnosis of Gastrointestinal Cancer in 150 Patients*

Number of Patients = 150	Mean Interval (Weeks)	
1. Before diagnosis was made	25	
2. Between onset of symptom and reporting to general practitioner	9	Range = one week
3. Between patient consulting general practitioner and being referred to hospital	10	to over two years
4. Between date of referral to hospital and histological diagnosis	6	

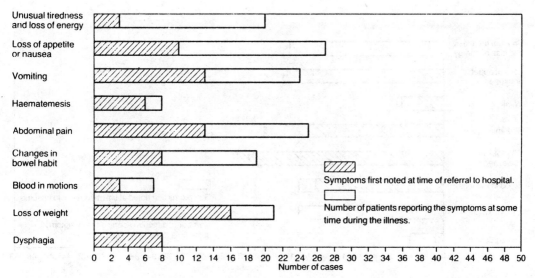

Fig. 1. Symptoms of carcinoma of stomach (n = 31).

referring the patient to a hospital physician or surgeon. At the time of this study in Leeds a general practitioner was able to request a barium meal but no other contrast radiography, and the interval before the investigation was completed might be a few weeks. The large majority of patients in this series were referred direct to surgeons. Investigations, such as blood counts, ESR, and occult blood tests, might have been requested by general practitioners before referral to hospital, but this information was not requested.

The footnotes to each figure show the

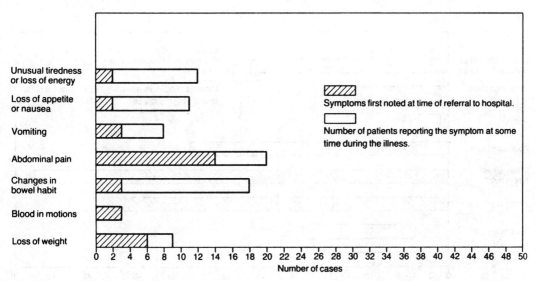

Fig. 2. Symptoms of carcinoma of caecum and ascending and transverse colon (n = 22).

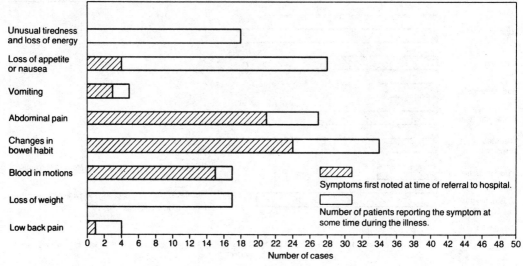

Fig. 3. Symptoms of carcinoma of sigmoid colon (n = 40).

intervals of time which occurred before a diagnosis was made after the patient had recognized that something was wrong. This time is subdivided into the time that passed owing to patient delay in reporting to the doctor, the time that passed before the general practitioner referred to hospital after the patient had first consulted him, and that which passed after the patient had been referred to hospital.

Consulting Rates

An analysis of the 127 records available showed that in 23 patients (18 percent) there was an increased consulting rate in

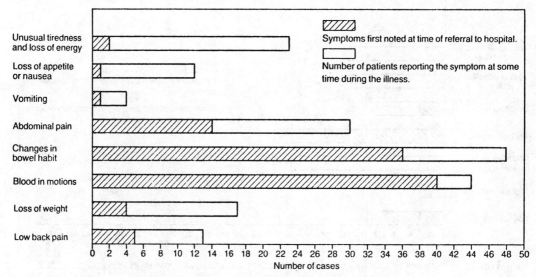

Fig. 4. Symptoms of carcinoma of rectum (n = 57).

the 12 months before the onset of symptoms which were regarded by the general practitioner as related to the final diagnosis. This increased rate was obtained by comparing it with the consulting rate per year of the particular patient during the previous five years. The increased rate was not due to screening tests initiated by the general practitioners.

Delay and Its Relation to Socio-Economic Class, Age, and Isolation

There was no significant difference in the socio-economic class, age, or social isolation of those patients who experienced delay compared with those who experienced no delay in referral. (Figures can be supplied on request.)

Discussion

It is possible that the information from general practitioner records in this study is inadequate owing to failure of the general practitioner to make records of consultations. There is also likely to be considerable selectivity in what the general practitioner records. What has been established is that a consultation occurred and that a date was entered on a record even though few symptoms may have been recorded. If a general practitioner failed to make any record then this would have tended to reduce the number of weeks elapsing between symptoms first being reported to the general practitioner and referral to hospital. It is impossible to exclude this error but patients might be expected to recall situations where they have frequently consulted their doctor before being referred to hospital. Whilst there is no way of checking this retrospectively, Table 2 shows the patient recall of frequency of consultation with their general practitioner compared with the doctor's recorded consulting rates.

These figures show that patients frequently underestimated their consulting rate when compared with the rate noted by the general practitioner.

Such a finding suggests that inadequate record keeping is not likely to distort grossly the delays which are reported in this study when they occur between a patient first going to the general practitioner and a referral being made to hospital. The close correlation between the differences in consulting rates during a period of 12 months and five years as recalled by the patient compared with the doctor's record suggests some consistency, despite the impossibility of validating such a retrospective study.

Symptoms and Diagnosis

In analysing the early symptoms of gastrointestinal cancer a distinction is necessary between those which occur singly and

Table 2. *A Comparison Between Patient's Recalled Consulting Rate and the General Practitioner's Recorded Consulting Rate*

	Patient's Recall Compared with General Practitioner's Records		
	Less Than General Practitioner	Same As General Practitioner	More Than General Practitioner
For five years before present illness	38	76	10
In 12 months before present illness	37	73	14

those which are clustered into symptom patterns. No attempt has been made here to examine the doctor's selectivity in recording symptoms, or the probability that symptom clusters are more significant than symptoms in isolation. In Figures 1 to 4, the association of symptoms is not indicated and the non-specific symptoms, like tiredness and loss of weight or appetite, may have preceded or been presented at the same time as the more indicative symptoms such as pain, blood in motions, dysphagia, or haematemesis. Horrocks and de Dombal (1975) have shown the accuracy of diagnosis on symptom data using a digital computer. This work was done in a surgical outpatient clinic where the patients had already been selected by the general practitioner. A similar approach using a computer might help the general practitioner to select symptom clusters indicative of disease and requiring further hospital investigation. Nevertheless, in almost 50 percent of cases there was immediate referral to hospital by the general practitioner when the patient first reported symptoms.

The histograms of the recorded symptoms (Figures 1 to 4) illustrate the difficulty for the general practitioner in selecting at first presentation those patients with serious pathology. Symptoms such as tiredness, loss of appetite, and vomiting occur frequently when no life-threatening underlying pathology is present.

Those patients with bleeding and pain were likely to be referred to hospital with the least delay. If it could be shown that one or two symptoms presenting together to the general practitioner in certain age/sex groups were associated with a high probability of serious disease, then the delay in diagnosis might be reduced. Such knowledge of indicative symptoms might also answer the question of whether or not early gastrointestinal cancer is frequently symptomatic or asymptomatic; it would also help in educating patients to recognize those symptoms which require immediate medical advice.

Delay in Patient Reporting Symptoms to the Doctor

Further studies are required to correlate early diagnosis after symptoms have developed with survival, and it is not known whether or not early diagnosis, dependent on symptoms, affects the prognosis. It has yet to be shown that there is benefit to be gained by making the diagnosis as early as possible after symptoms have developed. If this benefit is assumed, then the challenge to health education is to indicate to patients those symptoms which should be reported immediately to the doctor. This is not just a matter of knowledge as patient fears, denials, and expectations will influence the decision to be taken. In almost 50 percent of cases in this study many weeks elapsed between the patient realizing that "something was wrong" to the time when the patient consulted a doctor. Patient education must follow the doctor's first being convinced of the value of early diagnosis of symptoms, and secondly knowing which symptoms or groups of symptoms are indicative of serious disease. It may be that presymptomatic screening by endoscopy and cytology is the only way of improving survival rates from gastrointestinal cancer.

Delay Between the Patient Reporting Symptoms to the General Practitioner and Being Referred to Hospital

Those patients who delay before reporting symptoms to the general practitioner may be referred immediately to hospital when the first consultation occurs. Conversely those patients who report early to the general practitioner may suffer delay before being referred.

The findings of this survey do not reveal any correlation between age, sex, social status, or normal frequency of doctor/patient contact, and the delay before a patient is referred to hospital. Inevitably a general practitioner sees few new cases of gastrointestinal cancer in a year, and it is easier to allocate resources to those parts of the health service where diseases are concentrated—the acute medical and surgical wards of hospitals—rather than to the community where early diagnosis may lead to cure. By the time such concentration has been achieved this study shows that many weeks may have elapsed since symptoms first started. The delays in diagnosis are often due to patient delay in reporting to the general practitioner and to delay at hospital after referral has been made, but the longest delays occur when the general practitioner does not recognize the potentially serious nature of the patient's condition.

Pereira Gray (1966) made a comprehensive analysis of the role of the general practitioner in the early detection of malignant disease. He indicated the need for a retrospective analysis of cases of cancer such as has been attempted here, and he indicated reasons for delays in diagnosis in addition to the three discussed in this paper. He also considered the time elapsing before treatment was started and included patients diagnosed radiologically.

I have discussed only cases where the diagnosis was made histologically and where surgical treatment was given. A retrospective study of the delays in diagnosis, which includes all cases of gastrointestinal cancer, is necessary to determine whether the patterns of delay differ in those patients receiving surgery, compared with those patients who have gastrointestinal cancer at death, but who never have surgery. It is possible that when there is more delay the neoplasm has become so widespread by the time diagnosis is made that surgery is not attempted. Such further studies would need to include patients seen by consultant physicians at hospital.

Increasing the technical skill of hospital diagnosis and surgery is very expensive and probably has a strictly limited benefit unless ways can be found of achieving early detection of cancer at the primary care stage. A general practitioner with a list size of 2,500 patients can expect to see 200 to 250 patients per year with new episodes of gastrointestinal symptoms (OPCS *et al.*, 1974). The symptoms of tiredness and loss of appetite will occur even more frequently. It is important for the general practitioner to analyse and select accurately those patients who require the sophisticated technology of a modern hospital. Indeed, the computer potential which is seen dramatically in the images produced by the 'whole body scanner' can appropriately be applied to analysing the vast number of variables which confront a general practitioner listening to a patient's symptoms. The small desk-top computers now available make detailed research into symptoms possible, and it would be a mistake to consider the use of computers in general practice only in terms of data storage.

Conclusion

I have investigated one aspect of clinical research in general practice, the analysis of symptoms, which requires exploration with adequate resources. Perhaps the most important question is: "Does early treatment, once symptoms have developed, lead to increased life expectancy?" To concentrate research into cancer cure in the hospital is not only very expensive but in terms of benefit to the patient may be extremely wasteful. By comparison, research into the selection of patients who should appropriately and quickly be seen at hospital promises to be cost effective.

Acknowledgments

The interviewing was done by Mrs Valerie Lazenby, whose work is acknowledged with much appreciation. This study would not have been possible without Miss K. Edwards' secretarial work. The cooperation of the following surgeons: Professor G. R. Giles, Professor J. C. Goligher, Mr T. G. Brenna, Mr D. B. Feather, Mr G. Hill, Mr R. C. Kester, Mr D. Pratt, and Mr G. Wilson, over 100 general practitioners, and the patients and hospital records staff in Leeds is recognized with thanks. The advice of Professor I. D. G. Richards, Dr M. W. Sutcliffe, and Dr H. J. Wright was also a great help.

REFERENCES

Elster, K., Kolacyek, F., Shimamoto, K., & Freitag, H. (1975). Early gastric cancer—experience in Germany. Endoscopy, 7, 5–10

Gray, D. J. Pereira (1966). The role of the general practitioner in the early detection of malignant disease. Transactions of the Hunterian Society, 25, 121–175

Hodgkin, G. K. (1973). Evaluating the doctor's work. Journal of the Royal College of General Practitioners, 23, 559–567

Holland, J. F. & Frei, E. (1973). Cancer Medicine. Philadelphia: Lea and Febiger

Horrocks, J. C. & de Dombal, F. T. (1975). Computer-aided diagnosis of 'dyspepsia'. American Journal of Digestive Disease, 20, 395–406

Lim, B. S., Dennis, C. R., Gardner, B. & Newman, J. (1974). Analysis of survival versus patient and doctor delay of treatment in gastrointestinal cancer. American Journal of Surgery, 127, 210–214

Office of Population Census and Surveys, Royal College of General Practitioners & Department of Health and Social Security (1974). Morbidity Statistics From General Practice. Second National Study 1970–1971. London: HMSO

Rubin, P. (1974). Cancer of the gastro-intestinal tract. Journal of the American Medical Association, 228, 883–896

Waterhouse, J. A. H. (1974). Cancer Handbook of Epidemiology and Prognosis. London: Churchill Livingstone

ABSTRACTS

Heyden S, Bartel AG, Hames CG, McDonough JR: Elevated blood pressure levels in adolescents, Evans County, Georgia. JAMA 209(11):1683–1689, 1969

The significance of elevated blood pressures in young adults is still a subject of controversy. Two schools of thought have evolved regarding the prognosis of a condition that has been delineated as "prehypertensive" by some authors and "labile hypertensive" by others. In view of these conflicting observations, it was decided not to label a group of young persons as prehypertensive, labile, transient hypertensive, or borderline hypertensive who, seven years ago, were found to have elevated blood pressures in the Evans County (Georgia) Epidemiologic Study. The objective was to study the significance of blood pressure elevations at a young age *without treatment*.

The total representative sample of 15- to 25-year old adolescents examined in the initial phase of the Evans County Epidemiologic Study between 1960 and 1962 (abbreviated 1961) consisted of 435 persons (129 white males, 120 white females, 90 black males, and 96 black females). Fifty persons (20 white and 30 black) had an average blood pressure of three readings either greater than 140 mm Hg systolic or 90 mm Hg diastolic. The remaining 385 adolescents were normotensive. This study deals with the 50 persons found to have elevated blood pressures in 1961.

At the second examination seven years later, 20 of the 50 persons could not be reached since they were either in the armed services overseas, were on working assignments out of town, or had moved to other cities. Each of the remaining 30 individuals was matched with a normotensive person for age, sex, and race. The first 30 controls

meeting these criteria were used. In addition to several laboratory determinations, a sociological questionnaire was administered. None of the adolescents found to have elevated blood pressure levels in 1961 underwent any form of antihypertensive therapy.

The following criteria were used for the three categories of blood pressure levels in the 7 year follow-up study:

Normotension—at all three readings
   systolic   <140 mm Hg and
   diastolic   <90 mm Hg
Borderline hypertension—mean of three readings
   either systolic   140–159 mm Hg
   or diastolic   90–94 mm Hg
Sustained hypertension—all three readings
   either   ≥160 mm Hg
   or   ≥95 mm Hg

Clinical evaluation of the 30 adolescents with elevated blood pressures and their 30 normotensive controls during the 1968 reexamination are summarized in Table 1. Seven years after the diagnosis was made, sustained hypertension developed in five persons, and six had sustained hypertension with vascular complications. Two of the black females in this group died from cerebral hemorrhage, both verified by autopsy. In 12 of 30 young persons with elevated blood pressures, the seven-year follow-up revealed a decrease of their blood pressure to normotensive levels. No vascular complication was encountered in this group. Blood pressures in seven persons remained below the sustained hypertensive level, but should be called borderline

115

Table 1. *Clinical Evaluation of 30 Adolescents with Elevated Blood Pressures and 30 Normotensive Controls in 1961 and 1968*

1961	1968				
	Unchanged	Sustained Hypertension, Asymptomatic	Sustained Hypertension with Vascular Complications	Blood Pressure* L	E
30 Adolescents—elevated blood pressures	7	5	6	12	...
30 Adolescents—normal blood pressures	26	0	0	...	4

*L indicates lowered; E, elevated.

Reprinted by permission from Heyden, et al: JAMA, 209(11): 1683–1689, 1969.

hypertensive. Again, no vascular complication was found in this group. In the normotensive control population, no sustained hypertension was detected, no death occurred, and only four individuals had to be placed into the borderline hypertensive category at this time, while 26 individuals remained normotensive.

The important finding of this longitudinal study is that in 11 individuals previously with elevated blood pressures, either sustained hypertension or vascular complications, including death, developed. Blood pressures in seven more persons remained unchanged from 1961, and sustained hypertension or vascular complications are particularly likely to develop. In contrast, of these 18 subjects, blood pressures in only 12 returned to normotensive levels.

In summary, the clinical significance of elevated blood pressure levels in adolescents needs to be emphasized. This follow-up study extended over a seven-year period during which none of the 30 individuals was treated. It is suggested that if they had been under constant medical care, the outcome of the study might have been different. In view of the close association of overweight and subsequent weight gain in those in whom sustained hypertension eventually developed, one would recommend a strict weight reduction regime as well as antihypertensive therapy after thorough diagnostic evaluation.

Hames CG: Natural history of essential hypertension in Evans County, Georgia. Postgrad Med 56(6):119–125, 1974

Hypertensive disease, with its sequelae, is the primary cause of death in blacks and a major cause of death in whites. Increased knowledge concerning the natural history of the disease before target organs are involved is essential if appropriate methods for detection as well as preventive and therapeutic intervention are to be developed.

The long-term epidemiologic study of cardiovascular disease in Evans County, Georgia, has offered a unique opportunity to observe the natural history of essential hypertension in a total community with a biracial population and to assess in adolescents the predictive value in hypertension of such factors as elevated blood pressure, race and sex differences, excess weight, changes with age, morbidity, and mortality. The study population, identified by census, consisted of all persons 40 through 74 years old and a 50 percent random sample of

Table 1. *Changes in Mean Blood Pressure as Seen in Seven-Year Follow-Up, Evans County [Georgia] Cardiovascular Study*

Age Group	Black Males (mm Hg)		White Males (mm Hg)		Black Females (mm Hg)		White Females (mm Hg)	
	1960-1962	1967-1969	1960-1962	1967-1969	1960-1962	1967-1969	1960-1962	1967-1969
15-19	127.3/78.1	130.1/83.9	124.8/72.4	130.3/79.3	126.6/79.0	124.3/80.5	118.4/72.1	116.8/77.3
20-24	128.5/81.2	132.5/84.3	130.4/77.7	127.1/82.5	124.1/80.1	126.5/85.3	122.0/78.4	121.3/79.2
25-29	133.6/83.9	134.6/88.6	127.3/78.6	129.2/82.5	139.0/90.4	136.7/92.8	120.4/78.9	123.8/83.1

Reprinted by permission from Hames; Postgrad Med, 56(6):119-125, 1974.

those 15 through 39. Medical examinations were performed by two internists on 3102 subjects (92 percent) from the target population. A mercury sphygmomanometer with a cuff width of 14 cm was used. Measurements were obtained from the left arm with the subject seated. First and fifth phases (disappearance) of Korotkoff sounds were employed to designate systolic and diastolic pressures. In the 15 through 29 age group, 546 subjects were examined. Approximately 7 years later, 436 were available for reexamination; 20.2 percent were not available because of death, migration, or refusal to participate. To study morbidity and mortality in the same population but with a slightly younger cutoff point (ages 15 through 25), 435 subjects (129 white males, 120 white females, 90 black males, and 96 black females) were followed.

The prevalence of elevated blood pressure (1960-1962) in the age group 15 through 29 (criteria, 140 mm Hg systolic or 90 mm Hg diastolic) suggested that 22.7 percent of this population is hypertensive. The well-known fact concerning greater prevalence of hypertension in blacks was clearly demonstrated. The prevalence rates were as follows: black males, 34.9 percent; black females, 31.6 percent; white males, 19.0 percent; and white females, 12.7 percent. Data from the 1967-1969 exam-

inations on incidence of hypertension were next studied using the same criteria for hypertension as used in the 1960-1962 study. The incidence was as follows: black males, 36.2 percent; white males, 27.8 percent; black females, 24.6 percent; and white females, 12.1 percent. Table 1 compares the mean blood pressures obtained in the early and late studies.

In summary, a long-term epidemiologic study of 546 young people 15 through 29 years old was begun in 1960-1962. Race and sex differences in blood pressure levels were immediately apparent, even in this young age group. The association of weight with blood pressure was a highly significant feature in the white males, white females, and black females, but the relationship in black males was more obscure. In the first three groups, weight is related to the initial blood pressure as well as to its subsequent natural history. The data suggest that maintaining an ideal weight from early youth may be an important preventive means in the control of hypertension.

A seven-year follow-up of morbidity and mortality demonstrated a surprising amount of pathologic involvement in an adolescent group. The findings graphically point up the need to consider hypertension as an adolescent problem that demands early diagnosis and vigorous treatment.

Forsyth RA: Hypertension in a primary care practice.
J Fam Pract 10(5):803–807, 1980

Very little information is available on the characteristics of patients with hypertension who are seen in the usual office practice. Physicians are forced to base their decisions on data from studies of hypertensive patients who are seen in specialty clinics or in county, veterans, or university hospitals. Such populations may not be representative of the general population in that they are usually drawn from a low socioeconomic group, have an atypical prevalence of hypertension, may contain a large number of alcoholics, tend to contain a disproportionate number of complicated or noncompliant patients, and often do not include representative numbers of women.

The data compiled in this study were obtained from a population mix similar to that encountered in many office practices. Nine family physicians at a primary care office in the Los Angeles metropolitan area were asked to record data on all individuals with current or previously documented hypertension who were seen at the office over a period of six months. The study population was drawn from individuals enrolled in a prepaid insurance plan. The majority of the participants were in the lower-middle-income range. Two percent of the study population was black, 6 percent was Oriental. The standard procedure in the office was to measure the seated individual's blood pressure on the right arm. Blood pressure was measured at the beginning and end of each visit. The lower of the two pressures was recorded on the flow sheet.

At the end of 6 months, the charts were reviewed by the author to assess the severity of the individuals' hypertension and their response to medication. Only those individuals who had three recordings in which either the systolic blood pressure exceeded 159 mm Hg or the diastolic exceeded 94 mm Hg were included in the study. Severity was estimated by recording the highest systolic blood pressure and the associated diastolic blood pressure found on each patient's chart. These were retrospective data since they included blood pressures taken in months or years past. This approach usually made it possible to obtain a blood pressure that was taken before the patient started on medication or while the patient was off medication and was therefore representative of his/her untreated blood pressure. The magnitude of an individual's response to medication was estimated by recording the most recent blood pressure that was taken while the individual was on medication. The difference between the maximum pressures and the latest pressures obtained while the individual was on medication was used to measure the magnitude of the response to therapy.

This study reports on 490 patients (238 men and 252 women). The highest recorded blood pressure of hypertensive male patients averaged 177/113 mm Hg. The most recent blood pressure of males under treatment for hypertension averaged 144/92 mm Hg. For female patients, the corresponding figures were 179/112 mm Hg and 146/91 mm Hg. The average diastolic blood pressure for male hypertensives rose until age 54, then fell; the average for females rose until age 64 years, then fell.

Diuretics were used in 88.6 percent of males and 95.0 percent of females. Reserpine and methyldopa were the most common second-step drugs in use at the time of this study. Hydralazine was generally a third step drug, and guanethidine was generally a fourth-step drug. Propranolol and clonidine were used as either second- or third-step therapy in most instances but occasionally were used alone. Table 1 shows the percent of the patients who received single, double, triple, and quadruple therapy. Based on the average dosages and the prevailing costs, the average cost of medication for one year was $80. When all age groups are considered, blood pressures

Table 1. *Hypertensive Medications per Patient (Percent)*

	One Drug	Two Drugs	Three Drugs	Four Drugs
Male	38	52	9	1
Female	38	48	12	2

Reprinted by permission from Forsyth: J Fam Pract, 10(5): 803–807, 1980.

in treated hypertensive patients declined to 144/92 mm Hg in men and 146/91 mm Hg in women.

The age group 55 to 64 years contained 32 percent of the female hypertensive patients over 35 years of age and 26 percent of the male (i.e. hypertension was 23 percent more frequent in males at this age). Under age 35 years, however, hypertension was recorded eight times more often in males than in females (24 per 289 vs. 3 per 265). If the severity of hypertension is based on diastolic blood pressure, hypertension is severe in men more often than in women (9.7 vs. 3.2 percent). An unexpected finding in this study was the greater use of triple or quadruple therapy in women as compared to men (14 vs. 10 percent).

On the basis of these findings, it would seem appropriate to recommend that (1) in screening a young population for hypertension, greater emphasis be placed on males than on females; (2) the level of the diastolic blood pressure receive primary consideration when a determination is made as to whether or not an individual should be treated; (3) the diastolic blood pressure be used to monitor the response to medication; and (4) the use of triple or quadruple therapy be critically evaluated.

Medalie JH, Goldbourt U: Angina Pectoris Among 10,000 Men (2). Am J Med 60:910–921, 1976

Angina pectoris, known since antiquity, has been the subject of many anecdotal, clinical, and research publications. Despite this, there are still many puzzling features related to its physiology, pathology, etiology, and prognosis. In an attempt to elucidate some of the factors associated with the development of angina pectoris, 10,000 adult Israeli men, 40 years old and over, were followed intensively for five years.

The multivariate analysis reported in this paper examines the role of the significant "risk factors or variables" identified by the univariate analysis when all the other variables are taken into account. In this way, the most important variables in the screening and prediction of angina pectoris can be delineated.

Table 1 displays the follow-up results of 9764 men after five and seven years that bear on the natural history of angina.

The multivariate analysis revealed the following seven variables as the "significant" ones: age, blood pressure (systolic or diastolic), anxiety, psychosocial problems, serum cholesterol, diabetes, and electrocardiographic abnormalities (myocardial ischemia or nonspecific T wave changes). These seven variables were significant whether the patients with an infarct were included or not.

In the univariate analysis of angina pectoris in a previous study, it was found that of all the psychosocial problems, that of family problems showed the strongest association with the subsequent development of angina pectoris. A major finding arising from this study is the important independent role played in the development of angina pectoris by emotional and social problems, exemplified by anxiety and severe psychosocial problems of whatever nature but es-

Table 1. *"Natural History" of Chest Pain (in Subjects without Myocardial Infarction*)*

		Results Up To and Including 1968 (5 Years)						Up to April 15, 1970 (7 Years)			
				Myocardial Infarction Developed				Died			
								of Myocardial Infarction		of All Causes	
		Alive and Well		Alive		Died					
1963 Diagnosis	N = 100%	No.	%	No.	%	No.	%	No.	%	No.	%
Definite angina	256	219	85.5	18	7.0	10	3.9	14	5.5	30	11.7
Suspect angina	426	389	91.3	20	4.7	7	1.6	13	3.1	26	6.1
All other chest pain	1,316	1,241	94.3	52	4.0	10	0.8	19	1.4	43	3.3
No chest pain	7,744	7,310	94.4	269	3.5	41	0.5	71	0.9	295	3.8
Unknown	22	22	100.0	...	...	...	...	...	...	...	...
Total	9,764	9,181	94.0	359	3.7	68	0.7	117	1.2	394	4.0

*Free of myocardial infarction on electrocardiogram; and/or of a verified history of heart attack; and/or of left bundle branch block on electrocardiogram at intake (1963).
Reprinted by permission from Medalie, Goldbourt: Am J Med, 60:910–921, 1976.

pecially those related to the subject's family. With low anxiety, high cholesterol and blood pressure cause a rise in the incidence of angina pectoris from 12 to 39; with high anxiety, from 57 to 97/1000.

The beneficial effects of the wife's love and support as perceived by the male subjects is demonstrated in Table 2. In looking at this factor as related to anxiety, it appears that with high levels of anxiety, the incidence rate for angina is significantly reduced from 93 to 52/1000 by having a loving and supportive wife.

The presence of all seven risk factors (at a high level) increases the probability of angina pectoris developing within five years to 289/1000 from 14/1000 when these factors are low or absent. The wife's love and support are an important balancing factor, which apparently reduces the risk of angina pectoris even in the presence of high-risk factors. The implications of these findings

Table 2. *The Association of Five Year Incidence of Angina Pectoris (Cases of Myocardial Infarction Excluded) with Anxiety and Wife's Love/Support*

Anxiety Score	Wife's Love and Support	No. at Risk	No. Angina Pectoris Cases	Rate 1,000	
0-1	3+	4,110	88	21	
	2+	1,090	31	28	
	±	460	11	24	
	−	714	18	25	N.S.
2-3	3+	637	33	52	
	2+	242	11	45	
	±	150	11	73	
	−	183	17	93	$0.01 < p < 0.05$*

*p values are for significance of the incidence slope with rising scores for "wife's love."
Reprinted by permission from Medalie, Goldbourt: Am J Med, 60:910–921, 1976.

for clinicians lie in two directions. In the one, preventive measures, like antismoking, reducing cholesterol and blood pressure levels and weight, will probably help to reduce the incidence of myocardial infarction and, to a lesser extent, angina pectoris. But in the other, no matter how well this is done, the major sources of risk for angina pectoris will be missed unless it is accompanied by a detailed investigation of the subject's personal, family, and occupational life situations. The latter will allow the physician to assess the strengths and stresses in order to help the patient solve or adjust in a more satisfactory way to recurrent problems and thus reduce his anxiety. It again stresses the often mentioned need for, but rarely performed, coverage of the physical, emotional, and social aspects of the patient's life in order to prevent, delay, or diminish his angina pectoris.

Medalie JH, Goldbourt U: Unrecognized myocardial infarction: five-year incidence, mortality, and risk factors. Ann Int Med 84:526–531, 1976

In the spectrum of ischemic heart disease, the role played by unrecognized myocardial infarctions has assumed more importance as population group surveys have been added to clinical experience. Various population surveys and necropsy studies have shown that 20 to 60 percent of all myocardial infarctions were unrecognized by the subjects themselves, their physicians, or both. The importance of these findings can only be assessed if we know (1) the relation of unrecognized infarcts to clinically overt ones; (2) the relation to mortality, that is, the prognosis of subjects with unrecognized infarcts; and (3) the risk factors associated with their development—are they the same or different from those of clinical infarcts?

This paper reports the results of a five year prospective study in Israel of almost 10,000 adult men who were examined in 1963 and 1968. The study population consisted of permanent government and municipal employees 40 years old and older at the onset of the study. The coverage of the mortality follow-up was 100 percent and was extended to 1970 (7 years). Men at risk for this study were subjects who showed no evidence of myocardial infarction or left bundle branch block on ECG and had no suggestive history of infarct in 1963. The diagnosis of unrecognized infarction was made when the ECG in the 1963 or 1968 follow-up examination revealed evidence of myocardial infarction and when no history or other evidence was obtained that there had been a heart attack since the 1963 examination. The ECGs were read independently each time and were not compared with the previous ones.

In the course of five years, 9509 healthy adult subjects had an average annual incidence of 3.6 unrecognized infarcts per 1000 persons and 5.3 clinical ones per 1000 persons. There were 427 infarcts, of which 170 were unrecognized, that is, 39.8 percent of all infarcts.

A multivariate analysis showed that the most significant risk factors were age, left axis deviation, left ventricular hypertrophy, cigarette smoking, systolic or diastolic blood pressure, and peripheral vascular disease. Some of the known risk factors of clinical infarct, angina pectoris, or both, such as cholesterol, diabetes, anxiety, and psychosocial problems, did not play a significant role in unrecognized infarcts.

The general study population, without any signs of infarct at any stage during the follow-up period, had an average annual mortality rate of 4.6/1000 (Table 1), whereas those with unrecognized infarcts had 3.8 times this rate, that is, 17.3/1000. The pooled mortality rate for clinical in-

Table 1. *Mortality Associated with Unrecognized Infarcts: Comparison with Clinical Infarcts and the Rest of the Study Population (1963–1970)*

	At Risk for Average Period of 6 Years* (Diagnosed Between 1963–1965)			At Risk for Average Period of 3½ Years* (Diagnosed Between 1965–1968)			Total		
	At Risk	Died	Annual Rate/ 1000	At Risk	Died	Annual Rate/ 1000	At Risk	Died	"Pooled" Annual Rate/ 1000
	←──────────────────────── no. ────────────────────────→								
Study population without infarct (1963–1968)							9337	301	4.6
Subjects with myocardial infarct on ECG at 1965 or 1968 examination									
Unrecognized infarct	54	7	22	116	4	10	170	11	17.3
Clinical infarct	36	9	42	84	8	27	120	17	36.3
All clinical infarcts from 1963–1968, including sudden deaths < 1 h	86	35	68	171	52	87	257	87	74.8

*Follow-up was to mid-1970. Those diagnosed from 1963 through 1965 are assumed to have had their infarct midway between examinations I (1963) and II (1965); that is, from 1964 to mid-1970 = 6 years follow-up. Similarly, those diagnosed from 1965 through 1968 are assumed to have 3½ years of follow-up.
Reprinted by permission from Medalie, Goldbourt: Ann Int. Med, 84:526–531, 1976.

rate of the infarct-free section of the population.

On many occasions, it has been shown that diagnostic electrocardiographic evidence of myocardial infarction can disappear, sometimes in as short a period as six months; thus, a calculation of incidence rates based on examinations at two- or three-year intervals might considerably underestimate the "true" incidence. While it is impossible to make an accurate prediction of the "real" incidence, the experience of the American, Finnish, and Israeli studies suggests that for every clinical infarct detected, there is probably at least one unrecognized one in the same population group. In addition to missing a silent infarct by ECG, there is also the occasional rare case in which a positive ECG infarct finding has not been corroborated at necropsy.

The importance of these findings and the differences between the epidemiology of unrecognized infarcts and clinical infarcts rests on the outcome or prognosis of those people with unrecognized infarcts. It is on this point that the Framingham and Israeli experience diverge. The Framingham Study has shown that its subjects with unrecognized infarcts have the same mortality experience as those with clinical infarcts. In this study, analysis comparable to that of the Framingham Study shows that survivors of clinical infarcts had a 2:1 estimated relative risk of mortality as compared with the unrecognized infarcts (36.3 to 17.3/1000). However, when all clinical infarcts in the analysis are included, a method that brings this more "in line" with clinical practice, the mortality rate was 4.5 times the rate of the unrecognized infarcts.

Heyman A, Wilkinson WE, Heyden S, Helms MJ, Bartel AG, Karp HR, Tyroler HA, Hames CG: Risk of stroke in asymptomatic persons with cervical arterial bruits. N Engl J Med. 302:838–841, 1980

Some vascular surgeons recommend that asymptomatic persons with prolonged, high-pitched, midcarotid bruits have arteriographic examinations of the cervical and intracranial vessels and that if atherosclerotic stenosis is found in the internal carotid artery, endarterectomy should be carried out. There are no controlled clinical studies to support this opinion, and it is not certain whether prophylactic arterial surgery will reduce the likelihood of stroke in such patients. The current controversy on the management of such cases cannot be resolved until data are available on the natural history of this condition and on the results of medical and surgical therapy.

Useful information regarding the prognosis of asymptomatic cervical arterial bruits is now available from large population studies. In the Framingham Study, cervical arterial bruits were found to make an important independent contribution to the risk of stroke even when age, associated hypertension, and coronary heart disease were taken into consideration. This paper reports the results of a five- to seven-year period of observation on 72 stroke-free persons with asymptomatic cervical arterial bruits detected during a population survey of a biracial Southern community.

Persons selected for this study were residents of Evans County, Georgia, a small rural community in the "stroke belt" of the Southeastern United States. The initial survey of this community, which contains approximately 40 percent blacks, was carried out in 1960 and included all residents 40 years of age and older and a 50 percent sample of those 15 to 39 years of age. A follow-up survey was made between August 1, 1967, and August 31, 1969, to determine the incidence of heart disease and stroke. A multiple logistic model was used to evaluate the association of cervical bruits with each

of the outcome events (i.e., stroke and death due to vascular disease) and at the same time take into account other known risk factors.

Table 1 shows the age, sex, and race distribution of persons with cervical arterial bruits among the 1620 persons examined in 1967 to 1969 who were free of stroke and ischemic heart disease and 45 years of age or older. The relation of these bruits to the presence of hypertension is also shown. There was a progressive increase in frequency of bruits in each age decade of this population, with frequency ranging from 2.3 percent in persons 45 to 54 years of age

Table 1. *Relation of Cervical Bruits to Demographic Characteristics and Hypertension*

Feature	No. of Persons Examined	No. with Bruits	Prevalence (%)
Age (yr)			
45–54	564	13	2.3
55–64	592	25	4.2
65–74	354	25	7.1
≥75	110	9	8.2
All age groups (≥45)	1620	72	4.4
Sex			
Women	919	54	5.9
Men	701	18	2.6
Race			
White	1016	43	4.2
Black	604	29	4.8
Hypertension*			
Absent	1087	33	3.0
Present	533	39	7.3

*Systolic blood pressure ≥ 160 mm Hg.

Reprinted with permission from Heyman et al: N Eng J Med, 302: 838–841, 1980.

Table 2. *Relation of Stroke to Presence or Absence of Cervical Bruits According to Age and Sex*

Age at 1967–69 Examination (Yr)	Bruits Present			Bruits Absent		
	No. at Risk	No. with New Strokes	% with New Strokes	No. at Risk	No. with New Strokes	% with New Strokes
Men						
45–54	3	0	0.0	256	2	0.8
55–64	9	2	22.2	260	8	3.1
65–74	4	2	50.0	127	10	7.9
≥75	2	1	50.0	40	5	12.5
All age groups (≥45)	18	5	27.8	683	25	3.7
Women						
45–54	10	1	10.0	295	6	2.0
55–64	16	0	0.0	307	5	1.6
65–74	21	3	14.3	202	7	3.5
≥75	7	1	14.3	61	9	14.8
All age groups (≥45)	54	5	9.3	865	27	3.1
Men and women						
All age groups (≥45)	72	10	13.9	1548	52	3.4

Reprinted by permission from Heyman et al: N Eng J Med, 302:838–841, 1980.

to 8.2 percent among those 75 years of age or older. Of the total group of 1,620 persons, 72 (4.4 percent) were found to have cervical arterial bruits. The prevalence of these murmurs was 5.9 percent in women, 2.6 percent in men, 4.8 percent in blacks, and 4.2 percent in whites. Among persons with systolic blood pressure measurements of 160 mm Hg or greater at rest, 7.3 percent were found to have cervical arterial bruits, as compared with 3.0 percent of persons without this degree of hypertension.

In the six-year average period from the survey examination to the end of follow-up observation, stroke occurred more often among persons with cervical bruits than among those without such murmurs (Table 2). During this time the first episode of stroke occurred in 10 (13.9 percent) of the 72 men and women with bruits, as compared with 52 (3.4 percent) of the 1548

without bruits. Stroke also appeared much more frequently among men with cervical bruits than among women with bruits (27.8 percent and 9.3 percent, respectively).

The presence of asymptomatic bruits was associated with a significantly higher risk of stroke in men but not in women, with odds ratios of 7.5 and 1.6, respectively. Despite the high risk of stroke among men with bruits, the correlation between the location of the bruits and the type of subsequent stroke was poor. Moreover, cervical bruits in men were a risk factor for death from ischemic heart disease. These findings suggest that asymptomatic cervical bruits are an indication of systemic vascular disease and do not themselves justify invasive diagnostic procedures or surgical correction of underlying extracranial arterial lesions.

Medalie JH: Risk factors other than hyperglycemia in diabetic macrovascular disease. Diabetes Care 2(2): 77–84, 1979

This paper reports a 5 year prospective follow-up study done on 10,000 males in Israel. The end points of diabetes mellitus—clinical and unrecognized myocardial infarction, angina pectoris, sudden death, and hypertension—were examined.

After an initial examination, two further comprehensive examinations were performed at intervals of three and five years. Parallel to this, an efficient monitoring system kept the whole group under surveillance for serious illness and deaths through the five year period. At the final examination, 98 percent of those still living were reexamined, while the 100 percent mortality follow-up was extended for a total of seven years. In other words, the morbidity follow-up was for five years or approximately 50,000 person-years of observation, while the mortality follow-up of seven years gave approximately 70,000 person-years of observation. At the initial examination, all the dependent variables or disease conditions identified were included in the prevalence figures for that condition, and all those without signs of the condition were regarded as being at risk for the prospective follow-up. Any subject developing one of these conditions during the follow-up period or found at the final examination was classified as an incidence case. Efficient control and supervisory procedures were carried out throughout.

The average annual age-area-adjusted incidence rates and the variations between the birth areas for diabetes, clinical and unrecognized myocardial infarction, angina pectoris, and hypertension are shown in Table 1. In all cases, the incidence rates rise with age. Without considering variations in definition and methodology, it can be said that these figures are comparable to the rates of many European and North American studies.

The diabetic individuals in the study had twice the mortality rate from all causes than the nondiabetic individuals, with a little over 50 percent of this mortality being due to myocardial infarction and sudden death. Those with diabetes of longer duration (previously diagnosed) had more deaths from all causes than the newly diagnosed ones.

The age-adjusted mean values for a number of risk factors as related to previously and newly diagnosed diabetes are shown in Table 2. With the exception of uric acid, the other risk factors are all raised in those with diabetes as compared to those without diabetes (total population minus those with diabetes), but they are lower in the previously diagnosed than the newly diagnosed group. This unexpected finding is likely due to the results of medical management of the previously diagnosed group with a consequent reduction of weight, blood pressure, and cholesterol levels.

In this study population, the risk factors associated with the development of diabetes and its macrovascular complications are age, overweight, peripheral vascular dis-

Table 1. *Incidence of Cardiovascular and Related Manifestations in 10,000 Adult Males (5-Yr Prospective Study)*

Condition	Average Annual Adjusted Incidence Rate/ 1000	Variations between Birth Areas
Clinical myocardial infarction	5.3	3.6– 7.1
Unrecognized myocardial infarction	3.6	3.0– 4.6
All myocardial infarction	8.7	7.4–10.0
Angina pectoris	7.2	3.8–11.2
Hypertension	10.0	6.0–15.0
Diabetes	8.0	5.6–11.2

Reprinted by permission from Medalie: Diabetes Care, 2(2): 77–84, 1979.

Table 2. *Values of Selected Risk Factors in Diabetes (Age-Adjusted Mean Values)*

	Previously Diagnosed	Newly Diagnosed	Total Population
Cholesterol (mg/100 ml)	217	220	209
Systolic blood pressure (mmHg)	138	146	135
Diastolic blood pressure (mmHg)	84	87	84
Wt/ht^2	2.61	2.70	2.57
Uric acid	4.21	4.56	4.75

Reprinted by permission from Medalie: Diabetes Care, 2(2): 77–84, 1979.

ease, blood pressure, serum cholesterol (total and high density lipoprotein), uric acid, birthplace (Middle East and North Africa), education (low), hemoglobin, smoking, anxiety, severe psychosocial problems, and lack of social support. The prevention or alleviation of diabetic macrovascular disease needs a multifactorial approach against the major risk factors of the macrovascular complications as well as those related to diabetes in the individual, family, and community.

Fry J: Epidemic influenza. J R Coll Gen Pract 17:100–103, 1969

The features of influenza as the most extensive of recurrent epidemics are well known. Its regular periodic occurrences, affecting large sections of populations, are appreciated, as are problems of immunity and changing pathogenicity of the various strains of the causal influenza virus. Not so well known are some epidemiologic characters of the epidemics themselves. Features such as the age and sex distribution of those infected and individual susceptibility in successive epidemics and their severity when studied reveal some intriguing facts. Comparison of a series of epidemics enables a clinical profile to be defined, which is of some importance in developing therapeutic and preventive attitudes.

This paper summarizes and reviews eight successive epidemics of proven influenza over 20 years (1949 to 1968) in a single general practice. Special opportunities exist in general practice for such a study on account of the possibilities of following up and observing a relatively static and known population over many years.

The population studied was in a general practice sited in the suburbs of London. The size of the practice population averaged approximately 6000 persons. There was inevitably some movement of individuals in and out of the area, but the annual turnover did not exceed 7 percent. The study was based on a record system that enabled ready analysis of present and past morbidity within the practice. The diagnosis of "epidemic influenza" was made only when there was clear evidence of national or local epidemics during which virologic confirmation was available. During each epidemic analyses were made of its extent as determined by the numbers of persons seen by the physicians (patient-consultation rate); of those affected according to age and sex distributions; of severity, as shown by chest and other complications and deaths; and of individual susceptibilities.

The patient-consultation rates for each epidemic are shown in Table 1. The mean rate for the eight epidemics was 8 percent

Table 1. *Patient Consultation Rates During Influenza Epidemics 1949-1968*

Year	1950-1951	1953	1955	1957	1959	1961	1966	1967-1968
Strains of influenza virus	A	A	B	A	A/B	A	B/A	A
Patients consulting	223	264	150	930	849	203	544	675
Percentage of those at risk	6	6	3	17	14	3	7	8

Reprinted by permission from Fry: J R Coll Gen Pract, 17:100-103, 1969.

but within this there were some differences. Thus, the high rates during the "Asian" influenza epidemic of 1957 and the following one in 1959 were probably the result of relatively new strains of influenza virus to which there was little host immunity. The low rates of 1955 and 1961 are explained similarly—that there was good host immunity to "old" and well-known strains of virus. The age incidence in the eight epidemics showed a tendency for children to be most susceptible, but in some epidemics such as the most recent in 1967 to 1968, the elderly also were frequently infected. During the 20 years, there are records of ten individuals (now aged 44 to 68) who had suffered attacks of influenza in three epidemics, 415 in two epidemics and 2825 in a single epidemic.

As an illustration of the relative benign nature of influenza now, it is notable that during the eight epidemics with known infections affecting 3250 individuals, there were only seven *deaths* that could be attributed to influenza, and four of these occurred in an old ladies' home in 1967 to 1968. This is a fatality rate of 0.2 percent. *Chest complications* were not infrequent and occurred in 11 percent of attacks. The chest complication rates faded with the epidemic, but the reasons for high and low rates are not clear. The low rate of 3 percent for the

most widespread epidemic in 1957 may have been because it occurred in the autumn, whereas the other epidemics occurred chiefly in winter months. The usual clinical types of chest complications (Table 2) were acute bronchitis and segmental pneumonia. Acute bronchitis was noted chiefly in the young and the elderly. In the elderly (over 60), it was the chronic bronchitics who most often suffered from acute bronchitis. Complicating segmental pneumonias were distributed equally at all ages.

During 20 years in this practice, the extent of each of the eight epidemics ranged from 3 to 17 percent of the patients consulting (a mean rate of 8 percent). The true incidence was very much higher because by no means all patients who were infected needed to consult, and it is likely that twice as many were infected than consulted. Of 2950 persons who have been in the practice for 20 years, 1272 were seen for epidemic influenza at least once. With the exception of the epidemic of 1967 to 1968, the age distribution of influenza is that it tends to be an infection of children and teenagers and that the incidence falls with age, presumably because adults build up a natural immunity through contact with influenza over the years.

Any practical policy designed to prevent infection with influenza and to reduce

Table 2. *Clinical Types of Chest Complications in Influenza Epidemics (1949-1968) (Percentage of Attacks)*

Clinical Type	Acute Bronchitis	Segmental Pneumonia	Labor Pneumonia	All Chest Complications
Percentage of attacks	4	6	1	11

Reprinted by permission from Fry: J R Coll Gen Pract, 17:100-103, 1969.

complications must consider immunization and the use of broad spectrum antibiotics. There are special problems with each. Immunization is not completely successful because of the uncertainty of the causal strains of influenza virus in any epidemic, and there is no effective polyvalent vaccine available. It is impossible to undertake any scheme requiring regular immunization of the whole population, and the definition of "vulnerables" has not been a practical possibility in general practice. Prophylactic use of antibiotics also is impractical for the reasons of costs and the impossibility of selecting "vulnerables." The early use of broad spectrum antibiotics for chest complications certainly has improved the prognosis, and the fatality rate of 0.2 percent of all patients with influenza who consulted must be considered satisfactory.

Jolly DT: Acute tonsillopharyngitis in native and white families. Can Fam Physician 26:59–66, 1980

While streptococcal tonsillopharyngitis has been extensively investigated, tonsillopharyngitis as a clinical entity has not been the subject of as much attention. The relationship between environmental factors and host susceptibility in the development of tonsillopharyngitis remains to be investigated. In particular, the role of the family in determining the environmental conditions in which its members must function has only recently become the subject of medical interest. This study was conducted in an effort to assess the possible relationships between family smoking habits, the presence of allergic disorders within the family, crowding, and the presentation of tonsillopharyngitis in native and white families.

The Southwest Middlesex Health Centre (SWMHC) was opened in October 1974. It is a family practice teaching facility associated with the Department of Family Medicine of the University of Western Ontario. The SWMHC is located 25 km from London, Ontario, on the outskirts of Mt. Brydges, Ontario. The surrounding rural community as well as the Oneida settlement and Caradoc Reservation are served by this center. Consequently, the patient population has two distinct racial populations.

Patients given a diagnosis of pharyngitis, tonsillitis, or febrile sore throat during 1975 and 1976 were identified with the assistance of a computerized disease index. Native and white families in whom a diagnosis of tonsillopharyngitis had been documented during 1975 or 1976 were surveyed during 1978 whenever a family member presented

Table 1. *The Relationship between the Number of Cases of Tonsillopharyngitis per Family and Smoking*

| | | Native and White Families Combined | | | |
| | | Smoking Families | | Nonsmoking Families | |
Cases of Tonsillopharyngitis per Family during 1975 and 1976	Total No. of Families N	No. of Families	% of N	No. of Families	% of N
Three or more cases of tonsillopharyngitis	40	34	85.0	6	15.0
One or two cases of tonsillopharyngitis	119	90	75.6	29	24.4
No cases of tonsillopharyngitis	160	104	65.0	56	35.0

Reprinted by permission from Jolly: Can Fam Physician, 26:59–66, 1980.

Table 2. *The Relationship between the Number of Cases of Tonsillopharyngitis per Family and Allergic Disorders*

		Native and White Families Combined			
		Families with Allergic Disorders		Families with No Allergic Disorders	
Cases of Tonsillopharyngitis per Family during 1975 and 1976	Total No. of Families N	No. of Families	% of N	No. of Families	% of N
Three or more cases of tonsillopharyngitis	40	14	35.0	26	65.0
One or two cases of tonsillopharyngitis	119	34	28.6	85	71.4
No cases of tonsillopharyngitis	160	29	18.1	131	81.9

Reprinted by permission from Jolly: Can Fam Physician, 26:59–66, 1980.

to the center. Families registered prior to or during 1976 who had no computer record of tonsillopharyngitis during 1975 and 1976 were selected as controls. For the purpose of this study, a smoking family was defined as any family in which one or more of its members smoked cigarettes, cigars, or pipe tobacco. An allergic family was defined as any family in which one or more of its members received hyposensitization therapy or had a diagnosis of asthma, allergic rhinitis, or hay fever.

The average number of cases of acute tonsillopharyngitis per family was 2.3 and 2.1 for native and white families, respectively. Native patients had significantly more positive bacterial cultures than their white counterparts.

In both native and white families, smoking was reported more frequently by study families than by controls. Table 1 demonstrates the relationship between families that smoke and the number of cases of tonsillopharyngitis per family. This relationship was significant according to a chi trend linear analysis. As the number of cases of tonsillopharyngitis per family increased, the family was more likely to have members who smoked.

For both native and white families, allergic disorders were reported more frequently by study families than by their controls. Table 2 illustrates the relationship between families with allergic disorders and the number of cases of tonsillopharyngitis per family. As the number of cases of tonsillopharyngitis per family increased, the family was more likely to have allergic disorders. A significant linear trend was demonstrated for this relationship.

The average number of people per bedroom was used as an index of crowding. Native families tended to be larger than white families and so had more people per bedroom than white families. This, combined with a generally lower socioeconomic level, would contribute to crowded and substandard housing conditions that may have resulted in the increased number of cases of tonsillopharyngitis seen.

Fry J: Infectious mononucleosis: some new observations from a 15-year study. J Fam Pract 10(6):1087–1089, 1980

Although new developments have clarified somewhat the epidemiology and pathogenesis of infectious mononucleosis (IM), still there is much uncertainty. Most reports on IM have come from short planned field studies by physicians, epidemiologists, and virologists. General practice offers opportunities for observing and following up a fairly static population with families and individuals over long periods of time. This prospective study has been carried out in a family practice over a period of 15 years (1964 to 1979).

The practice is in a southeast London suburb, chiefly with social classes 2, 3, and 4. The population was stable at around 8500 during the period of study. An age/sex register recorded all the persons at risk. There was full access to pathology services at a nearby hospital (Beckenham Hospital). The diagnosis of IM was made on the basis of positive Paul-Bunnell or Monospot tests and on reported presence of abnormal mononuclear (glandular fever) cells on blood checks carried out at the local hospital laboratory. Prospective records were kept on all persons diagnosed as suffering from IM, and it was possible to relate subsequent family and personal course and history.

During the 15 years, the annual incidence rate was 1.6 per 1000 of the population (Table 1). This is much higher than the 0.2–0.6 per 1000 rates reported by others.

This suggests that in an average-sized practice of 2500, there may occur four new cases of IM in a year. Table 1 also shows the age distribution of the 214 persons with IM. (Four had two episodes.) There was no appreciable sex difference. The highest incidence was in the 10- to 19-year-old age group.

In no instance was there any reliable history of contact with any other known case of IM. There were, however, clusters of cases at times. Among the 214 persons with IM, there were 32 from families in whom more than one person was diagnosed with IM during the 1964 to 1979 period. In no family, however, was there any evidence of cross-infection.

Four persons apparently had two episodes of IM. On each occasion, the Paul-Bunnell or Monospot tests were positive, and there were atypical (GF) mononuclear cells in the blood. There was a lapse of nine months or longer between each episode. All but 2 of the 214 patients had unremarkable clinical courses and followed the recognizable pattern of illness with prolonged sore throat, tender palpable lymph glands in neck and elsewhere, and malaise and general disturbance that persisted for varying periods. One girl developed jaundice during her second attack of IM. One boy, 19 years old, was found dead in bed at home while being treated for IM. The autopsy report was that he died from "myocarditis

Table 1. *Infectious Mononucleosis: Numbers and Rates per 1000 in 1964 to 1979*

Age (Years)	0–4	5–9	10–14	15–19	20–29	30–39	40–49	50+	Total
Male	0	2	30	41	21	9	0	1	104
Female	1	2	28	48	20	9	1	1	110
Persons	1	4	58	89	41	18	1	2	214
(Incidence per 1,000 persons)	1.7	5.0	90.0	121.6	34.2	14.4	0.8	0.8	23.8*

*This represents an annual incidence of 1.6 per 1000.
Reprinted by permission from Fry: J Fam Pract, 10(6):1087–1089, 1980.

due to infectious mononucleosis." There were two remarkable cases in which an initial diagnosis of IM was made in the early course of the patient's illness, but both subsequently were found to have lymphoma.

These original findings from one family practice demonstrate the continuing value in modern times of what may have been old-fashioned recording of clinical observations as practiced by Sydenham and Mackenzie in the past. Such observations may not provide complete answers to current medical problems, but they do add important pieces of information.

Allhiser JN, McKnight TA, Shank JC: Lymphadenopathy in a family practice. J Fam Pract 12(1):27–32, 1981

The investigation of enlarged lymph nodes is frequently pursued with indecision, inconsistency, or lack of appreciation of relevant clinical and epidemiologic facts. In family practice, there are neither data on the incidence/prevalence of lymphadenopathy nor studies of the decision-making process in the clinical management of this problem.

The purpose of this report is fourfold. First, the annual incidence of lymphadenopathy is determined. Second, the paper analyzes the clinical spectrum and management of lymphadenopathy in a representative family practice setting, a family practice residency program. Third, based on this retrospective two-year audit and literature review, guidelines are suggested for the management of lymphadenopathy in family practice. And fourth, this report illustrates several aspects of one stimulating new area within family practice research—clinical decision making.

The study population was provided by the Cedar Rapids Family Practice Residency Program model office, an urban practice in a community of 110,000. At the midpoint of this study, there were 7483 active patients cared for by 24 resident physicians and by the full-time faculty. A printout was obtained of all patients being coded as having lymphadenopathy. Eighty patients were identified, and their charts were reviewed.

The annual incidence of the problem of enlarged lymph nodes was 0.5 percent in the study population. The sex ratio revealed 39 percent male patients and 61 percent female. In both sexes, this is a problem of children and young adults. Fifty-six cases (70 percent) were discovered by patients, and 15 cases (19 percent) were discovered by the physician (previously unknown to the patient). Thirty-seven patients (46 percent) reported pain, and 35 (44 percent) denied it.

Of 19 cases with more than one anatomic location of nodes, cervical nodes were included in 17 cases. The most common combination of enlarged nodes was cervical, axillary, and inguinal. Concerning etiology, as determined in this retrospective study, infectious or probably infectious was concluded in 55 (69 percent) of the cases. An unknown or not specified etiology was present in 23 (29 percent) of the cases.

It is interesting that nearly all the tests performed in this study were normal. The only positive findings were a positive Monospot in a patient with cervical adenopathy, one elevated white blood cell count in a patient with enlarged cervical/axillary nodes, and one positive PPD skin test in a patient with enlarged cervical/axillary/inguinal nodes. Three throat cultures were positive for β-hemolytic streptococcus. Despite not doing a sophisticated cost-effectiveness analysis, it appears that many unnecessary tests were performed. One might argue that the family physician should wait a period of time, such as two to three weeks, before launching into an investigation for lymphadenopathy. Notably, there were no cases of malignancy in this series of 80 patients.

The following levels of practical outpatient management are proposed (Table 1):

Level 1: an initial problem-directed history and physical examination, looking for evidence of localized infection, malignant primary (e.g., breast) mass, or systemic sign/symptoms (e.g., weight loss), is recommended.

Level 2: this would then include a throat culture for β-hemolytic streptococcus if there is cervical adenopathy (pharyngeal gonorrhea culture only if indicated by history). Antibiotics should be used if a culture is positive or if an obvious distal infection is noted. If the throat culture is negative and there is no evident infection, clinical observation is recommended for one to three weeks without further investigation and expense.

Level 3: should the node enlargement persist longer than three weeks, a complete blood count, a mononucleosis test, and perhaps a sedimentation rate are recommended to screen for mononucleosis, anemia, leukocytosis, leukemia, or evidence of other chronic disease. Should these be within normal limits and no new symptoms are present, again one to three weeks may pass before level 4 is reached. With symptoms of headache, malaise,

Table 1. *Levels of Work-Up*

Level 1
  History, physical examination

Level 2
  Throat culture, antibiotic if indicated, clinical observation 1-3 weeks

Level 3
  Complete blood count, mononucleosis test, sedimentation rate, clinical observation 1-3 weeks

Level 4
  PPD, chest x-ray film, biopsy and culture, serologic testing, skin testing

Reprinted by permission from Allhiser et al: J Fam Pract, 12(1):27-32, 1981.

and dry cough, screening for mycoplasma infection with a cold agglutinin titer could be considered.

Level 4: at this stage, a PPD skin test and chest x-ray film are recommended. (The chest x-ray film might be done earlier, i.e., in level 2, if the patient is an adult with a smoking history and has an isolated supraclavicular node.) The next critical decision is biopsy and culture vs. further serologic and/or skin testing. Conditions to be considered include toxoplasmosis, cytomegalovirus, lymphogranuloma venereum, cat scratch disease other fungal agents, and atypical mycobacterial infection.

Phizacklea S, Wilkins RH: The prevalence and diagnosis of headache in an urban practice. J R Coll Gen Pract 28:594-596, 1978

Headache was found to be the ninth commonest symptom in one British general-practice study. Another recent survey of a random group of females between 20 and 44 years old who kept health diaries showed that headache was the commonest symptom. Undergraduate medical education emphasizes the rare, serious diagnoses at the expense of the common, often trivial ones. Despite the significant contribution

that headache makes to the workload of a general practitioner, few studies of prevalence and diagnosis have been published.

A prospective study was designed to determine the prevalence of headache in a single-handed urban practice of 3000 patients from May 1, 1977 to October 31, 1977. During the study period, every consultation was recorded for a patient with headache either in the surgery or in the patient's home. The headache was recorded if it occurred alone or in association with other symptoms. Only headaches volunteered by the patient were included.

One hundred and twenty-five patients (4 percent of the practice population) made 192 consultations for headache (4 percent of the total consultations in the six-month period). The age and sex distribution of these patients is shown in Table 1. The age distribution of the practice population closely followed that for Great Britain as a whole except that there were fewer in the under-14 age group and more in the over-65 age group for both sexes.

The diagnoses are shown in Table 2. Ninety-seven patients were examined (77.6 percent of total), three patients were referred to outpatient clinics (2.4 percent of total), and two patients were admitted to hospital (1.6 percent of total).

In this study, headache was found to be commonest in females in the 20 to 40-year age group. The commonest diagnosis, ten-

Table 1. *Age and Sex Distribution of Patients with Headache*

Age (Years)	Males	Females	Males Percentage of Total	Females Percentage of Total
0–9	5	5	4	4
10–19	7	10	5.6	8
20–29	7	19	5.6	15.2
30–39	4	21	3.2	16.8
40–49	6	8	4.8	6.4
50–59	3	9	2.4	7.2
60–69	6	8	4.8	6.4
70–79	1	4	0.8	3.2
80–89	—	2	—	1.6
Totals	39	86	31.2	68.8

Reprinted by permission from Phizacklea, Wilkins: J R Coll Gen Pract, 28:594–596, 1978.

sion, that is, muscle contraction headache due to anxiety or depression, was four times more common in females than males. The diagnosis was based mainly on the history

Table 2. *Diagnoses Made in a Series of Patients Seen with Headache*

Diagnosis	Males	Females	Total	Diagnosis	Males	Females	Total
Tension (including depression)	7	31	38	*Drug Side Effects* Oral contraceptive	—	3	3
Migraine	4	12(a)	16	Dydrogesterone ("Duphaston")	—	1	1
Migraine and tension (requiring treatment for both)	—	3	3	Glyceryl trinitrate	—	1	1
				?Subarachnoid hemorrhage	1(d) (e)	—	1
Cervical arthrosis	1	2(b)	3				
Infections				Trauma	—	1	1
Sinusitis	7	5	12	Hypoglycemia	—	1	1
Upper respiratory tract	5	9	14	Cough	—	1	1
Tonsillitis	1	3	4	Noise	1	—	1
Bronchitis	1	2	3	Trigeminal neuralgia	—	1	1
Gastroenteritis	2	1	3	Vasomotor rhinitis	—	1	1
Labyrinthitis	—	2	2	"Periodic syndrome" of childhood	1	—	1
Influenza	1	—	1	Hiatus hernia	1(c)	—	1
Otitis media	1	—	1	Malingering	1	—	1
Pyelitis	—	1(c)	1	Unknown	3	5 2(d)	8
Herpes zoster	—	1	1				

(a) One patient also had headache due to trauma.
(b) One patient also had headache due to oral contraceptive.
(c) Patient admitted to hospital.
(d) Patient referred to outpatient clinic.
(e) Patient died.
Reprinted by permission from Phizacklea, Wilkins: J R Coll Gen Pract, 28:594–596, 1978.

and clinical examination. Investigations were few and the results often negative. In eight patients (6 percent of the total) no diagnosis could be made. Investigations were performed on two of these, and a further two were referred to outpatient clinics. All eight patients were further observed, and the headache subsided completely.

In two patients, serious causes were found. One was a 34-year-old woman who was admitted to hospital with clinical evidence of meningism and was found to be suffering from pyelitis. The second was a 69-year-old man who presented initially with classic features of tension headache—continuous tight pain in a hatband distribution only partially relieved by analgesics. Later, he developed diplopia and ataxia and was referred urgently to a neurologist.

Investigation revealed a lesion in one parietal region, but while in hospital he developed features resembling acute subarachnoid hemorrhage and rapidly died. Postmortem examination has failed to reveal the precise diagnosis, but further results are awaited.

Although diagnostic techniques have advanced during recent years, this study has shown that headache remains largely a problem for the general practitioner. Diagnosis is often extremely difficult and demands a high degree of clinical skill as well as a detailed knowledge of the patient's background. Most headaches, while troublesome, are self-limiting and not particularly serious. Nevertheless, the physician must be vigilant and recognize potentially catastrophic headaches at an early stage.

Morrison JD: Fatigue as a presenting complaint in family practice. J Fam Pract 10(5):795–801, 1980

The family physician is often faced with the patient who complains of fatigue. However, there is little true incidence data in the literature regarding this problem.

The medical records of 176 patients with

an isolated diagnosis of fatigue were reviewed. The study population represented the experience of four family physicians in private practice and of residents and staff of a university family medicine center in

Table 1. *Distribution of Fatigue Cases by Age, Sex, and Associated Diagnosis (N = 176)*

Age (Years)	Physical M	Physical F	Psychological M	Psychological F	Mixed M	Mixed F	Undetermined M	Undetermined F	Totals M	Totals F
<15	2	2	1	—	—	—	—	—	3	2
15–24	4	11	3	12	—	5	—	8	7	36
25–34	8	14	13	19	1	8	—	4	22	45
35–44	3	6	3	9	2	1	—	1	8	17
45–54	4	3	2	4	—	3	1	—	7	10
55–64	2	3	—	4	—	—	—	—	2	7
65–74	3	—	1	1	—	1	—	—	4	2
>75	—	4	—	—	—	—	—	—	—	4
Totals	26	43	23	49	3	18	1	13	53	123
Totals both sexes	69		72		21		14		176	
Percent	39		41		12		8		100	

Reprinted by permission from Morrison: J Fam Pract, 10(5):795–801, 1980.

Denver, Colorado, over a 12-month period. Variables included for study were age, sex, family structure, diagnostic testing, duration of symptoms, and associated final diagnosis.

Women outnumbered men in the study population two to one. Fatigue occurred most frequently in people 15 to 34 years old. Single people, both men and women, were represented in the study population at a higher rate than family members. Single women tended to have physical diagnoses

Table 2. *Associated Physical Diagnoses*

Physical Only (N = 69)	
Viral syndrome	27
Mononucleosis	9
Hypokalemia	5
Asthma/COPD	4
Hypothyroidism	3
Hypoglycemia	3
Hepatitis	2
ASHD	2
Hypertension	2
Allergy-fatigue	2
Diabetes mellitus	1
Hyperthyroidism	1
Anemia, iron deficiency	1
Rheumatic heart disease	1
Urinary tract infection	1
Strep pharyngitis	1
Mitral prolapse	1
Pregnancy	1
Antabuse ingestion	1
Physiologic	1
Mixed Physical and Psychologic (N = 21)	
Viral syndrome	4
Systemic lupus	2
Obesity	2
Allergy-fatigue	2
Hypoglycemia	2
Mononucleosis	1
Anemia, iron deficiency	1
Peptic ulcer	1
Congestive heart failure	1
Hypokalemia	1
Dietary-fasting	1
Menorrhagia	1
Sickle cell trait	1
Physiologic	1

Reprinted by permission from Morrison: J Fam Pract, 10(5): 795–801, 1980.

Table 3. *Associated Psychological Diseases*

Psychological Only (N = 72)	
Depression	31
Anxiety	19
Stress, acute	9
Adjustment reaction	4
Alcoholism	4
Other	5
Mixed Physical and Psychological (N = 21)	
Anxiety	9
Depression	8
Stress, acute	4

Reprinted by permission from Morrison: J Fam Pract, 10(5): 795–801, 1980.

associated with their fatigue, while women who were members of family units tended to have psychological diagnoses associated. Fatigue lasting longer than four months was more frequently associated with psychological problems, while symptoms less than four months in duration were more frequently associated with physical problems.

Case sorting according to a single physical or psychological diagnosis associated with the fatigue was attempted. The criteria for these diagnoses were those of the practicing physician, while the grouping of cases was carried out by the author alone. Several cases could not be clearly assigned to either category. Table 1 is a distribution of these categories by age and sex. Thirty-nine percent of the cases had associated physical diagnoses, 41 percent had associated psychological diagnoses, 12 percent had both kinds of diagnoses associated, and 8 percent had no discernible diagnosis associated. There were no significant differences between the sexes or among age groups in this distribution. Tables 2 and 3 delineate the specific diagnoses categorized as either "physical," "psychological," or "mixed."

Laboratory testing yielded relatively few positive results. More emphasis should probably be placed on the history and physical examination, while laboratory tests can be limited more than they were in this series. The complete blood count, serum potassium, and Monospot do appear to be useful tests, however.

A disturbing find was the high degree of failure to document "closure" in these patients. The picture drawn from this series was too often that of a single physician-patient encounter with the problem remaining unresolved. Subsequent laboratory testing may have suggested probable cause, but documentation of further discussion with the patient was frequently lacking. Certainly, the family physician owes his patients not only thorough evaluation of ill-defined problems but also communication regarding the possible causes of these problems.

Jones JG, Hazleman BL: Polymyalgia rheumatica and giant cell arteritis—a difficult diagnosis. J R Coll Gen Pract 31:283–289, 1981

Polymyalgia rheumatica has received increasing attention in recent years. It can lead to considerable morbidity, including sudden irreversible blindness, but effective treatment is available. Unfortunately, there is often considerable delay in making the diagnosis, partly because of the frequent absence of physical signs and lack of specific laboratory tests. In many patients an underlying vasculitis can be demonstrated; clinically, there is no clear distinction between giant cell arteritis (GCA) and polymyalgia rheumatica (PMR).

Early diagnosis and, as a consequence, early treatment are desirable if vascular complications are to be minimized. This study reviewed a group of patients with the intention of exploring the difficulties of diagnosis. The study group included 108 patients with GCA and/or PMR who presented at Addenbrooke's and Newmarket General Hospitals between January 1974 and March 1979.

The criteria for the diagnosis of PMR were (1) bilateral shoulder and pelvic girdle pain that was primarily muscular in the absence of true muscle weakness; (2) morning stiffness; (3) duration of at least two months; (4) ESR over 30 mm/hr or C-reactive protein (CRP) over 6 μg/ml; (5) absence of rheumatoid or inflammatory arthritis or malignant disease; (6) absence of objective signs of muscle disease; and (7) prompt and dramatic response (i.e., by the next day) to systemic corticosteroids. The criteria for the diagnosis of GCA were (1) a positive temporal artery biopsy or (2) cranial artery tenderness noted by a physician; (3) one or more of the following: (a) visual disturbance, (b) headaches, (c) jaw pain, (d) cerebrovascular insufficiency; (4) ESR over 30 mm/hr or CRP over 6 μg/ml; and (5) response to corticosteroids. The presenting features and the initial diagnosis of both general practitioner and hospital doctor were documented. In an attempt to define which features of the disease were responsible for misdiagnosis, the reasons for general practitioner referral and initial hospital diagnosis were assigned to five categories according to their most prominent feature. This depended on whether myalgia, arteritis, systemic symptoms, or abnormal laboratory tests caused the major diagnostic problem; a small number were assigned into a miscellaneous group.

Thirty-four patients fulfilled the criteria for diagnosis of PMR alone, 23 patients for GCA, and 51 had features of both disorders. The frequency of systemic symptoms is listed in Table 1. Ninety patients had one or more features. The ESR was raised in all patients, sometimes to a very high level.

A correct diagnosis was made by the referring doctor in 33 percent of patients and on initial attendance at hospital in 67 percent of patients. Symptoms were present for more than three months before referral to hospital in 39 percent of patients, and the delay before diagnosis at hospital was

Table 1. *Constitutional Disturbance
(Total Patients 108)*

Weight loss (3–20 kg)	63
Anorexia	64
Malaise	73
Night sweats	52
Fever (>37.5°C)	31
Depression	28

Reprinted by permission from Jones, Hazelman: J R Coll Gen Pract, 31:283–289, 1981.

greater than one month in 20 percent. Systemic illness (present in 83 percent of cases), anemia (33 percent), elevated alkaline phosphatase (73 percent) and raised immunoglobulin levels (48 percent) caused diagnostic problems in 28 patients at primary care level and in 23 patients at hospital.

Many patients with PMR and GCA are managed by their general practitioner and not referred to hospital. Those who are referred are more likely to be those with an atypical presentation and will consequently be more likely to cause diagnostic difficulty. Thus, no series of patients from hospital practice alone can be considered to present a typical picture of the disease. This survey, giving the experience of the disease in a district general hospital, is more likely to give a truer overall picture of the condition than a series from one department but does not include all patients who attended during the study period. Not all patients underwent temporal artery biopsy and therefore do not appear on the temporal artery list, and the diagnostic index does not cover outpatients.

Systemic effects and abnormal laboratory investigations caused difficulty with the referring doctor's diagnosis in 26 patients and with diagnosis at hospital in 23 patients. Weight loss, malaise, and anorexia (along with anemia, elevated ESR, and raised alkaline phosphatase) raised the suspicion of malignancy. Night sweats and fever suggested infection, including subacute bacterial endocarditis, viral illness, and meningitis. Endogenous depression was diagnosed in three cases. Arteritis caused headache, ophthalmoplegia suggested a brain tumour, and jaw pain a dental problem or trigeminal neuralgia. Femoral arteritis with local pain was diagnosed as inguinal lymphadenitis. When myalgia dominated the clinical picture, the diagnosis of clofibrate myopathy, postgastrectomy vitamin D deficiency, and polymyositis secondary to carcinomatosis were all considered. Local myalgia led to the mistaken diagnoses of osteoarthrosis, frozen shoulder, cervical spondylosis, and lumbar spinal disease.

Playfair HR, Gowers JI: Depression following childbirth—a search for predictive signs. J R Coll Gen Pract 31:201–208, 1981

Recent years have seen growing recognition that depression after childbirth occurs much more often than was formerly realized and that, although puerperal psychosis is rare and the "five-day blues" common, many mothers experience a condition less dramatic than the former but considerably more severe than the latter. This realization has stimulated many investigators to search for predictive features.

The aim of this study was to identify symptoms, signs, and other conditions presenting during the antenatal and perinatal periods that indicate, either singly or in combination, that depression is likely to occur after the birth. The investigation was carried out by 64 general practitioners in the British Isles. Each observer was asked to recruit up to a total of 15 mothers consecutively as they presented for antenatal care, for a period of 12 months, and to record information at four times: (1) at the initial

Table 1. *Presence of Depressive Symptoms (Percentages in Brackets)*

Symptom	R2	R3	R4
1. Tired, unable to cope	190 (30.7)	165 (26.7)	146 (23.6)*
2. Loss of appetite	47 (7.6)	92 (14.9)	46 (7.4)
3. Sleepless	184 (29.8)*	82 (13.3)	85 (13.8)
4. Tense, overanxious	109 (17.6)	116 (18.8)*	131 (21.2)*
5. Tearful	159 (25.7)	179 (29.0)	115 (18.6)
6. Irritable	192 (31.1)	111 (18.0)	158 (25.6)
7. Loss of interest	46 (7.4)	25 (4.0)	49 (7.9)
8. Sadness	50 (8.1)	52 (8.4)*	52 (8.4)*
9. Retardation	41 (6.6)	26 (4.2)†	33 (5.3)
10. Agitation	72 (11.7)	51 (8.3)	47 (7.6)
11. Discontent	39 (6.3)	29 (4.7)	48 (7.8)
12. Obsessional	34 (5.5)	27 (4.4)†	42 (6.8)
13. Guilt	28 (4.5)*	24 (3.9)	49 (7.9)*
Numbers	618	618	618

*1 patient not known.
†2 patients not known.
Reprinted by permission from Playfair, Gowers: J R Coll Gen Pract, 31:201–208, 1981.

antenatal appointment (R1), (2) during the second trimester (R2), (3) during the second week following the birth (R3), and (4) about 3 months after the birth (R4). A total of 618 sets of records were investigated. At each interview, the mood of the mother and the presence of the following 13 symptoms of depression were recorded: (1) tiredness/inability to cope, (2) loss of appetite, (3) poor sleep, (4) tense/overanxious, (5) easily tearful, (6) irritable/easily annoyed, (7) loss of interest, (8) sadness, (9) lack of response/retardation, (10) restlessness/agitation, (11) discontent, (12) tendency to obsessional behavior, (13) self-accusation/guilt feelings.

Of the 618 mothers, 150 (24.3 percent) had three or more symptoms of depression at, or about, three months after the birth (R4), and 62 (10 percent) had six or more symptoms.

The number of positive responses to the 13 symptoms at R2, R3, and R4 (as defined earlier) are given in Table 1. In general, the relative frequency of the symptoms remained very stable; at R2 and R4, the same group of five symptoms was most frequently reported, namely, irritableness, inability to cope, overanxiousness, tearful-

Table 2. *Potential Risk Factors, Correlations with the Symptom Score at R4*

*External stress after birth unrelated to confinement	0.40
Mood (R3)	0.32
Anxiety	0.28
*History of previous puerperal depression	0.26
History of psychiatric illness	0.21
Mood (R2)	0.20
Previous pregnancies of less than 28 weeks' duration	0.19
*Housing stress during pregnancy	0.17
Premenstrual tension	0.15
Painful menstruation	0.15
*Previous painful labours	0.15
*Adverse experience in previous pregnancies	0.14
*Financial stress during pregnancy	0.14
Previous pregnancies lasting at least 28 weeks	0.13
*Condition affecting baby sufficient to require medical attention	0.12
†Partner's employment status	0.12
†Partner's social class	0.11
Attitude towards pregnancy	0.07

R(0.05%) = 0.08.
*Dichotomous variable: the correlation is point-biserial.
†Lower class or status is associated with increased depression.
Reprinted by permission from Playfair, Gowers: J R Coll Gen Pract, 31:201–208, 1981.

ness, and sleeplessness. At R3, the same symptoms predominated except that loss of appetite ousted sleeplessness. At R2 and R3, guilt feeling was the symptom least frequently recorded, but its prevalence doubled at R4. This increase is significant at the 5 percent level.

Table 2 lists those factors whose correlation with the symptom score at R4 is significant at the 5 percent level. The most important factor is stress after the birth that is unrelated to the confinement. The kinds of stress reported included personal difficulties with the husband and in-laws, ill health of the patient or relatives, and financial and housing difficulties. Difficulties with the partner were caused either by his enforced absence because of his job or by problems in the personal relationship.

Five principal prognostic factors were identified: a history of previous puerperal depression at the initial antenatal examination; at the same stage, a history of previous miscarriage; during the pregnancy, the presence of six or more symptoms of depression; shortly after the birth, a severe attack of the "blues" with a symptom score of six or more; and, following the birth, external stress, in particular marital difficulties, housing problems, and physical ill health of the mother.

Three less significant but nevertheless ominous pointers to be noted at the initial antenatal examination are dysmenorrhoea, a history of psychiatric illness, and low employment status of the partner. The presence of these signs should alert the doctor to a greater probability of depression during the puerperium.

Stott PC: Contraceptive behaviour and fertility patterns in an Inner London group practice. J R Coll Gen Pract 30:340–346, 1980

The provision of contraceptive services is now undertaken by the majority of general practitioners and is increasingly coming to be accepted as a marker of good medical care. As a trainee in a busy Inner London practice, the author found that 7 percent of his consultations were for contraceptive advice. This study was undertaken in order to (1) define the contraceptive workload, (2) determine how effectively the services offered had enabled people to plan their families and control their fertility, and (3) discover what factors influenced the choice of contraception.

At the time of the study, the practice had a list size of about 7500 patients of whom about 3000 were women between 17 and 40 years old. They came from mixed ethnic origins, mostly English, Irish, Asian, and Greek, but a few were West Indians. During a period of nine months, between November 1977 and August 1978, a questionnaire was given by the doctors, nurse, and health visitor to 600 women attending the surgery for contraceptive advice. No woman completed the questionnaire more than once, and confidentiality was ensured. After the study period, an assessment was made of the relative proportions of patients seeking contraceptive advice from their general practitioner, a local authority clinic, both, or neither by examining the records of 400 alphabetically consecutive female patients in the age range 17 to 40 years. This sample is about 13 percent of the total number in the age/sex index for this group.

Of 600 questionnaires handed out, 458 were completed, a take-up rate of 76 percent. Of the 400 women whose records were examined after the study period, 46 percent had sought contraceptive advice from the general practitioner, 13 percent from a local authority clinic, and 5 percent from the two combined. No reference to contraception was found in 36 percent of records.

Table 1. *Contraceptive Method at Time of Survey*

	Number	Percentage
Oral contraceptive	281	61
IUCD	76	16
Nothing	31	7
Cap	17	4
Multiple methods	14	3
Sheath	12	3
Withdrawal	10	2
Sterilization	9	2
Rhythm	3	<1
Pessaries	2	<1

Reprinted by permission from Stott: J R Coll Gen Pract, 30: 340–346, 1980.

Sixty-one percent were using oral contraceptives and 16 percent the IUCD. These two methods constituted the greatest proportion of the recurrent workload. Four percent were using the cap (Table 1). The outcomes of pregnancy related to planning are shown in Table 2. Eighteen percent of all pregnancies miscarried; 29 percent of all pregnancies and 50 percent of all unplanned pregnancies ended in terminations. Table 3 displays the distribution of failures related to method of contraception.

In this practice, oral contraceptives are the most commonly used method, 92 percent of the women in the survey having tried them at some time. Of these, about 40 percent had never used anything else, 36 percent came to the pill after trying other methods (notably the sheath), and 23 percent had left it to try mainly the IUCD or the cap. The most common reasons for change were medical problems caused by the pill (38 percent) and fear of possible side effects (38 percent). In contrast, only 13 percent of the 123 women who had tried an IUCD had started with this method and stayed on it; 60 percent had come to it after trying other methods, and 27 percent had left mainly because of the medical problems it caused (35 percent) and failure resulting in pregnancy (24 percent). Sixteen percent of the women had tried the cap, but only two had used this solely; 48 percent were using it because other methods had proved unsuitable; and 49 percent had tried it and discontinued because it spoiled their sex life (18 percent), because they felt they needed better protection (26 percent), or because it was too messy (31 percent). Of the women who had used unprescribed methods (39 percent) such as withdrawal, the sheath, or pessaries, only a very small number had never tried anything else—the majority had progressed rapidly to more reliable methods.

The survey indicated that the population had used contraception reasonably effectively. At first sight, the proportion of unplanned pregnancies (58 percent) seems excessive. However, as has been shown, since 45 percent of these pregnancies oc-

Table 2. *Outcome of 373 Conceptions in Relation to Planning (Percentages in Brackets)*

	Planned	Unplanned
Live births	107 (29)	71 (19)
Pregnancies progressing	13 (3)	5 (1)
Miscarriages	38 (10)	31 (8)
Terminations		108 (29)

Reprinted by permission from Stott: J R Coll Gen Pract, 30: 340–346, 1980.

Table 3. *Number of Failures Related to Method of Contraception*

	Number of Failures	Percentage of Total Failures
Using no contraception at time	54	45
IUCD	17	14
Sheath	15	12
Oral contraceptive	13	11
Cap	9	7
Withdrawal	7	6
Rhythm	4	3
Temperature	1	<1
Pessaries	1	<1

Reprinted by permission from Stott: J R Coll Gen Pract, 30: 340–346, 1980.

curred while no contraception was being used, it represents a true contraceptive failure rate of 2.5 per 100 woman years.

The survey results confirmed expectations about patterns of contraceptive use and reasons for changing methods. The most common first choice was oral contraception, only a minority having used the sheath previously or needing to change subsequently.

Cameron AS, Barker M, Douglas RM: Symptoms and feeding patterns in the first year of life. Aus Fam Physician 8:1245–1253, 1979

Much debate has surrounded the question whether allergies to foods and cow's milk are commonly responsible for symptoms experienced during the first year of life. Many family physicians have the impression that elimination of cow's milk from an infant's diet often leads to an improvement in such symptoms as recurrent rhinorrhea, cough, bronchitis, skin rashes, and gastrointestinal symptoms. The Research Committee of the RACGP in South Australia has been interested in this question, and in 1977 a study was designed to document the prevalence of symptoms in the first year of life and to attempt to define the incidence of cow's milk allergy.

Cooperating physicians, widely distributed throughout South Australia in 34 one-man or group practices, undertook to distribute the diaries to mothers of newborn children confined by them. This study reports an analysis of symptom and food diaries maintained throughout the first 12 months of life of 482 infants.

In the large majority of cases, some symptoms were experienced in each of the four systems under review (Table 1). On average, each child experienced 4.4 separate episodes of respiratory symptomatology, 7.9 episodes of ENT symptomatology, 8.5 episodes of gastrointestinal symptomatology, and 6.3 episodes of skin symptomatology during the first year of life. During that year, also, the majority of children were taken to their family physician with symptoms in the ENT and skin systems; 62.7 percent of children experienced symptoms in the ENT system lasting more than 30 days.

Table 2 indicates the distribution of the children in four groups. Altogether, 77 of the 482 diaries have revealed symptomatology at some time in the year that could conceivably have been associated with cow's milk ingestion. However, in only 1 of these 77 children were withdrawal and challenge tests carried out to determine whether the symptomatology disappeared on withdrawal of cow's milk and reappeared on its reintroduction into the diet.

Table 1. *Symptomatology in 482 Children During the First Year of Life*

	Respiratory	ENT	Gastrointestinal	Skin
Percent with symptoms	85.3	97.1	84.6	88.2
Mean no. of separate episodes	4.4	7.9	8.5	6.3
Mean no. of morbidity days	29.3	56.2	23.6	50.1
Percent with symptoms for more than 30 days in the year	34.0	62.7	26.3	44.4
Percent with symptoms requiring medical attention and/or medication in this system	45.6	53.3	27.2	54.1

Reprinted by permission from Cameron et al: Aus Fam Physician, 8:1245–1253, 1979.

Table 2. *Distribution of Children in Symptom-Association Groups*

		No.	%
Group 1:	Symptoms minor and unrelated to foods or milk	103	21.4
Group 2:	Some symptoms conceivably related to food or formulae	39	8.1
Group 3:	Frequent or chronic symptoms unlikely on dairy evidence to be related to foods or milks	263	54.6
Group 4:	Some symptoms conceivably related to cow's milk ingestion	77	15.9
	Total	482	100.0

Reprinted by permission from Cameron et al: Aus Fam Physician, 8:1245-1253, 1979.

Most of the remaining 76 children had long periods of complete freedom from symptoms while taking cow's milk, and the evidence of any association with cow's milk was generally very tenuous. Soya substitutes were introduced in 13 cases, and cow's milk was temporarily discontinued in another 11 cases. Only 16 of these 77 children continued to experience chronic symptoms during the last two weeks of their first year.

This study underlines the extraordinary frequency with which children experience symptoms in their first year of life, most of which do not come to medical attention. It also emphasizes the fact that mothers make quite frequent modifications in their infant's formula or diet and that ascribing a causal role to a particular component of the diet is exceedingly difficult. From analysis of the information contained in the diaries, there appears to be a need for properly conducted challenge and exclusion tests before labeling a child as suffering from a milk or food allergy. Because these were only done on one occasion, it appears that only one child of 482 had symptoms that were probably related to cow's milk and that for 76 others the possibility of symptomatology being associated with cow's milk ingestion remains quite unproved. For 85 percent of the children whose diaries were studied, despite frequent symptomatology, there was no evidence even to suggest the possibility of such an association.

Walker RB, Hough JC, Brough JW: A survey of intestinal parasites in rural children. J Fam Pract 11(4):559-561, 1980

Intestinal parasites, while often representing asymptomatic infestations, may cause serious acute or chronic disease in children. This is more likely in the poorly nourished and those with multiple illnesses. These parasites are ubiquitous in the United States; however, clinical index of suspicion is rarely high outside areas of high prevalence.

Intestinal parasites are not generally considered a significant health problem in West Virginia. A study was undertaken to determine the prevalence of intestinal parasites in a group of rural, economically disadvantaged children in southern West Virginia.

History and physical examination, stature measurement, hematocrit, white blood cell count, and peripheral smears for differential white blood cell count were obtained on each child. An attempt was made to obtain at least two stool specimens on different days. Only a single stool specimen was obtained in 44 children. A total of 229 stool examinations were made. No attempts were made to identify pinworm ova.

Table 1. *Comparative Incidence and Clinical Findings for Intestinal Parasites*

Class	Number	Sex Distribution		Age (Years)	Height (T value)	Weight (T value)	Hematocrit	Eosinophils
		Male	*Female*					
Positive stool	37	18	19	3.4 ± .9	47.2 ± 8.3	48.3 ± 8.8	34.9 ± 2.6	5.9 ± 5.9
Negative stool	71	35	36	3.4 ± 1.0	48.9 ± 11.7	52.3 ± 10.4	35.9 ± 1.9	4.5 ± 5.0
Giardia	24	12	12	3.5 ± .9	44.0 ± 8.9	47.1 ± 9.4	35.0 ± 3.0	6.3 ± 5.7
Ascaris	17	8	9	3.3 ± 1.0	52.8 ± 8.0	50.8 ± 8.8	34.5 ± 2.4	7.0 ± 7.3
Trichuris	3	2	1	2.7 ± 1.2	47.2 ± 16.0	45.9 ± 16.9	33.0 ± 4.6	11.3 ± 11.4
Total	108	53	55	3.4 ± 1.0	48.3 ± 10.7	51.2 ± 9.9	35.5 ± 2.1	4.7 ± 4.8

Reprinted by permission from Walker et al: J Fam Pract, 11(4):559–561, 1980.

One hundred eight children, 1–6 years old, were included in the study. In 37 (34 percent), a clinically relevant intestinal parasite was diagnosed. Giardia lamblia (24 per 108), Ascaris lumbricoides (17 per 108), and Trichuris trichiura (3 per 108) were recovered and accounted for all organisms found except for a single subject with multiple (six) organisms (Table 1).

Stature did not differ significantly in infested vs noninfested subjects except in the case of Giardia. Giardia-infested patients had significantly lower means of height (P = .05) and weight (P = .05) than noninfested subjects. There were no significant differences in hematocrit, peripheral eosinophils, age, or sex distribution between infested and noninfested patients.

The children in this study were at high risk for intestinal parasite infection. Low socioeconomic status leading to poor sanitary facilities and resultant poor personal hygiene, little exposure to preventive education, and marginal access to safe water are probably responsible. High-risk groups such as this one are not uncommon in central Appalachia, and health care providers in such areas should maintain a high index of suspicion for the problem.

Giardiasis has been shown to cause chronic malabsorption in children. The cases represented in this study were largely asymptomatic, but decreased stature was noted in Giardia infested children. Even in areas of low prevalence, children at high risk for intestinal parasites should be screened by stool examination, if possible. Giardiasis should be vigorously treated, even if asymptomatic, because of possible chronic malabsorption.

Fiorini GT: Degenerative arthritis of the lumbar spine in laborers. Can Fam Physician 26:243–245, 1980

Low back strains are becoming the single most common cause of disabling injuries in construction and industry, and they are also causing the greatest number of lost work days. Repeated bending and lifting, irrespective of injuries, hastens the natural progression of wear and tear in the lumbar spine as manifested by degenerative changes. This study was undertaken in one family practice because the author had the impression that relatively minor back injuries, besides occurring quite frequently, seemed to result in disabilities extending over weeks or months.

The study included only injuries to the lumbosacral spine caused by overexertion, as in bending, lifting, and twisting. Other injuries to the back caused in any other fashion, such as falling, were excluded. The survey consisted of 171 workers divided into a study group of 82 and a control group of 89. The study group consisted of 82 construction and factory workers who had injured their backs at work in the process of lifting. The 71 men and 11 women were private patients eligible for Workmen's Compensation. Each patient in the study group was followed until recovery or for at least one year after the date of accident. When a patient returned to his original job or to some other lighter kind of work, that patient was considered recovered. All these patients had radiologic studies of the lumbosacral spine at least once, usually at the time of the injury. The radiologic findings were reported by a radiologist. Disabilities that continued for more than six to eight weeks were seen in consultation with an orthopedic surgeon. Longer-standing disabilities would usually be admitted to a hospital or to a rehabilitation centre for further investigation and work assessment. A control group consisted of 89 consecutive blue collar applicants to Dofasco Steel Company and various other industries. These 76 men and 13 women were required to have a physical examination and a routine x-ray of their lumbar spine as a prerequisite to employment. Their ages ranged from 20 to 50 years.

Table 1. *Patients Disabled More Than 1 Year, Compared to X-Ray Findings*

Age	No. of Pts.	% Disabled Over 1 Year	Abnormal X-Ray
15–19	0	0 %	0 %
20–29	3	13.6%	0 %
30–39	4	16 %	50 %
40–49	3	13.6%	100 %
50–59	6	86 %	100 %
60–69	3	75 %	100 %
Total	19	23.4%	73.7%

Reprinted by permission from Fiorini: Can Fam Physician, 26:243–245, 1980.

Table 2. *Average Duration in Weeks for Disabilities Less Than One Year*

Age	Normal X-Ray		Abnormal X-Ray	
	No. of Pts.	Average Duration of Disability in Weeks	No. of Pts.	Average Duration of Disability in Weeks
15–19	2	4	0	0
20–29	12	10	7	11.6
30–39	7	10	14	9.5
40–49	4	6	14	15
50–59	0	0	1	3
60–69	0	0	1	12
Total	25 (38%)		37 (42%)	

Reprinted by permission from Fiorini: Can Fam Physician, 26:243–245, 1980.

Disability of a year or more occurred in 23.4 percent of the study group (Table 1). Some of the older workers remained out of work permanently. Average duration of disability for those incapacitated less than a year was ten weeks (Table 2). Only 15.5 percent of patients in the age group 20–49 years sustained a low-back disability for one year or more, while 81 percent of patients over 50 years were disabled for one year or even permanently. Of the patients in the study group, 3.7 percent were suspected of having discogenic pain, yet myelograms and discograms demonstrated a herniated disc in only 1.2 percent of these patients.

These results in lost work days are more conservative than those described by others. Only lifting injuries were considered in this survey, while other investigators included every other kind of back injury such as those caused by falling or crushing, which may all result in more severe back injuries. In any event, the best therapy of these problems is prevention. This can be achieved through a concerted effort by the medical profession, industries, and government agencies to help workers move from one category of work to another.

Buchan IC, Deacon GLS, Ryan MP, Buckley EG, Irvine R: Problem drinkers and their problems. J R Coll Gen Pract 31:151–153, 1981

This paper attempts to define some of the characteristics of problem drinkers and their families, as perceived by seven general practitioners in England.

The seven physicians taking part in the study are single-handed general practitioners working in a health center. They have a total list of 9763 in a new town. Within each of the seven practices, a control, matched for age and sex, was identified for each problem drinker. This was done by random selection. Both the spouses and the controls of the problem drinkers proved to have a similar age range; there were a similar number of children in the control and study group. Active and inactive problems were recorded for all members of the family, and the total number of recorded consultations by each individual, both direct and indirect, was noted for the year 1978.

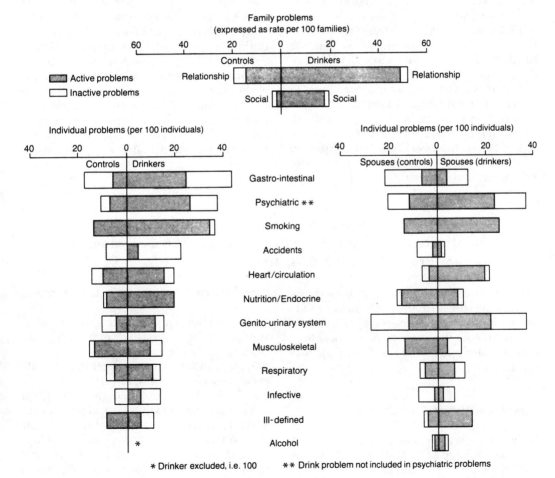

Fig. 1. Rates of main problem categories in controls and drinkers. Reprinted by permission from Buchan et al: J R Coll Gen Pract, 31:151–153, 1981.

It was found that the physicians used a variety of terms to describe problem drinkers and that it was difficult to differentiate fully between the "alcoholic" and the "problem drinker." One hundred and six patients out of a practice population of 9763 were identified as having a drinking problem. Ninety-two of these were male. The prevalence of those defined as having a drinking problem was, in males over 18, 3.3 percent and in females, 0.5 percent. The consultation rate for drinkers was almost twice that for controls. However, the consultation rate for spouses was only slightly higher than that for controls, and the rates for children of drinkers and controls were almost identical.

There was a higher average number of known casualty attendances among drinkers (1.3 for drinkers and 0.4 for controls). Intoxication with alcohol was observed in a quarter of their attendances at casualty departments. Almost two-thirds of attendances were for lacerations or soft tissue injuries. Assault was mentioned in one out of ten of the casualty reports. Spouses of drinkers also had a higher attendance rate at casualty departments.

Drinkers had more identified problems, other than alcohol abuse, when compared with controls. Spouses had more active but slightly fewer inactive problems than controls. When individual problems were classified using the WONCA code, the reason for the substantial difference in the total number of problems in drinkers and controls was a much greater prevalence of active gastrointestinal, psychiatric, smoking, and accident-related problems among drinkers (Fig 1). The most striking difference between the families of problem drinkers and those of controls was in joint family difficulties. There was almost a fourfold difference in the prevalence of social and interpersonal relationship problems.

Alcoholism, or problem drinking, can be defined in terms of the quantity of alcohol consumed. This definition may have the merit of apparent precision, but there is the additional need to quantify more clearly the effect of alcohol abuse on the individual and the family. The ultimate problem of alcohol is not the alcohol itself but its effect (poverty, marital disharmony, peptic ulcer, and so on).

Ramesar S, Schuman SH, Groh MJ, Poston JH: Detection of affective disorders in family practice: 126 assessments. J Fam Pract 10(5):819–828, 1980

In order to test the implied hypothesis (what is the true incidence/prevalence of affective disorders in a sample of adults in a family practice?), a protocol for data collection was designed with the following features:

Observer Blinded

Only the research assistant would have prior knowledge as to case/compeer status at the time of the interim home interview.

Standardized Psychiatric Interview

A comprehensive, semistructured interview was designed to cover major areas, including work, play, sleep, aggression, affection, sex, mood, appetite, self-esteem, life events, social supports, alcohol, and smoking. Home visits provided the setting for interim assessments by a clinical psychiatrist and a research assistant. During the home visit, questions were asked to assess any self-medication or prescription use that would be relevant to signs and symptoms under study.

Table 1. *Timing of Prospective Study and Selection of Patients for Home Visits*

Year	Activity	Population Characteristics
1972	Teaching practice opens	Recruiting from a broad range of census tracts (greater Charleston, South Carolina)
1975 (July–August)	First of a series of summer projects to acquaint each new resident (15–16) with his newly assigned families (300)	Approximately 10% of active enrolled families participated, including 298 adults. They received dental examinations, home visits, self-rating tests, and multiphasic screening tests
1977 (August)	First follow-up study estimates 5-year prevalence and 2-year incidence rates for affective disorders (men and women)	85 adults identified as cases by combining drug list and problem list to include all persons with one or more episodes of anxiety, depression, from 1972 to 1977
1978–1979 (December–April)	Second follow-up study utilizes a case-compeers, observer-blinded design with 126 assessments during 84 home visits, by two observers: a psychiatrist and a research assistant	Two major groups: $n_1 = 47$ cases* $n_2 = 47$ compeers Two minor groups: $n_3 = 14$ spouses of cases $n_4 = 18$ spouses of compeers

*Cases, representing sicker persons in the population, tend to be lost in long-term medical follow-up studies.
Reprinted by permission from Ramesar et al: J Fam Pract, 10(5): 819–828, 1980.

Table 2. *Frequencies of Eight Major Variables for Four Study Groups with Chi-Square Values* and Overall Frequencies, $N = 126$ Assessments*

Overall Frequency	Psychiatric Assessment	Frequency Among Cases/Compeers	Chi-Square	Frequency Among Spouses of Cases/Compeers	Chi-Square
Number %	No. & Variable	$N = 47/N = 47$	df = 1	$N = 14/N = 18$	df = 1
59/126 = 46.8	1. Diagnosis of anxiety, depression, or both	26/23	.1705	4/6	.0092
41/126 = 32.5	2. Sadness	16/17	.0000	5/3	.6772
48/126 = 38.1	3. Anomie	20/17	.1783	6/5	.2661
47/126 = 37.3	4. Personality deficiency	20/15	.7283	6/6	.0339
32/126 = 25.4	5. Unable to cope	17/10	.8706	4/1	1.6593
37/126 = 29.4	6. Anxiety only	14/17	.1925	2/4	.0130
7/126 = 5.6	7. Depression only	3/3	.1780	0/1	.0164
15/126 = 11.9	8. Both anxiety and depression	9/3	2.3882	2/1	.0525

*Chi-square statistic, one degree of freedom, Yates corrected for continuity; none are significant.
Reprinted by permission from Ramesar et al: J Fam Pract, 10(5):819–828, 1980.

The cohort of patients surveyed in this study (December 1978 to April 1979) can be traced back to the opening of the teaching practice in August 1972 (Table 1). For each case, a compeer was sought from the list of still active patients from the original cohort of 213 noncases. Each compeer was matched with an index case for sex, age within five years, and marital status. Two instruments were used: a standardized 61-question interview and a self-rating checklist.

Forty-seven cases of affective disorder, 47 age-sex-marital status-matched compeers, and 32 spouses participated. Results show little agreement between family practice records (drug and problem lists) and assessment at home visits. Over 46 percent of adults showed signs of anxiety, depression, or both. Eight major variables are listed in Table 2 for comparison between the major groups (47 cases and 47 compeers) and between the minor groups (14 case-spouses and 18 compeer-spouses).

Gaps in physician-patient communication account for some of the missed diagnoses. Prospective studies of these common disorders are handicapped by problems of (1) definition and criteria, (2) fluctuations in sick/well status over time, (3) changing levels of severity and levels of detection, and (4) losses of the sicker persons from the population for follow-up study. A generally useful model for affective disorders emphasizes the interaction between intrinsic factors (subjective stress) and extrinsic factors (objective stress). A flow sheet is presented to help the clinician assess the major components of stress, patient's ability to cope, and plan for management.

Herbst KG, Humphrey C: Prevalence of hearing impairment in the elderly living at home. J R Coll Gen Pract 31:155-160, 1981

The prevalence of deafness in the elderly population in the United Kingdom has not yet been accurately established, but it is generally believed that about one in three of all those over retirement age suffers from impaired hearing and that the proportion rises with age to about two in three among those aged 80 and over. However, the studies that have given rise to this assumption have based their estimates entirely on information given by respondents in answer to questions about their hearing, or on the observation of interviewers. They have not used audiometric testing.

Using pure-tone audiometry, the prevalence of hearing impairment was assessed

Table 1. *Type of Hearing Loss by Age (Percentages in Brackets)*

Type of Hearing Loss	Age in Years				
	70-74	*75-79*	*80-84*	*85+*	*Total*
	No (%)	No (%)	No (%)	No (%)	No (%)
Normal hearing	42 *(38)*	17 *(23)*	4 *(11)*	2 *(6)*	65 *(26)*
Unilateral loss	14 *(12)*	15 *(20)*	3 *(9)*	3 *(9)*	35 *(14)*
Bilateral loss	56 *(50)*	42 *(57)*	28 *(80)*	27 *(84)*	153 *(60)*
Total	112 *(100)*	74 *(100)*	35 *(100)*	32 *(100)*	253 *(100)*

Reprinted by permission from Herbst, Humphrey: J R Coll Gen Pract, 31:155-160, 1981.

in a sample of elderly people living at home aged 70 or more. Deafness was defined as an average loss over the speech frequencies at 1 kHz, 2 kHz and 4 kHz of 35 dB or more in the better ear. The initial sample consisted of all 365 persons aged 70 and over registered with the central surgery of one Inner London group general practice. Forty-eight refused to participate, and 46 were either untraceable, in hospital, or on holiday during the field-work period. Eighteen respondents were subsequently excluded for a variety of reasons ranging from poor English to inadequate audiometry. Thus, the final sample analyzed consisted of 253 people (69 percent of the initial sample). Nonrespondents did not differ significantly from respondents with regard to either age or sex. In all cases, the ears were examined for wax. The presence of wax was recorded only when the meatus was totally occluded.

It was found that 60 percent of the popu-

Table 2. *Bilateral Deafness by Age (Percentages in Brackets)*

Decibel Loss in the Better Ear	Age in Years		
	70-79	80+	Total
	No (%)	No (%)	No (%)
35-44	38 (39)	8 (14)	46 (30)
45-69	47 (48)	34 (62)	81 (53)
70+	13 (13)	13 (24)	26 (17)
Total	98 (100)	55 (100)	153 (100)

$X^2 = 10.387$ with 2 df p < 0.01.
Reprinted by permission from Herbst, Humphrey: J R Coll Gen Pract, 31:155-160, 1981.

lation under study were deaf and that the proportion who were deaf rose with age to 84 percent of those aged 85 and over. A further 14 percent of respondents was found to have a unilateral loss of 35 db or more (Table 1). In 25 percent (57), the

Table 3. *Estimates of Percentage Prevalence of Deafness in the Elderly Population Based on Self-Assessment*

Author	Date	60+	65+	70+	75+	80+	85+
		F	M				M F
Sheldon	1948	29	38	—	—	—	60 68
					M F		
Wilkins	1948	—	—	—	28 25	—	—
			M F				
Harris	1962	—	35 30	—	—	—	—
Kay et al.	1964	—	37	—	—	—	—
Richardson	1964	—	—	—	—	50	—
Townsend & Wedderburn	1965	—	30	—	—	—	—
Brockington & Lempert	1966	—	—	—	—	54	—
Goldberg	1970	—	—	31	—	—	—
Nottingham Social Services	1973	—	—	—	32	—	—
Milne	1976	39	—	44	—	53	—
Abrams	1978	—	—	—	36	—	—
Present study (self-estimate)	1980	—	—	38	39	54	69
Present study (based on audiometry)	1980	—	—	60	69	82	84

Reprinted by permission from Herbst, Humphrey: J R Coll Gen Pract, 31:155-160, 1981.

sample wax was blocking both ears, but the presence of wax was not significantly related to deafness.

Deafness was related to social class. Those in the registrar general's classes IIIm, IV, and V were significantly more likely to have impaired hearing (p < 0.01). There was no significant difference between the proiortions of men and women who were deaf. As regards age, the very old were not only more likely to be deaf than the "young old," but their deafness was also more severe (p < 0.01) (Table 2).

As was suspected, the prevalence found using audiometry is substantially higher than that noted in previous studies where estimates were based only on self-

assessment. However, these results are broadly comparable with earlier self-assessment studies (Table 3).

The findings of this study challenge conventional assumptions about the prevalence of hearing impairment in old age. These assumptions have led to a serious underestimate of the scale of the disorder. This study suggests that impaired hearing is, in fact, usual not only for those over eighty but for those in their seventies as well. The incidence of impairment uncovered in this study gives cause for concern; it should be given due consideration in the allocation of resources and in the practice of health professionals.

O'Sullivan J, Carson N, Forsell P: Screening in general practice (2). Aus Fam Physician 8:1109–1112, 1979

This paper presents the results of a 12-month screening survey for hypertension in an Australian group practice and includes early observations on therapeutic outcomes. The study was conducted at the Blackburn Clinic by seven full-time family physicians (including an FMP trainee), a part-time associate (two sessions), and an obstetrician and gynecologist. From patient records (numerically filed), the current practice population was conservatively estimated at over 30,000 patients. Excluding home and hospital visits, approximately 50,000 physician/patient contacts were recorded for that year.

After reviewing current literature and following discussion with clinicians and researchers, it was agreed to regard as abnormal a blood pressure that, after the patient's lying down for ten minutes, was greater than 150/100 mm Hg on three separate occasions. A standardized "blood pressure assessment" form and continuing care record sheets were designed. All patients diagnosed as having hypertension were referred to their own physicians for a detailed history, a full examination, and

certain routine investigations (blood pressure assessment form) prior to commencement of therapy.

Only 2 percent of the patients screened were identified as new cases of hypertension, which was less than expected. However, 383 patients (known and currently treated hypertensives) were counted during the screening process. When these cases are included, the total number of hypertensives is 470 and the total number of patients screened is 4,776; thus, 10 percent of patients suffered from hypertension (Table 1). No case of secondary hypertension was found or suspected by any physician.

The overall effects of treatment of the 72 patients were examined in two ways. First, the average pretreatment blood pressure was 180/106 mm Hg, and the average blood pressure after treatment (recorded at the last visit at least 12 months after treatment was initiated) was 156/92 mm Hg. Second, in the individual patient, 88 percent had their diastolic blood pressures successfully reduced to below 100 mm Hg, but only 53 percent had both systolic and diastolic pressures reduced below 150/100 mm Hg, set as

Table 1. *Patients Screened in 12 Months*

Total number of known hypertensives receiving therapy	383
Total number of "normal" persons screened	4,393
Total number of persons with normal B.P.	4,101
Number of patients with hypertension on first visit	292
Number of patients with hypertension on second visit	162
Number of patients with hypertension after third visit	87
Total number of patients screened	4,776
Total number of hypertensives (new and old cases)	470

Reprinted by permission from O'Sullivan et al: Aus Fam Physician, 8:1109–1112, 1979.

the upper limits of normal in this study. The medical records of all patients (47 percent) in whom optimum reduction had not been obtained were examined. This revealed that in the majority of cases the physician accepted the higher level as satisfactory despite good cooperation from the patient and in the absence of drug side effects.

The need to record the blood pressure on three separate occasions was confirmed again by this study. Of the 292 persons found to be hypertensive on the first visit, 162 were still hypertensive on the second visit, and only 87 were hypertensive on the third occasion. This serves as a reminder that unless this approach is taken, a large number of normal persons might be labeled as "hypertensive" and condemned to lifelong unnecessary therapy.

The outcome of therapy was surprisingly poor when compared with its objective. (Only 53 percent had a satisfactory post-treatment level of blood pressure.) It is recommended that practitioners should critically look at their own results in a similar way (a form of audit), and it may well be that results in general are poorer than believed. In addition, there is a need to know what are the true outcomes achieved by specialty clinics against which the general practitioner may measure the degree of success of his own interventions.

Woolnough KV, Domovitch E, Wilson D: Screening females for gonorrhea. Can Fam Physician 27:849–851, 1981

Routine screening for gonorrhea in the female population is an area that deserves scrutiny. The literature gives little direction for or against screening programs.

This study was undertaken at the Family Practice Unit, The Wellesley Hospital, whose patient population is a wide cross-section mostly living in the city core. Any patient receiving a pelvic examination had a cervical swab for Gram's stain, culture, and sensitivity. Those who specifically requested a VD test because of contact with a positive case were not entered in this study. Cultures were taken in the Family Practice Unit, which is adjacent to The Wellesley Hospital. All cultures were in the laboratory within six hours of being taken. The culture medium was charcoal, and a slide for Gram's stain was also included.

A total of 721 people entered the study: six were found to have gonorrhea by the method mentioned previously (Table 1).

In Ontario, the cost of Gram's stain and culture for gonorrhea was only $5.85. The cost of Gram's stain, culture, and sensitivity was $9.75. The least cost generated was thus $5.85 per patient for a screening program. Using this figure, the total cost of this study was approximately $4,200. The cost of detecting a case of gonorrhea in different subgroups within the study is outlined in Table 2.

The overall incidence of gonorrhea in this study was 0.83 percent, so that diagnos-

Table 1. *Results of Screening 721 Women for Gonorrhea*

All Patients	No.	%
Total patients	721	100.0
Sexually active	600	83.2
More than one partner	69	11.5
Partner more than one partner	87	14.5
Partner more than one partner, among those with more than one partner	49	71.0
Partner more than one partner, among those with only one partner	39	7.3
GC Positives		
Total number	6	0.83
Sexually active patients	6	1.00
Sexually inactive patients	0	0.00
More than one partner	2	2.9
Partner more than one partner	3	3.4
Answering yes to questions #2 and/or #3	3	2.8
Answering yes to questions #2 and #3	2	4.1
Reporting only one partner	4	0.75
Reporting partner having only one partner	3	0.58

Reprinted by permission from Woolnough et al: Can Fam Physician, 27:849-851, 1981.

ing an individual case of gonorrhea was very expensive. If only sexually active women reporting more than one partner and/or the partner having more than one partner had been screened, the positive rate would have risen to 2.8 percent. Fifty percent of the positive diagnoses in this study would have been made using a questionnaire alone.

A screening program with a positive rate of less than 4.3 percent is not felt to be cost effective. The primary method of surveillance should be identifying high-risk groups. Certain groups of women should still be cultured, including: (1) women who seem more likely to have more than one partner based on physician's knowledge. This group includes women whose regular sexual activity has been interrupted for reasons such as illness, physical separation, pregnancy or family dysfunction; (2) transients; (3) emotionally or mentally impaired people; (4) people with a history of venereal disease; (5) people who say they have had contact with venereal disease; (6) pregnant women; (7) women who have signs or symptoms suggesting venereal disease. The last group would include women with gynecologic complaints such as dyspareunia, discharge and irregular bleeding, or findings of discharge on examination.

Table 2. *Cost of Detecting Gonorrhea in Different Sub-groups*

All patients included	$700
Sexually active patient	585
Patient with one partner, partner one partner	960
Patient with more than one partner, partner more than one partner	210

Reprinted by permission from Woolnough et al: Can Fam Physician, 27:849-851, 1981.

MacAdam DB, Siegerstetter J, Smith MCA: Deafness in adults—screening in general practice. J R Coll Gen Pract 31:161–164, 1981

Many people have hearing difficulty, but estimates of the extent of the problem vary, partly because different criteria are used to define deafness and partly because hearing handicaps may be caused by failure of the brain to discriminate and interpret sounds as well as by failure of the sense organs in the ear to respond to noise. A recent review suggests that 15–20 percent of all those aged over 65 may be deaf. The most recent information, from the General Household Survey, gives an overall prevalence rate for "difficulty with hearing" of 14 percent in females and 17 percent in males aged 16 and over; only about 15 percent of those found to have hearing difficulties wore a hearing aid. The aims of this study were to (1) estimate the prevalence of deafness in adults using a random sample drawn from the lists of general practitioners, (2) assess the effectiveness of a simple question in screening for deafness, (3) identify variables associated with an increased frequency of deafness, and (4) discover the level of knowledge in the population about equipment and places of help for deaf people.

A random sample of 1083 people, drawn from the lists of two general practices in Leeds, England, was used to estimate the prevalence of deafness among adults. Children under 16 years old were excluded. A test for deafness (defined as failure to hear 35 dB at 1,000 Hz in one or both ears) using a portable audiometer proved simple to operate with little observer variation. The audiometers were standardized at the beginning and at the end of the study; no change was found. At each available frequency (250 Hz, 1000 Hz and 4000 Hz), the sound was produced at 20 dB, 35 dB, and 60 dB. Subjects could not see the apparatus during testing. The audiometry results were given to the general practitioners. Ears were not examined for wax or eustachian catarrh.

Sixty-four percent (1083 out of 1697) of the adult sample agreed to take part and were interviewed and tested. The refusal rate was similar in the two practices. No approach was made to 4 percent because they were severely ill, bereaved, or suffering from some other recent distress known to their doctor. The data for both practices were combined. The age-sex distribution of the nonresponders did not differ from that of the sample as a whole. The prevalence of deafness by age is shown in Table 1. There was no evidence of a different prevalence among those nonresponders who were tested later.

The prevalence of deafness increased with age and was lowest in social classes I and II; there was no significant difference between the sexes. Audiometry showed that 17 percent of those who thought their hearing was abnormal had no recorded loss of hearing using the stated test and that 18 percent of those who are deaf would be overlooked if the question "Do you think your hearing is normal?" was used for initial screening in general practice.

Twenty-six percent of those who were deaf wore hearing aids (23 out of 90). Only 14 percent of the sample (152 out of 1069) knew about equipment for the deaf other than hearing aids—for example, amplifiers for the telephone, television, and record player; flashing lights for the telephone or door bells; audio teaching aids. Of all of these, telephone accessories were the most widely known.

Hearing difficulties in at least one close relative over two generations were reported by just over a third of the sample. This aspect of family history was similar whether or not the subject had normal hearing, was deaf in one ear, or was deaf in both ears. Fifty percent of the sample (541 persons) had worked in a noisy place. Eight percent (34 out of 436) of those who had spent up to 25 years in a noisy place were deaf; 14 per-

Table 1. *Deafness by Age (Percentages are Given in Brackets)*

		Age			
		16–44	*45–64*	*65 and over*	*Total*
Deafness	Present	12 *(2)*	25 *(7)*	53 *(24)*	90 *(8)*
	Absent	481 *(98)*	348 *(93)*	164 *(76)*	993 *(92)*
Total		493	373	217	1,083

Reprinted by permission from MacAdam et al: J R Coll Gen Pract, 31: 161–164, 1981.

cent (15 out of 105) of those who had spent longer in such conditions were deaf.

This study has described the payoff that could be expected if screening for deafness were carried out in general practice using simple methods and equipment. While the general practitioner is likely to refer for specialist opinion those who are identified as deaf, much general information and advice about deafness is available that is at present not known by the majority who visit their doctor.

Miller SL, Norcross WA, Bass RA: Breast self-examination in the primary care setting. J Fam Pract 10(5):811–815, 1980

Despite its strong appeal as a noninvasive, cost effective, and simple procedure for early detection of breast carcinoma, very little is currently known about regular breast self-examination (BSE) among adult females in the United States. Where interest in breast cancer prevention has been shown, it has most typically been in the area of early diagnosis using radiologic techniques (eg, mammography) rather than in behavioral control methods such as self-examination. Given the cost differential between these two approaches and the fact that the former has not been proved effective in the early detection of the disease, this situation is not ideal.

This paper investigates the association between several medical and nonmedical factors and self-reported rates of BSE in a selective sample of women. At three primary care centers, 260 women completed the BSE survey over the two-month period. The sample was, for the most part, white (83 percent), Christian (67 percent), and highly educated (23 percent college graduates or higher, 34 percent reporting some college). Moreover, the sample was skewed in favor of younger women despite the fact that one of the data-collection sites was a local senior citizen's health center. While only 12.6 percent of the subjects was over age 55, some 69 percent was 30 years or younger. The sample bias favoring white educated respondents was probably a function of (1) the fact that the other collection sites were University Hospital primary care clinics and (2) self-selection.

Table 1 reports the mean year frequency of self-reported BSE among sample members classified in terms of three selected background characteristics. While the yearly rate of self-reported BSE was only slightly higher for blacks than for either whites or Orientals, it was considerably lower for Mexican Americans than for all other groups. A statistically significant trend ($P < .05$) indicating that the level of self-reported BSE is less for Catholic sample members than for their Protestant and Jewish counterparts is also found in Table 1.

The pattern of findings from this study suggests that BSE behavior may be conditioned more by culturally determined attitudes than by "rational" factors such as a woman's "objective" risk for, and knowledge of, the disease. Sample members who performed well on the risk factor examination were not significantly more likely than those performing at moderate or low levels to report self-examining on a regular basis. In addition, no significant differences in the rate of self-examination between high-risk women and women at a lower level of risk, measured in terms of age and known factors, were found.

In contrast, the general pattern and relative strength of the association between rates of BSE and the background factors considered does indicate that a differential sociocultural response to BSE is likely to exist in the asymptomatic population. Put differently, the considerably lower rate of self-examination for Mexican-Americans, and the significantly lower rate for

Table 1. *Breast Self-Examination Rates of the Primary Care Sample by Selected Background Characteristics*

Selected Characteristics	Average Number of Yearly Breast Self-Examinations	Number of Subjects	F-Ratio
Ethnicity			
Black	7.4	20	
White	7.0	207	
Oriental	7.0	4	.57
Mexican-American	5.0	12	P > .05
Religion			
Jewish	7.5	6	
Protestant	7.3	101	2.72
Catholic	5.3	65	P < .05
Level of Education			
>College Graduate	7.9	24	
College Graduate	7.8	31	
Some College	7.4	86	1.5
≤High School Graduate	6.1	105	P > .05

Reprinted by permission from Miller et al: J Fam Pract, 10(5): 811–815, 1980.

Catholics, found to obtain in this study, may represent differences in attitudes pertinent to BSE practices on the part of women in these groups.

The findings of this study point to the possibility that socioculturally based attitudes may be at work to inhibit BSE among certain groups of women in this society. However, given the selective nature of the sample, this thesis needs to be verified using data from a population based sample. The results of further research may be useful in designing programs to educate health practitioners in the primary care setting to be more sensitive to differences in BSE practices among adult females, thereby helping to increase the rate at which they are likely to self-examine.

Keller K, George E, Podell RN: Clinical breast examination and breast self-examination experience in a family practice population. J Fam Pract 11(6): 887–893, 1980

The breast is the most prevalent site of cancer incidence and mortality among women. Indeed, breast cancer will develop in nearly 1 out of every 13 women, and it is the leading cause of all deaths among women aged 40 to 44 years. Breast cancer has a more favorable prognosis if detected at an early stage. If breast cancer is discovered before lymph node metastases have occurred, the five-year survival rate is 84 percent. Unfortunately, only about 45 percent of breast cancers are found before they have spread to the axillary nodes. When there is nodal involvement, the five-year survival rate is 56 percent.

It is therefore essential to promote methods that can help detect breast cancer in its early stages. Some have argued that routine screening by self-examination and clinical examination lead to the discovery of breast cancer at a clinically more localized stage. In this study, a patient questionnaire, chart audit, and resident questionnaire were used to assess clinical breast examination and breast self-examination experience in a family practice patient population. a questionnaire was mailed to a sample of 772 female patients, 25-65 years old, surveying their knowledge, attitudes, and behavior concerning breast self-examination and routine clinical examination during the five-year period 1974 through 1978. The sample was generated using systematic, stratified sampling, and it represented 53 percent of the population of 1460 "regular" female patients. From the sample of 772 women, the authors randomly audited 185 of their charts for documentation of clinical breast examinations, breast cancer risk factors, and breast self-examination teaching by family practice residents.

Despite the fact that 99 percent of the respondents were aware of breast self-examination, only 19 percent said they practiced it every month. The majority said they practiced breast self-examination, but irregularly. Fifty-one percent practiced it at least four times a year. Eight percent said they never examined their breasts. Of those who practiced self-examination, 55 percent felt confident that they were performing it correctly.

Two factors seemed to be related to routine practice of breast self-examination. Women whose physicians had discussed breast self-examinations with them and demonstrated the procedure were more likely to practice breast self-examination monthly. In the group that had the procedure demonstrated, 21 percent practiced self-examination monthly and only 3 percent said they never practiced self-examination. Whereas in the group with no discussion or demonstration from a physician, only 14 percent practiced breast self-examination monthly, and 21 percent said they never practiced self-examination. The group that had a physician discuss breast self-examination but who had not demonstrated it did almost as well as the group

Table 1. *Patient Report of Reason(s) for Not Practicing Monthly Breast Self-Examination (BSE)*

Reason	Percent Reporting
Forget to do it every month	57
Do not know why	19
Not sure if correctly practicing BSE	18
Feel I do not have to worry	6
Too busy	5
Do not know how to do BSE	4
Think it is frightening	4
Did not know it should be done every month	2
Did not know about BSE	1
Think it is embarrassing	1
Other	7

Reprinted by permission from Keller et al: J Fam Pract, 11(6): 887-893, 1980.

with demonstration; 21 percent said they practiced breast self-examination monthly, and 7 percent said they never practiced breast self-examination. The second factor related to routine practice of breast self-examination was confidence in one's ability to do it correctly. Patients who were confident that they were practicing it correctly were more likely to practice it monthly.

When asked why they did not practice breast self-examination monthly, 57 percent of the respondents said they "forget" to do it each month. Other reasons for not practicing monthly breast self-examination are shown in Table 1.

The low number of annual clinical examinations and low performance of BSE may be explained partially by the physician's setting too narrowly the parameters of when a clinical breast examination and BSE teaching could be done appropriately, that is, a Pap smear/pelvic or general examination. A more aggressive approach by the physician may increase the number of women who get routine clinical breast examinations and who supplement them by monthly BSE.

English EC, Geyman JP: The efficiency and cost effectiveness of diagnostic tests for infectious mononucleosis. J Fam Pract 6(5):977–981, 1978

Pharyngitis with fever, adenopathy, and fatigue is commonly encountered in everyday practice, often raising the question of infectious mononucleosis. Concern over the degree of accuracy of diagnosing infectious mononucleosis raises the issue of cost effectiveness of relevant laboratory procedures and, consequently, cost benefit to the patient.

Two patient populations were surveyed. The first consisted of 1712 patients between 14 and 30 years of age, seen over a 3½-year period at the University Hospital, Harborview Medical Center, and other affiliated hospitals in Seattle, Washington. The initial test used in patients suspected of infectious mononucleosis in this group was the Ortho Monospot test. Criteria for use of the Monospot test were based entirely on clinical grounds, such as pharyngitis, fever, adenopathy, fatigue, and occasionally splenomegaly. Whenever a positive Monospot agglutination occurred, a presumptive heterophil was titered. The second population consisted of 1969 university students, 18 to 25 years old, seen at the Hall Health Center, University of Washington, Seattle, Washington, over a four-year period. The tests on these students were performed at the Hall Health Laboratory and followed a different format. The first screening procedure for any student with a sore throat and lymphadenopathy consists of an initial leukocyte count and differential as well as a blood smear. Serologic testing with the "monoscreen" was performed only when the following criteria were met: an absolute increase in mononuclear cells in the blood greater than 4000/cu mm or a relative increase of greater than 50 percent, with atypical lymphocytes of at least 15 percent of the total leukocyte count.

The efficiency of these two approaches to diagnosis is summarized in Table 1:

The calculation of cost effectiveness is based on WBC, differential, and blood smear; Monospot/"monoscreen"; and heterophil titering costs. The average charge in the community is $10 for WBC, differential, and blood smear, $6.50 for Monospot or "monoscreen," and $6.50 for heterophil titering or $23 for hematologic, slide agglutination, and serologic evaluation. Table 2 shows the results of this calculation.

When infectious mononucleosis is suspected clinically, diagnosis is made most efficiently when a leukocyte count is first performed to demonstrate the presence of increased numbers of atypical lymphocytes. This study indicates that by such hematologic selection of patients before serologic testing (whether by Monospot or "monoscreen") a fivefold increase in degree of accuracy of diagnosis can be achieved with corresponding gains in cost effectiveness. A confirmatory heterophil titer adds negligible benefit.

Table 1. *Efficiency of Diagnosis*

Method I	Number of Patients	Method II	Number of Patients
Selected on clinical grounds	1,712	Selected on clinical and hematological grounds	1,969
Monospot positive	104	'Monoscreen' positive	558
Differential heterophil positive	97	Heterophil positive	553
% positive	5.6	% positive	28.1

Reprinted by permission from English, Geyman: J Fam Pract, 6(5):977–981, 1978.

Table 2. *Cost Effectiveness of Diagnosis**

Diagnostic Method I	Number of Patients	Cost per Positive without Confirmatory Serologic Titering	Cost per Positive with Confirmatory Serology
Patients clinically selected with concurrent WBC, differential, smear, and Monospot†	1,712	$272	$298
Incidence of Positives		6.1%	5.6%

Diagnostic Method II	Number of Patients	Cost per Positive without Confirmatory Serologic Titering	Cost per Positive with Confirmatory Serology
Patients selected by an initial screening based on hematologic criteria in patients suspected of IM. 'Monoscreen' conditional to hematologic criteria.†	1,969	$ 58	$ 63
Incidence of Positives		28.3%	28.1%

*Based upon assumed costs of $10.00 for WBC, differential, blood smear; $6.50 for Monospot/'monoscreen'; $6.50 for differential heterophil titering.
†According to Table 1, confirmatory serologic titering was performed only when the Monospot or 'monoscreen' was positive.
Reprinted by permission from English, Geyman: J Fam Pract, 6(5): 977–981, 1978.

Tucker JB, Barasz D, Greenfield S, DeSimone JP: Throat culturing techniques in the family practice model unit. J Fam Pract 12(5):925–931, 1981

Since many graduates of any family medicine residency will practice without accessible laboratory facilities, a program was begun to teach residents basic throat-culturing techniques. Since pharyngitis is seen so frequently by the family physician, throat-culturing techniques were one of the first projects undertaken. This study was designed to show that office throat-culturing techniques can be taught to family medicine residents and that accurate results can be achieved.

A literature review was completed, and in conjunction with the head microbiologist at the hospital laboratory, a protocol for culturing, plating, and reading throat cultures was developed. The residents and nursing staff were taught in didactic sessions, in laboratory demonstrations, and one on one with faculty preceptors in the model unit. Cultures from the same patients were plated and read in both the residency laboratory and the hospital microbiology laboratory. The posterior pharynx and tonsils of patients with symptoms of pharyngitis were swabbed by the residents and transported by Culturette (Marion Scientific Corporation) to the residency laboratory. The same Culturette was used in both the residency and hospital laboratories. The hospital laboratory processed the Culturette in the usual manner, which was identical to and the model for the protocol used in the residency laboratory. The St.

Joseph's Hospital Health Center laboratory is under strict quality control by the New York State Health Department and consistently has been found to be 95 to 100 percent accurate in frequent periodic evaluation of unknown specimens.

Cultures from 1290 patients were studied. The residency laboratory reported 225 to be positive for group A streptococci and 1065 to be negative. Concurrently, the hospital laboratory found 261 cultures positive. Data are presented in Table 1. The false positive rate was 0.047 (48/1029) and the specificity of the residency laboratory was 0.953 (981/1029). Most importantly, the false negative rate was 0.322 (84/261), and the sensitivity of the residency laboratory was 0.678 (177/261). Thus, about one in three patients with streptococcus went undiagnosed by the residency laboratory.

The results are disappointing but nonetheless important. The false-negative rate and sensitivity of the residency laboratory are poor. A correct diagnosis of only 67.8 percent of patients with streptococcal disease is unacceptable when the potential sequelae are considered. The results of this study question both the simplicity and accuracy of office throat culturing. The study

Table 1. *Comparison of Hospital and Resident Laboratories*

	+Hospital	−Hospital	
+Residency	177	48	225
−Residency	84	981	1,065
	261	1,029	

$\chi^2 = 9.28$ P < 0.01.
Reprinted by permission from Tucker et al: J Fam Pract, 12(5):925-931, 1981.

shows that office bacteriology is not to be undertaken lightly and that the delicacy of materials and techniques cannot be underestimated. Such poor results in an educational setting with formal preparation and ongoing supervision prompt great concern for the private physician's office.

It is strongly suggested that those physicians currently relying on office cultures periodically review and validate their findings with an accredited laboratory. Furthermore, those physicians planning to begin office throat culturing should obtain initial consultation, ongoing supervision, and confirmation of results from a qualified microbiologist.

Robson J, Lurie N, Hart JT: Ten years' experience in general practice of dip-slide urine culture in children under five years old. J R Coll Gen Pract 29:658–661, 1979

By the age of 5, as many as 20 percent of children with significant bacteriuria already have radiologic evidence of infective damage to the renal tract. Early diagnosis of bacteriuria is therefore important for two reasons. It may be an indicator of surgically correctable urinary tract anomalies that might otherwise end in irreversible renal failure, and failure to control bacteriuria can lead to reduction of kidney growth and renal scarring.

The dip-slide method of urine culture is a reliable discriminator of significant bac-

teriuria. It has been found to be cheap, simple, and well suited to general practice. This paper describes 10 years' experience of the application of dip slides to children under 5 years of age at times of ill health in one general practice in South Wales.

The study was based in Glyncorrwg, a geographically isolated industrial village in the South Wales valleys. Ninety-seven percent of the population is registered with a single practitioner with a list size of 2,081. Of this population, 94.2 percent are drawn from the Registrar General's Social Classes

3, 4, and 5. The study was retrospective, using the practice records of children for whom the principal was responsible.

Practice policy aimed to obtain at least one dip-slide urine culture from all children in the first 5 years of life, preferentially using times of ill health. Dip-slides were to be obtained from all children with specific urinary tract symptoms, or those with nonspecific symptoms not satisfactorily accounted for. Follow-up after treatment of bacteriuria was to be continued until negative cultures were obtained and repeated at any subsequent episode of ill health. The criterion for a positive dip slide and significant bacteriuria was a single count of $\geq 10^5$ bacteria per ml. All cases of balanitis were excluded and no dip slides were attempted in the first month of life. In the event of recurrent bacteriuria, a new episode was defined either by an intermediate negative culture or a change of organism.

A total of 567 children under 5 registered with the practice in a ten-year period, of whom 559 presented with symptoms of ill health during the first five years of life. Dip-slide urine culture was obtained from 158 (27.9 percent) of those registered. Thirty-four (12.3 percent) girls and 23 (7.9 percent) boys had at least one episode of bacteriuria. Of these, ten (29.4 percent) girls and six (26.1 percent) boys had more than one episode.

Out of a total of 123 positive dip slides, 91 (73.7 percent) yielded a significant pure growth, five (4.7 percent) yielded a significant mixed growth, and 27 (21.9 percent) yielded an unidentified bacterial count of $\geq 10^5$ per ml. Pure *Escherichia coli* was grown in 59.7 percent of episodes of bacteriuria in girls and 53.1 percent of episodes in boys. Pure growths of *Proteus* were recorded in 6.4 percent of episodes of bacteriuria in girls and 28.1 percent of episodes in boys (p < 0.05).

Forty-nine (85.9 percent) children with bacteriuria had their first detected episode under the age of 3. Of the 57 children with bacteriuria at some time, ten girls and four boys were followed up by radiologic investigation. Abnormalities were detected in two boys (one megaureter with stones and one abnormal calyceal system) and three girls (one urethral stenosis, one vesicoureteral reflux, and one duplex kidney). The two obstructive lesions were amenable to surgery.

Symptoms usually ascribed to the urinary tract in older children and adults were not found to be discriminating for bacteriuria in this age group, and the symptoms associated with the request for a dip slide (at patient-initiated consultation rather than doctor-initiated follow-up), could not be used to predict the presence or absence of bacteriuria. Of those children with symptoms "specific" to the urinary tract (frequency, dysuria, enuresis, smelly or cloudy urine, loin or abdominal pain, haematuria) 26.9 percent had bacteriuria. In those with "nonspecific" symptoms (sore throat, cough, misery, nappy rash, anorexia, or vomiting) 29.2 percent had bacteriuria. Out of a total of 440 dip slides requested, 27.9 percent yielded significant bacteriuria. This high yield suggested that a greater degree of suspicion among those with nonspecific symptoms was necessary. In a cohort followed for the first five years of life, 36 percent of children were tested with dip slides at some time. Twelve (12.0 percent) girls and 14 (12.8 percent) boys had at least one episode of bacteriuria, and of these a quarter had recurrent episodes.

Because of the relatively small numbers of patients, the results of this study should be treated with some caution. However, if confirmed by more rigorous studies, the high incidence of bacteriuria, the failure of traditional symptoms to discriminate between the presence or the absence of bacteriuria, multiple episodes in a quarter of those with bacteriuria under 5 years, and a preponderance in boys under 3 years have considerable implications for diagnostic policy and follow-up. Dip-slide culture is a valuable tool in the diagnosis, management, and follow-up of urinary tract infection and should be used widely.

Steffan WC, Schneiderman LJ: Contribution of unexpected serum thyroxine (T_4) abnormality to detection of thyroid disease. J Fam Pract 11(6):873–875, 1980

It is generally recognized that unexpected screening laboratory abnormalities rarely lead to diagnoses and are often ignored by physicians. On the other hand, there is little information about how these procedures compare to the history and physical examination in uncovering new cases of disease. In this study, the authors sought to evaluate the screening T_4 as a diagnostic tool in comparison with the history and physical examination.

The screening serum thyroxine (T_4) was compared to the history and physical examination as a means of detecting new cases of thyroid disease in a university hospital outpatient population. Of 2,257 T_4 results obtained during a six-month period, 219 represented patients whose values fell outside the laboratory's range of normality (4.5 μg/100 ml to 12.0 μg/100 ml) on their initial medical evaluation. Of these, 11 patients could not be further studied because of inadequate medical documentation. The remaining study population of 208 patients contained 87 with elevated T_4 values and 121 with reduced T_4 values.

Table 1 summarizes the results. Of the 13 new cases of hyperthyroidism in the six-month study period, ten were suspected on the basis of history and physical examination; three were diagnosed as a result of following up the elevated screening T_4. Of

the 32 new cases of hypothyroidism, 23 were diagnosed on the basis of history and physical examination, nine only after the observance of a low screening T_4. Thus, approximately one-quarter of new diagnoses of thyroid disease were made not by history and physical examination but by the unexpected appearance of a deviant T_4 on the screening laboratory panel.

From this study, the authors conclude that the screening T_4 in the outpatient setting is a useful "extender" of the physician's diagnostic skills, a fact that the physicians themselves seem to recognize. Indeed, in reviewing the follow-up of the abnormal T_4 values, it was noted that physicians were almost always able to record signs and symptoms of thyroid disease in retrospect.

Further assessment of the diagnostic value of the screening T_4 will require data concerning the cost of the test, the cost of follow-up studies both to rule in and rule out thyroid disease, and the ultimate health benefits to be gained by recognition of the disorder in the absence of overt clinical signs and symptoms. At this time, however, the authors believe that in the general medical ambulatory setting, the T_4 component in a biochemical screening panel uncovers a substantial number of patients with thyroid disease who would otherwise go unrecognized.

Table 1. *New Cases of Thyroid Disease Diagnosed by History and Physical Examination vs Screening T_4 Determinations*

	Number of Patients	Mean Age (Years)	Mean T_4 Value
Hyperthyroidism (N = 13)			
Detected by history and physical examination	10	35	23.3
Detected by screening T_4	3	55	17.8
Hypothyroidism (N = 23)			
Detected by history and physical examination	23	43	2.8
Detected by screening T_4	9	44	2.5

Reprinted by permission from Steffan, Schneiderman: J Fam Pract, 11(6):873–875, 1980.

Hahn DL, Baker WA: Penicillin G susceptibility of "rural" Staphylococcus aureus. J Fam Pract 11(1):43–46, 1980

It is generally well known by practicing physicians that the incidence of resistance to penicillin G among strains of *Staphylococcus aureus* (*SA*) isolated from within the hospital environment is quite high. Many physicians, however, remain under the impression that strains of *SA* isolated from the community at large are still relatively susceptible to penicillin G. Insofar as the authors are aware, the question of differences in susceptibility of "urban" vs "rural" community staphylococci has never been addressed directly in the American literature. As a practicing physician in Madison, Wisconsin, one of the authors had the opportunity to compare the penicillin susceptibility of *SA* isolated from outpatients in a Madison multispecialty group with that of similar isolates from a rural practice in Wisconsin. These antibiograms (patterns of antibiotic susceptibility) were further compared with those of the three community hospitals in Madison and with isolates from predominantly nonurban sources processed at the Wisconsin State Laboratory of Hygiene.

Since 1974, a registered specialist microbiologist has kept records of antibiograms of all pathogens isolated from patients at the East Madison Clinic (EMC), a multispecialty group practice located in Madison, Wisconsin (population 175,000). In 1975, East Madison Clinic became associated with a three-physician general practice located in Sun Prairie, Wisconsin, a town of approximately 10,000 people about 10 to 15 miles from Madison. Subsequently, all bacteriologic specimens from the Sun Prairie Clinic (SPC) were processed and recorded at East Madison Clinic. Antibiograms were obtained using conventional media and commercially available antibiotic discs by the Kirby-Bauer method.

From September 1, 1974, to June 30, 1978, a total of 50,169 specimens were processed at East Madison Clinic of which 1752 (3.5 percent) yielded *SA* in pure or mixed culture. Antibiograms were available for 1,575 (90 percent) of these isolates. Most specimens of *SA* not subjected to susceptibility testing were felt to be incidental organisms, such as *SA* isolated in conjunction with Group A, β-hemolytic streptococci on throat culture.

Table 1. *Penicillin Susceptibility of Staphylococcus aureus*

	1974		1975		1976		1977		1978	
	No.	*%*	*No.*	*%*	*No.*	*%*	*No.*	*%*	*No.*	*%*
EMC/SPC	103 (4 Months)	25.7	413	20.8	384	25.3	429	19.6	246 (8 Months)	16.3
Hospital A	532	20.0	510	20.0	503	16.0	435	16.0	121 (6 Months)	19.0
Hospital B	470	23.0	445	22.6	619	18.0	544	19.0	213 (4 Months)	15.8
Hospital C	—	—	—	—	79	21.0	145	14.0	82 (8 Months)	17.0
	7/71 to 6/72		7/72 to 6/73		7/73 to 6/74		7/74 to 6/75			
Wisconsin State Laboratory of Hygiene	853	31.9	1001	26.9	988	29.4	840	26.9		

EMC = East Madison Clinic.
SPC = Sun Prairie Clinic.
Reprinted by permission from Hahn, Baker: J Fam Pract, 11(1):43–46, 1980.

162

Table 2. *Susceptibility of Staphylococcus aureus to Selected Antibodies*

	Number	EM %	TCN %	KF %	OX/M %
East Madison Clinic (1977–1978)	580	97.4	95.1	100.0	99.7
Sun Prairie Clinic (1977–1978)	95	98.9	97.9	100.0	98.9
Hospital A (1977–1978)	556	96.5	93.7	100.0	98.9
Hospital B (1977–1978)	757	96.4	92.3	99.8	99.6
Hospital C (1977–1978)	227	95.9	91.8	100.0	97.6
State Laboratory of Hygiene (7/1/74 to 6/30/75)	840	97.5	93.6	99.2	99.3

EM = Erythromycin.
TCN = Tetracycline.
KF = Cephalosporin.
OX/M = Penicillinase Resistant Penicillin (Either Oxacillin or Methicillin).
Reprinted by permission from Hahn, Baker: J Fam Pract, 11(1):43–46, 1980.

From July 1, 1971, to May 31, 1975, the Wisconsin State Laboratory of Hygiene reported susceptibility data for 3682 isolates of *SA*. (No compilation was available after May 31, 1975.) Table 1 tabulates the penicillin G susceptibility of a total of 9955 *SA* isolates from all locations on a yearly basis. There is a clear trend toward decreasing susceptibility of *SA* to penicillin G in both hospital and office settings in Madison. For the years 1974 and 1975, when comparable data were available, 21.7 percent of 516 *SA* isolates from EMC-SPC were penicillin G susceptible. Although this difference is statistically significant ($\chi^2 = 8.4$, $P < 0.01$), it is of no clinical significance because susceptible strains from both sources are in the minority.

These data present strong evidence that at least in the state of Wisconsin isolates of *SA* are generally resistant to penicillin G irrespective of the source of the isolate: similar patterns of resistance were found from rural, urban, and hospital sources alike. Specifically, there was no evidence to suggest that a clinically useful difference in penicillin G susceptibility separates rural from urban "community" staphylococci in the 1970s.

Effective alternate drugs are available for office use in *SA* infection. Table 2 displays further antibiotic susceptibilities of *SA* from this study. Although data are shown only for selected time periods, no differences or trends in susceptibility for any Wisconsin location were present for any of the four antibiotics shown during the period 1974–1978.

Semmence A, Kynch J: Hernia repair and time off work in Oxford. J R Coll Gen Pract 30:90–96, 1980

Although for most causes of incapacity for work in Great Britain there was no significant increase in median duration if 1962 to 1963 is compared with 1967 to 1968, there was such an increase for four groups of disorders: varicose veins, silicosis, and occupational pulmonary fibrosis; synovitis; bursitis and tenosynovitis; and hernia of the abdominal cavity. Repair of hernia is the most common operation in men and is the third most common in British hospitals. There is much to be said for trying to find out why some men get back to work more quickly than others.

In this study, the variation in time off work was investigated in 261 men between

18 and 65 years old whose inguinal herniae were repaired in Oxford hospitals in 1971 to 1972 and 1974 to 1975.

The average length of hospital stay was 4.9 days. Age, civil status, social class, hospital, smoking habits, presence of cough on admission, sick pay, and type of operation did not appear to influence its duration. The average length of time off work was 51 calendar days (compared with 70 calendar days nationally), and 236 men claimed sickness benefit from the day they entered hospital, which was usually the day before operation. The remaining 25 were off work before operation for periods up to 71 days. Postoperative complications, type of job, amount of sick pay, social class, smoking habits, the hospital, whether an estimate of time off work had been given, who gave the estimate, and previous frequency and duration of sickness absence all significantly af-

fected time off work. Postoperative complications, particularly chest complications, were associated with more time off. The heavier the job, the longer the time off, and the higher the sick pay and social class, the shorter. The six men who stopped smoking, having been asked to do so at their initial outpatient appointment, took an average of 38 days to return to work. Complications, a heavy job, low sick pay, and family worries were found to be the main factors associated with increased time off.

The value of this study lay in reemphasizing the effect of medical opinion on men's expectations and the importance of explaining to a candidate for operation the implications from the point of view of absence from work. Doctors may often be unaware of the consequences of too cautious a prognosis.

Buchan PC, Nicholls JAJ: Pain after episiotomy—a comparison of two methods of repair. J R Coll Gen Pract 30:297–300, 1980

Episiotomy is a very common operation, but little is known of its short-term or long-term morbidity. This prospective study was designed to investigate both the postpartum perineal discomfort and the coital problems of primigravidae following vaginal delivery with episiotomy and to compare perineal skin sutured with either nonabsorbable (silk) or absorbable (Dexon) sutures, with the silk sutures being interrupted and the Dexon suture subcuticular.

One hundred and forty primigravidae were admitted to the study. Each had a spontaneous vertex delivery and mediolateral episiotomy performed by the delivering midwife. No patient who had an extended episiotomy or any additional lacerations was included. The episiotomy was repaired by one of the four senior house officers within one hour of delivery. In all cases, a continuous chromic catgut suture (Ethicon 761) was used for the vaginal epithelium,

interrupted sutures of the same material were used for the muscle layers, and the patient was randomly allocated to have her perineal skin repaired with either interrupted black silk sutures (Ethicon 562) or a subcuticular Dexon suture (Davis and Geck 6441-78). The black silk sutures were removed on the fifth postpartum day, and the Dexon suture was left to be absorbed spontaneously. Postpartum perineal pain was assessed by monitoring the patients' analgesic requirements. Four months after delivery, each patient was sent a questionnaire about the delay in resumption of coitus, any dyspareunia experienced, and its severity and duration.

Eighty-five percent of the 140 primigravidae took analgesics in the early puerperium because of perineal pain. Patients whose perineal skin was sutured with Dexon had significantly less perineal pain the third, fourth, and fifth postnatal days.

Patients who had epidural analgesia in labor suffered significantly more pain during the first five postnatal days. One hundred patients (71 percent) returned the postal questionnaire. There was a significantly greater number of patients in the 30- to 40-year old age group who had dyspareunia lasting for longer than four weeks. The timing of first coitus after delivery did not influence the presence or persistence of dyspareunia. Dyspareunia was more common and lasted longer in patients sutured with Dexon, and it was also more common in older primigravidae irrespective of the suture technique.

That 85 percent of the patients studied had to take regular analgesics for perineal pain and that there was an 85 percent incidence of dyspareunia show a considerable problem with both short-term and long-term morbidity following episiotomy.

This study shows the short-term advantage of using a subcuticular suture in episiotomy repair. Although Dexon may cause less immediate inflammatory reaction than either silk or catgut, the delayed absorption of Dexon leads to increased dyspareunia. Dexon sutures should be removed on the fifth postnatal day to avoid this problem. Particular care should be taken with the elderly primigravida who is in even greater risk of developing dyspareunia. The high incidence of post-episiotomy morbidity revealed in this study indicates the need for further and more prolonged study of the indications for and repair of episiotomy in obstetric practice.

Leavesley JH: A study of vasectomized men and their wives. Aus Fam Physician 9:8–10, 1980

A 1971 study by the Australian National University showed the ratio in Australia of female to male sterilizations to be 18 to 1. By 1974, the ratio was down to two to one, and if the trend evidenced in other parts of the world is followed, a one to one ratio will ensue. This study was intended to define and appraise the background, attitude, and feelings of the men and their wives who have contributed to this rapid escalation of demand for vasectomy.

The survey was carried out with the aid of two questionnaires sent to 50 men on whom vasectomies had been consecutively performed by the author, not more recently than six months and not longer than 5 years previously. The survey was also sent separately to their wives and a control group of 50 couples using other methods of contraception. These 50 couples were selected at random by the appearance in the author's surgery of either husband or wife for any reason during a two-week period in October 1975 who were known to be using fertility control other than sterilization and

who would cooperate. They were also contacted separately, and an 83.5 percent response was obtained.

The average age of men having the operation was found to be 37.8 years; that of their wives was 34.9 years. The average length of marriage was 13 years. From comparative figures, it seems that vasectomy is undergone at an earlier stage of marriage in America than in Australia. The average number of children per family was found to be 2.5, which is slightly lower than figures produced in other studies throughout the world, including Australia. Unlike some Eastern countries, the sexes of the children have no statistical relationship as to whether a vasectomy was carried out or not. Comparatively more professional men had the operation in this survey than in similar studies.

Perhaps the most striking of the numerous results was that the general health of 43.6 percent of the wives of vasectomized men had improved following their husband's operation. Only 2.5 percent of the men felt their health was better. Half the men had no time off from work, and almost three-quarters none or one day off; the average time of resumption of intercourse was 8 days.

Areas of sexual health were comparatively examined, and libido and sexual satisfaction were found to be significantly improved in the vasectomy sample when compared with users of other methods of contraception. In contrast, about a quarter of the control women reported loss of libido with the use of their chosen contraceptive method. Harmony of marriage and frequency of intercourse improved, but not significantly, in the vasectomy sample compared with the control. The major reason for choosing vasectomy was completion of the family, and the wives of the vasectomized men were, without exception, enthusiastic in their endorsement of the operation in that they would agree again to their husbands being sterilized and would recommend it to others.

Agrawal RL, Alliott RJ, George M, Gomez G, Trafford JAP, Jequier PW, Lishman JD, Turner JRB, Baber NS, Dawes PM: The treatment of hypertension with propranolol and bendrofluazide. J R Coll Gen Pract 29:602–606, 1979

Propranolol and bendrofluazide have been used, both together and separately, for the treatment of hypertension for over 10 years. However, although the two drugs are commonly used together, no report has been published comparing the effect of combined treatment with both drugs with that of each agent separately.

In this study, the doses were fixed at an optimal level of 160 mg/day propranolol and 5 mg/day of bendrofluazide. A double-blind, crossover study was performed to compare the antihypertensive effect of each drug alone and in combination. One hundred and forty patients, 19 to 66 years old, entered the study from six centers. Three general practices entered 25, 25, and 23 patients, respectively, and three hospitals entered 31, 12, and 24 patients, respectively. Patients were excluded if there was a history of recent myocardial infarction, angina, evidence of cardiac failure, airway obstruction, the presence of heart block, creatinine clearance below 50 ml/min, diabetes mellitus requiring insulin or oral hypoglycemic treatment, gout, grade 3 or 4 retinopathy (Keith-Wagener), or any drugs likely to interfere with antihypertensive therapy.

After a placebo introductory period of two weeks in general practice or four weeks in hospital, patients were randomly allocated to treatment with either propranolol 80 mg twice a day, bendrofluazide 2.5 mg twice a day, or propranolol plus bendrofluazide twice a day, provided the diastolic blood pressure (phase 4) was between 100 and 130 mm Hg. Matching placebo tablets were given during the single drug periods to ensure maintenance of double blindness. At the end of each treatment period, which lasted four weeks (general practice) or six weeks (hospital), treatment was changed according to a random code. Patients were seen every two weeks throughout the trial, and blood pressure was measured after lying or sitting for three minutes, standing for two minutes, and also, in most cases, after three minutes' exercise. Three recordings of systolic or diastolic (phase 4) blood pressure were made on each visit by the same observer, with a standard mercury sphygmomanometer.

One hundred and forty patients satisfied the entry criteria, and of these patients, 101 (45 men and 56 women) with a mean age of 51.8 years and with a mean weight of 72.1 kg (158.6 lb; range 44.9–116.1 kg [98.8–

Table 1. *Standing Means ± Standard Error*

	Placebo	Bendrofluazide	Propranolol	Propranolol + Bendrofluazide
Systolic blood pressure				
Centre 1 n = 23	183.3 ± 3.43	165.6 ± 2.71	162.9 ± 2.71	151.9 ± 2.71
Centre 2 n = 23	175.8 ± 3.86	157.4 ± 2.77	153.0 ± 2.77	148.4 ± 2.77
Centre 3 n = 19	172.4 ± 6.85	149.6 ± 3.61	146.8 ± 3.71	134.5 ± 3.81
Centre 4 n = 10	195.7 ± 8.44	171.7 ± 6.85	189.5 ± 6.13	150.0 ± 6.13
Centre 5 n = 14	177.4 ± 5.52	147.9 ± 4.90	153.3 ± 4.90	138.8 ± 4.90
Centre 6 n = 12	174.2 ± 5.79	152.9 ± 4.26	153.5 ± 4.08	141.5 ± 4.08
Diastolic blood pressure				
Centre 1 n = 23	104.0 ± 1.44	97.0 ± 1.16	93.9 ± 1.16	87.3 ± 1.16
Centre 2 n = 23	109.4 ± 2.91	97.2 ± 1.90	95.5 ± 1.90	92.2 ± 1.90
Centre 3 n = 19	114.2 ± 2.80	105.0 ± 2.21	101.7 ± 2.27	94.0 ± 2.34
Centre 4 n = 10	106.4 ± 2.72	91.2 ± 3.70	96.2 ± 3.31	81.5 ± 3.31
Centre 5 n = 14	107.1 ± 3.78	94.9 ± 2.89	98.5 ± 2.89	89.0 ± 2.89
Centre 6 n = 12	114.3 ± 3.46	102.4 ± 3.07	99.0 ± 2.94	96.4 ± 2.94
Pulse rate				
Centre 1 n = 23	73.6 ± 1.41	77.3 ± 1.64	67.9 ± 1.64	67.7 ± 1.64
Centre 2 n = 23	83.4 ± 2.07	83.5 ± 1.75	76.3 ± 1.75	74.0 ± 1.75
Centre 3 n = 19	90.2 ± 2.56	84.7 ± 2.37	72.9 ± 2.44	73.7 ± 2.51
Centre 4 n = 10	57.8 ± 5.18	77.5 ± 2.58	70.1 ± 2.16	63.5 ± 2.16
Centre 5 n = 14	91.1 ± 2.33	80.3 ± 2.11	72.2 ± 2.11	75.1 ± 2.11
Centre 6 n = 12	81.7 ± 3.13	81.6 ± 1.71	67.6 ± 1.63	67.7 ± 1.63

Reprinted by permission from Agrawal et al: J R Coll Gen Prac, 29:602–606, 1979.

255.4 lb]) completed the study. No patients were withdrawn because of the effects of treatment, and two centers (one from general practice and one from hospital) accounted for 25 of the withdrawals, mainly for nonattendance. Table 1 gives placebo and adjusted treatment means and standard errors for blood pressure and pulse rate measured in the standing position for each of the six centers.

The results show that the combination of 80 mg propranolol and 2.5 mg bendrofluazide is more effective than either drug alone and that this effect is independent of the order in which the drugs are given. The antihypertensive effect of the combination and propranolol alone was fully developed within two weeks of starting treatment. Side effects were minimal, and the combination was well accepted by patients.

Michal R, Gehlbach SH: An evaluation of potassium usage in ambulatory hypertensive patients. J Fam Pract 10(4):621–624, 1980

Diuretic-induced hypokalemia in ambulatory hypertensive patients is a major concern. It has been estimated that the incidence of hypokalemia in patients can increase from 2 percent to over 23 percent after treatment with diuretics. Among clinical consequences of hypokalemia, which include muscle weakness, polyuria, and fatigue, the most feared is the development of arrhythmias, especially in patients on concurrent digoxin therapy.

A chart review was conducted in a family

medicine group practice to examine habits of potassium monitoring and supplement prescribing for patients receiving diuretic therapy for control of hypertension. Eighty-four percent of the 134 patients studied were monitored for serum potassium. Hypokalemia was defined as a serum potassium less than 3.5 mEq/liter.

For those with values obtained both before and after institution of diuretic therapy, mean potassium fell from 4.1 mEq/liter to 3.8 mEq/liter, and 29 percent of patients had potassium levels fall to 3.5 mEq/liter or less. Almost half of patients received some type of potassium therapy, with diet enrichment and pharmacologic supplementation being the most common. Approximately 54 percent of the patients on potassium were treated prophylactically. In only 1.5 percent of patients was potassium used to treat symptoms alone.

It appears that physicians in this practice do respond (either by reevaluating serum potassium or instituting potassium therapy) to laboratory evidence of hypokalemia, especially when potassium falls below 3.2 mEq/liter. A trend toward early monitoring of geriatric patients was seen.

In this practice, there was no important difference between the mean potassium values (postdiuretic therapy) regardless of whether or not the patient was placed on potassium therapy. Several factors may explain this finding. Since the number of observations in this sample is small, it is possible that a real difference between the average potassium levels of patients receiving and not receiving supplements exists but was not recognized. There are also problems in potassium administration that must be considered. There has been no attempt in the practice to standardize dosage of potassium supplements, and it is possible that patients were receiving inadequate supplementation. It is also very likely that many patients prescribed potassium were not following physician advice. In any event, without better supporting guidelines for use of potassium and without clear evidence for efficacy of supplementation as it is practiced, the widespread, routine use of potassium supplements for uncomplicated hypertensive patients may not be warranted.

Webb PA: Effectiveness of patient education and psychosocial counseling in promoting compliance and control among hypertensive patients. J Fam Pract 10(6):1047–1055, 1980

Poor patient compliance with physician recommendations is a major problem in treating chronically ill patients. Poor compliance represents a particularly difficult challenge in treating hypertension since only about 50 percent of hypertensive patients comply with their physicians' recommendations for keeping appointments, consuming medications, or attempting new dietary regimens. Uncontrolled hypertension poses a serious health threat; thus, hypertension represents a model system for studying methods to improve patient compliance.

This study evaluated the relative effectiveness of additional patient education and psychosocial counseling in improving patient compliance. At a family practice clinic, 123 low-income, rural, black hypertensive patients were pretested on several psychological characteristics and randomly assigned to one of three groups: vigorous, group patient education and family physician appointments; supportive, individualized psychosocial counseling and family physician appointments; or family physician appointments only, which was the baseline medical care. Intervention and

Table 1. *Postintervention Diastolic Blood Pressure and Compliance Scores by Group*

Group	Mean Diastolic Blood Pressure (mmHg)			Kept Appointments (max = 12)	Bringing and Consuming Medications (max = 18)
	Preintervention*	*Postintervention**	*Difference*		
Education	95.7	88.9	6.8	10.1	4.6
Counseling	93.2	87.4	5.8	11.2	5.0
Control	91.6	88.1	3.5	10.2	4.8

*Average of averages.
Reprinted by permission from Webb: J Fam Pract, 10(6):1047–1055, 1980.

follow-up each lasted three months, and the intervention was in addition to the patients' baseline medical care. Compliance was measured by keeping follow-up appointments; bringing antihypertension medications to each appointment; consuming these medications; and diastolic blood pressure.

The compliance and pre- and postintervention blood pressure scores for each intervention group are shown in Table 1. The return for follow-up appointment rates did not differ significantly between the groups.

Blood pressure levels improved in all three groups, and the rate of improvement was greatest within the education group (Table 2). For example, at postintervention compared to preintervention, almost 21 percent more patients within the education group had a diastolic blood pressure of 90 mm Hg or lower vs 8.1 percent more for the counseling group and 4.2 percent more for the control group. However, by a chi-square analysis there were no significant differences in these rates of improvement between the groups or within the groups between the patients of different family physicians or different social workers (P > .10).

Neither vigorous patient education nor psychosocial counseling, both in addition to high-quality baseline medical care, was found to improve compliance or diastolic blood pressure control better than the baseline medical care alone among a sample of low-income, black, rural hypertensive patients. These results suggest that psychosocial counseling by itself may be an ineffective strategy for improving compliance or diastolic blood pressure control. At the same time, education and counseling may enhance patient compliance among chronically uncontrolled hypertensive patients who are already receiving high-quality medical care when these patients also receive more individualized follow-up care.

Table 2. *Percentage of Patients within Group with Controlled Diastolic Pressure: Preintervention and Postintervention (Six-Month Period)*

Diastolic Blood Pressure	Group (Percentage of Patients)		
	Education	Counseling	Control
90 mmHg or lower at preintervention = controlled	43.2	45.2	61.8
90 mmHg or lower at postintervention = controlled	63.9	53.3	66.0
Stayed below 90 mmHg from pre- to postintervention	33.3	40.0	50.9
Dropped below 90 mmHg from pre- to postintervention	30.6	13.3	15.1
Increase in control from pre- to postintervention	20.7	8.1	4.2

Reprinted by permission from Webb: J Fam Pract, 10(6):1047–1055, 1980.

Williams K: Chest pain among oral contraceptive users.
J R Coll Gen Pract 30:33–34, 1980

The association between fatal thromboembolism and the use of the oral contraceptive pill is well known, and the increased incidence of certain nonfatal thromboembolic events is also on record. Comparatively little work has been published, however, on minor thromboembolic episodes manifesting as chest pain, which might also be related to oral contraceptive use. This study of chest pain was undertaken in women of childbearing age to determine whether or not an association exists with oral contraceptive usage.

Five hundred and fifty women known to be taking the pill were randomly selected from the age/sex and contraceptive registers of two general practices, one in a Derbyshire industrial town and one in a middle-class suburb of Nottingham, and matched for age with 550 women thought not to be using oral contraception. Each woman was sent a general health questionnaire (later to be used by the practices) containing over 50 questions of general interest. One of these asked what form of contraceptive (if any) was being used, and another asked whether patients had suffered from chest pain severe enough to cause concern during the previous year. These two questions were given no particular prominence among the others.

Women who reported chest pain were sent a follow-up questionnaire that asked in simple terms about the severity of the pain, its nature (stabbing, burning, or a dull ache), its speed of onset and duration, and whether there had been any difficulty in breathing or pain on inspiration during the attack. Patients were also asked whether they had seen a doctor about the pain and, if so, what the diagnosis had been. They were asked to state, as nearly as possible, when the episode occurred. An arbitrary system was adopted for "scoring" the responses to this follow-up whereby pains resembling embolic episodes would score high and those not doing so would score low.

A response rate of 77 percent was obtained. In the final analysis, there were 489 pill users but only 289 controls (many women originally thought to be controls admitting to being oral contraceptive users). The frequency of chest pain of any type during the 12-month recall period was 7.3 percent (57 patients). In pill users, it was 6.3 percent (31 patients) and in controls 9 percent (26 patients). The difference was not statistically significant ($0.5 > p > 0.25$).

There was still no significant difference when the results had been standardized for age and when women with a previous history of relevant medical complaints had been excluded from the study (Table 1). If consideration is directed to those people not so excluded who had pains likely to be of an embolic nature, the frequencies in the two groups become even closer to each other.

From this study, there is no evidence to implicate oral contraceptives with chest pain in women of childbearing age. Therefore, there appears to be no justification to change current prescribing habits and little reason to embark on an extensive prospective study of chest pain in relation to pill use, not least because the publicity arising from such a study before the results were known could well lead to unnecessary anxiety among women using the pill and a decrease in the popularity of the most effective method of contraception at present available.

Table 1. *Conditions Causing Patients to Be Excluded from the Study*

Malignant or unspecified neoplasms
Surgical operation within 90 days
Hospital inpatient treatment within 90 days
Pregnancy
Hypertension
Heart disease
Cardiovascular disease
Blood dyscrasias
Deep venous thrombosis and pulmonary embolism

Reprinted by permission from Williams: J R Coll Gen Pract, 30:33–34, 1980.

Andrewes DA, Dawson MJ, Moore RMA, Morris CA, Chuter PJ, Eden BW, Freestone DS: Trimethoprim and co-trimoxazole in the treatment of acute urinary tract infections: patient compliance and efficacy.
J R Coll Gen Pract 31:274–280, 1981

Patient compliance with prescribed treatment for acute illness depends on a number of factors: the presence of symptoms, the occurrence of side effects, the number of drugs administered concurrently, the number of treatments required in a day, the comprehension of the patient, the clarity of treatment instructions, and the convenience of administration. Treatment that is highly effective in the control of an acute infection may lead to poor compliance during the last days of the treatment course; paradoxically, a less effective treatment may enjoy better compliance in these circumstances. Compliance may also influence the occurrence of side effects since a higher level of compliance leads to larger doses of the drug being taken.

In this study, the compliance of drug regimens of a single daily tablet of trimethoprim and two tablets twice daily of co-trimoxazole was compared, both prescribed as seven-day courses for women with symptoms of acute lower urinary tract infections. The study also gave an opportunity to compare efficacy and the occurrence of side effects associated with these two regimes.

Fifty-three female patients over 18 years old with symptoms of acute lower urinary tract infections (dysuria and/or frequency) attending group practices in Telford or Shrewbury were included in this investigation. Patients who were pregnant, with known abnormalities of the urinary tract, with a history of urinary calculus or urinary tract infection within the preceding month, or with any severe chronic disease requiring treatment with prescription-only medicines, or who showed evidence of impaired renal or hepatic function or blood dyscrasias, were excluded. Midstream samples of urine were collected. Immediately following collection of the first urine sample, patients were allocated by random selection for treat-ment with either co-trimoxazole 960 mg (equivalent to two tablets, each containing 80 mg trimethoprim and 400 mg sulpha-methoxazole), twice daily, or trimethoprim 300 mg (equivalent to a single tablet) daily for seven days. Patients were asked to complete a card each day for seven days from the start of treatment to record details of the occurrence and severity of symptoms of dysuria, frequency, fever, malaise, rash, nausea, vomiting, indigestion, and sore mouth/tongue. Fourteen days after the start of treatment, patients provided a second midstream urine sample for microscopy and culture, returned their symptom card and their treatment jar for assessment of compliance, and were questioned about any other symptom events occurring in the interval. Recurrence of infection within six weeks of entry into the study was recorded.

Of the 53 patients entered into the study, 27 were treated with co-trimoxazole and 26 with trimethoprim. The two groups did not differ significantly (5 percent level), comparisons being made by t-tests, appropriately modified where necessary, to account for inequality of variance. *Escherichia coli* was isolated from 23 (79 percent) of the 29 infected urines, of which five (22 percent) isolates were resistant to sulphafurazole. All isolates of *E. coli* were sensitive to trimethoprim. *Staphylococcus albus* and *S. aureus, Streptococcus faecalis,* and *Proteus* species were isolated from the other six infected urines. The spectrum of infecting organisms was similar in the two groups of patients. Second urine samples were collected from 27 of the 29 patients with bacteriuria. All 12 patients who received trimethoprim and 12 of 15 patients treated with co-trimoxazole were bacteriologically cured regardless of the infecting species of bacteria or its antibiotic sensitivities.

Patient compliance was significantly

greater with trimethoprim: corrected percentage compliance rates were 97.5 percent for trimethoprim and 79.1 percent for co-trimoxazole (p < 0.05). Trimethoprim and co-trimoxazole were of equivalent effectiveness in the control of symptoms. Side effects were more frequent with co-trimoxazole, but the difference was not significant.

Coope J: Is Oestrogen therapy effective in the treatment of menopausal depression? J R Coll Gen Pract 31:134-140, 1981

Depression is a common disabling condition in general practice and is particularly prevalent at the menopause. It has been an open question whether oestrogen therapy is effective in the treatment of this problem.

This study was a randomized controlled trial including tests of blood coagulation, biochemistry, and hormone profiles. In carrying out this trial, the severity of depressive illness was examined in patients around the menopause, and correlations were sought between this and hot flushes or hormone profile. The response of depressive illness to oestrogen therapy was measured and compared with the response to matching placebo tablets. Compliance was measured by serum oestrone levels. Effectiveness of the oestrogen preparation used was estimated by the reduction in patients' hot flush counts, compared with that obtained in a previous similar controlled trial by the same author using a different standard oestrogen preparation.

The patients were all on the NHS list of a semirural group practice of 7500 between 1976 and 1978. A notice in the surgery waiting room asked women who were 40 to 60 years old and suffering from flushes or depression to see the doctor. When they attended, they were asked about contraindications to oestrogen therapy such as breast or genital cancer, thromboembolism or thyroid, hepatic or renal disease; if there was no contraindication, patients were accepted for inclusion in the trial. Those who had previously taken any type of hormone preparation ceased therapy for six months before starting treatment. They were in-formed that they would be receiving oestrogen but that their treatment would be inactive for part of the time; the design of the trial was not disclosed. Patients were given a code number and were allotted at random to one of two groups. Group 1 (29 patients) received piperazine oestrone sulphate 1.5 mh b.d., 21 days out of 28 for six months, followed by nonmatching placebo tablets for two months, then placebo tablets that matched the oestrogen, twice daily 21 days out of 28 for six months. Group 2 (26 patients) received the treatments in reverse order. Treatment given in the first and last six months was double blind. Neither the patients, their doctor, nor the laboratory staff knew whether the patient was taking oestrogen tablets or matching placebo. Treatment given during the seventh and eighth months was single blind. Thus, there was a two-months gap between the two halves of the trial, which allowed withdrawal flushes to settle in patients taking estrogen for the first six months. Patients were shown how to complete the short form of the Beck depression inventory, and the score was assessed by the doctor. Patients also completed a diary card for each month, recording the number of hot flushes and sweats experienced during each period of 24 hours. Severely depressed or suicidal patients were referred to a psychiatrist or admitted to hospital and did not take part in the trial.

Fifty-five patients completed the trial. Two died, one of recurrence of gastric carcinoma, one after epileptic seizures following withdrawal of barbiturate therapy.

These were not included in the analysis. There was no evidence of thromboembolic disease in either case. The following side effects were attributed to therapy with piperazine oestrone sulphate: severe breast swelling (one case); fluid retention and left ventricular failure with gallop rhythm, basal crepitations, and sacral edema that resolved on withdrawing oestrogen and treatment with frusemide (one case); two patients developed severe depression after three months on oestrogen therapy and were admitted to hospital. No patient on matching placebo deteriorated sufficiently to be admitted to hospital. Although randomized, the groups appeared to be comparable with regard to age, hysterectomy status, flush accounts, depression scores, and hormone levels at the beginning of the trial.

Hot flushes improved significantly on oestrogen compared with placebo. Depression scores and well-being showed significant and equal improvement on oestrogen and placebo. Significant improvement in flushes in patients on placebo was observed in the first half of the trial but did not occur in the second half in patients who had previously taken oestrogen. No significant changes occurred in biochemistry. Coagulation tests showed acceleration of the prothrombin time in patients taking 'Harmogen' compared with those on placebo.

The conclusions of this study, which was carried out in general practice by the patients' own family doctor, are that oestrogen therapy is no more effective than placebo in the treatment of menopausal depression in middle age and that there is insufficient evidence to support the view that 'Harmogen' is the preferred preparation at the menopause.

Lambert IJ: A comparison of the treatment of otitis externa with 'Otosporin' and aluminium acetate: a report from the services practice in Cyprus. J R Coll Gen Pract 31:291–294, 1981

Otitis externa is a common problem in UK general practice, but is more prevalent in a hot climate and in association with swimming and diving, particularly in dirty water. The problem of a substantial number of cases during the summer months prompted a review of the diagnosis and management of this condition in this practice.

The study population consisted of all servicemen and dependents looked after by the garrison medical center at Episkopi and the families' medical center at Berengaria. These are a few miles apart on the southern coast of Cyprus. At the time of the study, the combined population was 4200; there were many children and young adults. The diagnosis was made on what the meatus looked like, whether there was inflammation (with or without discharge) and pain on pressure on the tragus, and if there was no history or symptoms of middle-ear pathology. If infected wax or discharge blocked the meatus, the ear was cleaned to inspect the eardrum, but no other cleaning was routinely attempted. Swabs were sent directly to the laboratory in transport medium; fungal as well as bacterial infection was looked for. Cases were allocated at random to one of two treatment groups, one being given ear drops of polymixin, neomycin, and hydrocortisone (Otosporin), the other aluminium acetate ear drops BP. In the absence of complications, patients were seen at least every seven days, and the initial medication continued for 14 days unless a marked deterioration in symptoms made further action necessary, or the ear was healed. The ear was considered to be healed if it was free from symptoms and appeared normal on examina-

Table 1. *Organisms Isolated from Swabs Taken*

	Cases	Percent
Ps. pyocyanea	42	*34*
Staph. aureus	25	*20*
Coliforms	10	*8*
Bacillus spp.	1	*0.8*
Proteus spp.	1	*0.8*
B-haemolytic strep.	1	*0.8*
Mixed growth	2	*1.6*
No growth	40	*32*
Monilia	2	*1.6*
Total	124	

Reprinted by permission from Lambert: J R Coll Gen Pract, 31:291–294, 1981.

tion. If there was no improvement after two weeks, the medication was changed and further treatment begun as necessary.

During the seven months of the study, a total of 126 cases were seen in 270 consultations, a rate of 30 per thousand of the population. Twenty-seven said they had had a similar episode in the previous year, but there was little recurrence during the study period, and only two people had more than one attack. Nearly 80 percent of cases had been swimming the week before onset of symptoms, but no single beach or pool could be incriminated. The organisms isolated from the swabs taken are shown in Table 1. *Pseudomonas* was the most commonly isolated species; it has already been noted that *Pseudomonas* is more common in swimmers and has caused outbreaks in populations exposed to contaminated pool water. The incidence of nonswimmers in the *Pseudomonas* group was significantly lower in this study.

All cases were entered in the trial. In a closed community with one practice, the follow-up rate was high, and only nine cases were lost. Of the 117 remaining, 108 (92.3 percent) were successfully treated with the initial medication (Table 2). There was no significant difference in the failure rate of the two drops or in the time taken to effect a cure. Response to treatment was usually rapid with either medication, with few cases of persistent infection. Aluminium acetate is one of several nonantibiotic applications that may be used; it is effective, cheap, and safe. The antibiotic/steroid preparations, which are more commonly used and expensive, should be kept for more severe or resistant cases.

Table 2. *Results of Initial Treatment*

	Aluminium Acetate	'Otosporin'	Total
Cured	59	49	108
Treatment changed	3	6	9
Lost to follow-up	3	6	9
Total treated	65	61	126

$P = 0.2924 \gg 0.05$.
Reprinted by permission from Lambert: J R Coll Gen Pract, 31:291–294, 1981.

Russo PM, Schneiderman LJ: Effect of topical corticosteroids on symptoms of clinical sunburn. J Fam Pract 7(6):1129–1132, 1978

Anti-inflammatory agents are an obvious choice as a remedy for sunburn symptoms, and topical corticosteroids have been evaluated with varied results. These studies have several shortcomings. Either they were carried out in laboratory settings using ultraviolet lamps to produce the condition or lacked appropriate controls. The present study was undertaken to evaluate the effectiveness of topical corticosteroid therapy in relieving the subjective and objective symptoms of sunburn in a natural setting. This was done by combining clinical (natural sunlight) sunburns with double-blind protocol and using subjects as their own controls.

The subjects for this study, all young, white, healthy adults, were recruited at the beaches in and around San Diego, California, or solicited through an ad in a local newspaper. Of the sunbathers who entered the study, 42 did so on the day they obtained their acute sunburn, and another eight started the day after sun exposure. They showed varying degrees of erythema and generally complained of soreness and burning at this time. Each subject was given two identical jars of topical creams, labeled A and B, following a double-blind format. One jar contained fluocinolone (Synalar), and the other contained the cream but lacked the active ingredient. Therapy was evaluated by means of a random, double-blind study in which subjects who had ac-

quired acute natural sunburn served as their own controls. Subjects applied fluocinolone cream to an acutely exposed area of their body and the inert carrier base to a symmetrical, similarly exposed area twice a day for five days while avoiding further exposure. The subjects recorded by means of a rating scale the progression, at both sites, of redness, pain, blistering, swelling, and peeling.

Of the 50 persons who were asked to join the study, 30 returned the results form. Seven forms were not completely filled out. The remaining 23 subjects (11 males, 12 females) had filled out the form according to the format and were used in the analysis that followed. Some pruritus on both sides (steroid and control) was noted by two subjects. No other adverse reactions or side effects occurred.

No significant differences were noted in relief of pain or redness between the steroid-treated and the inert cream (placebo)-treated areas of sunburn. In all subjects, resolution of sunburn symptoms occurred within three to five days following exposure.

Baxter R: Research committee report on Varihesive and the treatment of chronic leg ulcers. Aus Fam Physician 9:599–601, 1980

This trial sets out to compare Varihesive with tulle gras in the treatment of chronic leg ulcers.

All members of the Royal Australian College of General Practitioners were invited to participate in the trial; 132 general practitioners responded. All surgeries were visited and the doctor interviewed in 75 percent of cases. Follow-up reminder letters were issued on two occasions, and telephone contact was made to those taking part. The criterion for an ulcer to enter the trial was those ulcers not responding to regular treatment for at least four weeks. The treatment group (tulle gras or Varihe-

sive) was allocated by opening consecutively numbered envelopes with previously randomized instructions. Elastocrepe compression bandage was used for both Varihesive and tulle gras. Varihesive is a hypoallergenic adhesive of pectin, gelatine, polyisobutylene, and carboxymethylcellulose used in stomal therapy under the name Stomahesive. It was cut to the shape and size of the ulcer and applied weekly.

Overtly infected ulcers were excluded until treatment of infection was completed. The details of duration, previous treatment, and etiologic factors were obtained, and the ulcers were assessed at weekly intervals using a transparent grid to gauge size. Pain was assessed as either moderate to severe, slight discomfort, or nil. The trial ran over a 12-month period.

Despite the large number of practitioners taking part, there were only 35 cases meeting the trial criteria. Therefore, it can be concluded that nonhealing leg ulcers are a rare condition, and several general practitioners expressed this opinion when contacted. The use of diuretics was one of the most common reasons for nonhealing in the opinion of the participating practitioners. There were 27 females and 8 males with a mean age of 66 years. Varicose veins were an aetiologic factor in 68 percent of cases, trauma in 45 percent, oedema in 42 percent. Multiple aetiologies, that is, varicose veins, trauma, arterial insufficiency, diabetes melitus, oedema and infection, were present in some cases, especially the long-standing and large ulcers.

There were 12 cases treated with tulle and 23 with Varihesive. Table 1 shows the

Table 1. *Comparison of Healing Rates*

	Tulle	Varihesive
Patient number	10	14
Mean ulcer size	1.83 cm^2	2.16 cm^2
Mean duration	10.5 weeks	8.0 weeks
No. of ulcers healed	8[(80%)]	11[78%)]
Mean time to fully heal	7.6 weeks	6.2 weeks

In this group, it was not possible to show any significant difference in the rate of healing.

Reprinted by permission from Baxter: Aus Fam Physician, 9:599–601, 1980.

comparison of healing rates for Varihesive and tulle:

Nonresponding leg ulcers are not common in general practice, and there are many difficulties with conducting a controlled trial using these methods. Varihesive is an effective treatment for refractory ulcers. Healing can be expected even in very chronic large ulcers provided infection is not a problem.

Lister G: Rhesus incompatibility and a survey of the care of rhesus negative pregnant women in one general practice. J R Coll Gen Pract 30:35–39, 1980

The effectiveness of the administration of anti-D immunoglobulin for preventing Rh-immunization in pregnancies of rhesus-negative women and also in cases of rhesus mismatched transfusions is now recognized and has been in use since 1966, but only on a wide scale since 1971. However, there is still a failure rate of 1–2 percent following prophylaxis.

This study was carried out in a group practice with a list size of about 12,000 in women who were delivered during the first ten months of 1977. There were 106 deliveries (including one set of twins) and 16 rhesus-negative mothers (one of whom had the twins). Of 17 infants delivered to these mothers, eight were rhesus negative, seven rhesus positive, and two were not grouped. None of the mothers developed antibodies,

and all the rhesus-negative mothers at risk received anti-D. However, the survey showed discrepancies between hospital and practice records.

This small survey shows a discrepancy between hospital and practice records and a need for better communication between hospital and office practice. The notes show that all hospital deliveries are carefully monitored, and that rhesus-negative women bearing rhesus-positive infants receive anti-D. However, there is a loophole where women, especially primigravidas where the blood group may be unknown, miscarry early in pregnancy, particularly if treated at home.

The following recommendations are made for better record keeping in the pregnancies of rhesus-negative women:

1. Ensure that blood is taken for blood group and antibodies, in addition to other routine specimens, from all pregnant women at booking (around 12 weeks).
2. Ensure that any woman who has a miscarriage, especially one treated at home, has her blood group checked and anti-D given if required. Perhaps the midwife could be asked to do this. The same applies to any woman having a termination.
3. A colored sticker indicating a rhesus-negative group should be put on the main record envelope and on the antenatal card for easy recognition. In addition, RH.NEG should be written in red on the notes and antenatal card, as stickers sometimes peel off.
4. For rhesus-negative women, the husband's group and genotype should be recorded. This is relevant if the mother develops antibodies, but if the father is rhesus negative, there will be no need for anti-D to be given.
5. Maternal antibodies should be checked at 12, 28, and 36 weeks during the antenatal period; if antibodies appear, more frequent assessment is required. Maternal blood should be taken after delivery for antibodies and screening for fetal cells. The results must be recorded on the postnatal discharge form and antenatal record card.
6. Cord blood should be taken for the baby's group, hemoglobin, direct Coombs' test, and serum bilirubin. If the infant is jaundiced, any treatment should be recorded.
7. Ensure that anti-D is given to all rhesus-negative women who give birth to a rhesus-positive infant. This is particularly important after early hospital discharge.
8. If the baby is stillborn or a neonatal death, cord blood should be taken if possible for the usual tests, and these should be recorded with the infant's weight, condition, presence or absence of jaundice, congenital abnormalities, and condition and weight of the placenta.
9. Follow up for antibodies 6 months after delivery.

Burns P, Jenkinson D: Hazards from the use of child-resistant drug containers. J R Coll Gen Pract 30:555–556, 1980

The use of child-resistant drug containers for dispensing prescription drugs is widespread as a voluntary measure practiced by the pharmaceutical profession. Safety packaging has been legally required in the United States for prescription drugs since 1974, and in the United Kingdom it has been mandatory for all drugs containing aspirin and paracetamol sold over the counter for children since January 1976 and for adults since January 1977. Accidental child poisoning has declined since these measures were introduced, and it has been suggested that the use of these containers should be extended to all drugs.

The authors suspected that the elderly and others lacking dexterity found difficulty using these containers and that the solutions they adopted created hazards. Sixty-five consecutive patients applying for repeat prescriptions for antirheumatic drugs in a semirural Nottinghamshire practice were visited at home without warning by a medical student (P.B.) attached to the practice. They were shown a Snap-Safe child-resistant container (arrows on lid and body aligned and lid pushed off) and asked if they had had drugs dispensed in any. Patients then usually produced their own drugs for inspection spontaneously; if they did not, they were asked to do so. If they had experienced Snap-Safe containers, they were asked to demonstrate how they used them, and if they were able to do so, a note was made of whether or not they had found it easy. Those patients unable to use them were asked how they overcame the problem by demonstrating with their own drugs. A note was also made of the types of container the drugs were stored in, whether they were correctly labeled, and whether it was the original container.

Fifty-nine patients had been supplied with drugs in Snap-Safe containers. Their ages ranged from 42 to 90 years, the largest number being in the 70- to 79-year-old group. Forty-one (70 percent) patients were unable to use the containers. They either asked somebody else to open them, left the lid loose, or put them in another container. Eighteen (30 percent) patients were able to use the containers, but only 13 (22 percent) of them did so with ease, these being predominantly the younger patients (modal age group 40 to 49 years). The remaining five (8 percent) patients either used an implement to assist them or persisted in spite of difficulty.

It is not entirely clear why the containers were not being used. Some patients blamed poor eyesight, and others admitted to being confused by the instructions. The effort and concentration required by the elderly to open the containers appeared to be problems. Thirty-five (59 percent) patients adopted methods of tablet storage that removed the child-resistant property of the containers, and 27 (46 percent) of them stored them in a way that was hazardous to themselves. The latter group of patients sometimes transferred the tablets to another container such as a tumbler or a container with tablets of another type already in it, but usually to an empty conventional container inappropriately labeled.

Pharmacists will usually comply with a patient's request for a conventional container, although most patients appear to be unaware of this or are unwilling to ask. Physicians should be aware of this potential source of medication error, and pharmacists should try to identify patients who cannot use child-resistant containers and supply a satisfactory alternative. Physicians could help by writing the necessary instructions on the prescription. An abbreviation such as "SC" would save time.

Gross H, Caplan C: Cholesterol in preteen children of parents with premature coronary disease.
J Fam Pract 6(3):495–499, 1978

Premature coronary artery disease is promoted by three major risk factors: high serum cholesterol, high blood pressure, and cigarette smoking. The atherosclerotic process is known to begin early in life, and the pathologic changes may be irreversible once they are established. Therefore, if the predisposing traits could be identified in childhood, early intervention could be possible.

This study suggests a simple solution to a potentially complex problem, a problem that community physicians may otherwise be tempted to leave to the lipoprotein research laboratory. Families containing a parent who had manifested coronary heart disease before the age of 50 were identified, and the preteen children underwent a single serum cholesterol estimation. The presence of disease in the parent before the 50th birthday clearly establishes the early onset of the pathologic process, which presumably, therefore, is both more severe and more apt to be familial than when the disease occurs in more senior citizens.

Using a simple and inexpensive protocol, serum cholesterol determinations were performed on 50 children 12 years old and younger. These children were taken from 28 families in which one parent had suffered a myocardial infarction before the age of 50.

Eight of the 50 children were found to have significant elevation of serum cholesterol. This was an incidence of 16 percent—twice that of the general pediatric population. The eight children (age range 8 to 12 years) had cholesterol levels above 200 mg/100 ml. There were four boys and four girls. Of these eight children, four had readings over 240 mg/100 ml (8 percent).

The patient with a single random elevated serum cholesterol, once identified, must be evaluated to confirm the diagnosis of hypercholesterolemia and to exclude secondary causes such as diabetes mellitus, thyroid, renal or hepatic disease, or the use of birth control pills in older girls. With the diagnosis confirmed, the whole family should be investigated. However, such testing was beyond the intent of this study.

Families affected by premature coronary artery disease readily accept screening and advice about habits and diets. Intervention is controversial. No long-term studies are available, and decisions have to be made on the basis of incomplete evidence.

It would appear reasonable to say that if there is to be prophylaxis of coronary heart disease, then it may begin in these easily identified preteen children with both an adverse family history and an elevated serum cholesterol level. Such children may be found among the patients of every family physician.

Woods JO, Cullen MJ, Dorman RH: The prevention of coronary heart disease in general practice. J R Coll Gen Pract 30:52–57, 1980

Coronary heart disease is now the chief single cause of death in Britain. In men 45 to 54 years old, 52 percent of all deaths in 1973 were due to cardiovascular disease, and more than three-quarters of these were due to coronary heart disease. The mortality from coronary artery disease in younger men has doubled in the last 20 years. Despite all the advances of modern medicine, life expectancy for a man who reaches the age of 40 is very similar to what it was at the turn of the century. The prevention of coronary heart disease is thus one of the major challenges in medicine today.

Four hundred and eighty-one (75 percent) of the male patients between 35 and 55 years of age in a health center group practice were screened for risk factors for coronary heart disease. An attempt was made to alter these factors, and the effectiveness of the intervention was later assessed.

Participants were informed of the dangers of cigarette smoking and on the advisability of taking regular exercise and maintaining ideal weight. Where appropriate, patients were given diet sheets. Health education literature relating to the risks of coronary heart disease was distributed to all participants. If a patient had a diastolic blood pressure over 100 mm Hg at initial examination, he was subsequently recalled for at least two further readings, and treatment was begun if the diastolic blood pressure was persistently above 100 mm Hg. If the serum cholesterol was over 7.0 mmole/1 (270 mg/100 ml) at initial examination, he was recalled for a full lipid analysis. If he was more than 20 percent overweight, he was given an appointment to attend a clinic in the health center run by the dietitian and the local community medical officer.

The number of patients with the various risk factors is shown in Table 1:

The effect of the authors' advice was assessed at least six months after initial examination. Forty-five patients had diastolic blood pressures 100 mm Hg or more. In 21

Table 1. *Risk Factors Identified*

	Number	Percentage
Smokers	265	55
Diastolic blood pressure 95 mm Hg or over	71	15
Diastolic blood pressure 100 mm Hg or over	45	10
Cholesterol more than 7.0 mmol/l	47	10
Weight		
Ideal	270	56
0–9% overweight	77	14
10–19% overweight	92	19
More than 20% overweight	41	9
Family history positive	87	18
Major electrocardiographic changes	30	6
Number of patients screened	481	100

Reprinted by permission from Woods et al: J R Coll Gen Pract, 30:52–57, 1980.

Table 2. *Effects on Blood Pressure*

	Number	Percentage
Diastolic blood pressure persistently 100 mm Hg or over	24	100
Diastolic blood pressure improved at review	22	92
New hypertensives discovered/total number in practice	14/29	48

Reprinted by permission from Woods et al: J R Coll Gen Pract, 30:52–57, 1980.

patients, the blood pressure settled (at least two subsequent readings were under 100 mm Hg) and did not receive treatment. This left 24 requiring treatment, including ten who were known to be hypertensive and under treatment and five other known hypertensives under treatment whose diastolic blood pressure was below 100 mm Hg at the time of screening. Fourteen of these 29 patients (48 percent) were discovered by this screening to have blood pressure persistently over 100 mm Hg requiring treatment (Table 2). This group included three severe hypertensives who, unknown to us, had stopped treatment. At review, there was an improvement in the diastolic blood pressure in 22 of the 24 patients, the average pressure improving from 108 to 91 mm Hg, a fall of 17 mm Hg.

Of the 32 patients with raised blood cholesterols, all of whom were treated by diet alone, 15 were checked 12 months after the initial reading and the remaining 17 after six months. Thirty-one patients (96 percent) had a lower cholesterol at review than at initial examination. Within this group, the average cholesterol was lowered from 7.82 to 6.69 mmole/1, a 14 percent reduction. Two hundred and ten patients were overweight, and they were all given a reducing diet sheet and, where appropriate, advised to take more exercise. The 41 patients who were more than 20 percent overweight were given an appointment to attend the dietitian. The 23 who attended lost an average of 2.8 kg (6.3 lb) (3 percent) during an average period of attendance at the clinic of between four and five months.

This study suggests that a screening program can be carried out as part of general practice and shows that an improvement in risk factors can be achieved.

Heyden S, Heyden F, Heiss G, Hames CG: Smoking and coffee consumption in three groups: cancer deaths, cardiovascular deaths and living controls. A prospective study in Evans County, Georgia. J Chron Dis 32:673–677, 1979

Among some lay persons and in a few lay publications over the past ten years, the opinion has been perpetuated that coffee consumption may be associated with carcinogenesis. Scientific evidence to support this hypothesis has not been reported. Previous and also more recent animal experiments make a causal relationship between administering caffeine and development of cancer unlikely. Studies in man, exclusively conducted *retrospectively,* have been summarized in 1971. The results have, for the most part, denied any association between coffee consumption and carcinogenesis. The Evans County Study in Georgia for the first time offers the opportunity to study this problem *prospectively* since the Evans County population in 1967–1969 was questioned about their coffee drinking and smoking habits. All deaths occurring over the subsequent ten years have been ascertained and the causes of death coded. The question addressed in this study is whether coffee consumption and smoking habits are prospectively related to the risk of cancer mortality in a total community sample.

The 2530 adults (60 percent whites, 40 percent blacks) living in Evans County were interviewed about their daily coffee consumption during the examinations in 1967–1969. Nonconsumers of coffee and those who usually drank less than five cups a day were allotted into one group, while those who consumed five or more cups a day throughout the entire year were allotted to the second group. Since habitual coffee drinking is usually correlated with smoking, we also took the latter into consideration. Ex-smokers were grouped together with nonsmokers; a small number of pipe and cigar smokers who did not inhale were excluded from the analysis. Physical exam-

inations of the 2530 adults were carried out by two physicians, including chest x-rays, prostate and breast examinations, Pap smears, and hematocrit determinations. The study population reported on here was free of any manifest or symptomatic cancer as ascertained by these physicals.

All cancer deaths of the Evans County population between July 1, 1969 and April 1, 1978, were registered. Only definite cases with biopsy or with hospital records were used in this study, and "possible" cancer cases were excluded. Thus, the total number of cancer deaths was 74. The choice of study design was influenced by the relatively small number of cancer deaths (3 percent of 2530 persons over 10 years of follow-up) and the large pool of potential controls. A case-control design was elected to ascertain the frequency of coffee drinking and cigarette smoking as exposures in cancer decedents and comparends. Age, sex, and race were established as potential confounding factors in the Evans County population, as they were associated both with coffee drinking and smoking and predictive of the outcome independently of the putative exposures. A matched case-control design was then chosen as the option for the control of these confounding factors. One source of controls was those persons who died of cardiovascular disease during the same observation period. Since there was an average of three cardiovascular deaths for each cancer death, each of the 74 cancer patients was matched randomly with one patient of the same age, race, and sex who had died from cardiovascular disease. In addition, each cancer patient was randomly matched with a living examinee of the same age, race, and sex. In this manner, the coffee consumption and smoking habits of three subgroups could be contrasted prospectively over nearly 10 years (1968–1978).

The 74 cancer patients died an average of 4.4 years after the examinations; 33 (45 percent) were regular cigarette smokers in 1967–1969. In the cardiovascular group, there was a slightly smaller number of smokers, 27 (36 percent), while the living group contained only 22 (30 percent) smokers. The difference in smoking habits between the white men of the cancer group, which had more smokers than any other group, and those of the living group was statistically significant ($p < 0.05$). Similarly, there was a significant difference in smoking habits between the white males combined with the black males of the cancer group as opposed to the white males and black males in the living group. In contrast, the difference in smoking habits of the cardiovascular group as opposed to the living group is less evident. It should be noted, however, that in the total study population as well as in all race and sex categories, the number of smokers in the cardiovascular group exceeded that of the smokers in the living group.

When compared to deaths from cardiovascular diseases, the deceased cancer patients were 1.7 times more likely to be smokers during the 1967–1969 interview. This association of smoking with mortality due to malignancies does not reach statistical significance. However, when cancer decedents are contrasted to living controls, the cancer cases were twice as likely to be smokers (significant at the level of 0.05) in 1967–1969.

The coffee drinking habits of the cardiovascular and the living groups were identical. This observation supports previously reported results from the Evans County Study inasmuch as the general mortality was the same in light and heavy coffee drinkers.

In summary, cigarette smoking was related to mortality from cancer, but no evidence was found to associate heavy coffee drinking with cancer death in this population sample from Evans County, Georgia. While these results do not prove conclusively that heavy coffee consumption is unrelated to carcinogenesis, the data support a cocarcinogenic effect of cigarette smoking in certain organ systems.

Chu FZ, Day RG: Smoking recognition by family physicians. J Fam Pract 12(4):657–660, 1981

Cigarette smoking is the single most important preventable cause of illness, disability, and death in the United States today. Cigarette-produced illnesses result in more than 350,000 deaths annually and directly generate $5-$8 billion in excess heatlh care costs.

Previous studies have attempted to measure the effectiveness of physician advice and counseling in smoking-cessation programs. These studies appear to have tacitly assumed that physicians routinely recognize and document the smoking habits of their patients and have an intimate knowledge of their patients' specific health risks. This study was designed to evaluate this as-

sumption by examining the recognition of smoking patients by family physicians.

This study was conducted at the family medicine center at the University of Colorado, Denver. The charts of 187 patients who had been seen at the A. F. Williams Family Medicine Center within the previous year were randomly selected and reviewed. For each smoker, the amount smoked and whether the smoking habit was recognized by the physician were also determined.

With the results of the initial study, an educational program was presented to all of the residents and faculty. This program consisted of two consecutive one-hour noon

Table 1. *Summary and Comparison of the Smoking Studies*

	1979 Percent (Number)		1980 Percent (Number)
Smokers	36 (67/187)		40 (202/505)
Nonsmokers	33 (62/187)		39 (197/505)
Smoking status unknown	31 (58/187)		21 (106/505)
Smokers recognized	18 (12/67)	P < 0.001	51 (103/202)
Males	26 (5/19)		49 (42/85)
Females	15 (7/48)		54 (63/117)
Smokers recognized by residents			
Class of 1980	17 (4/23)		34 (10/29)
Class of 1981	27 (3/11)		43 (29/68)
Class of 1982			59 (43/71)
Smokers recognized by faculty	43 (3/7)		62 (21/34)
Smokers recognized			
with associated diagnoses		P < 0.05	56 (76/136)
without associated diagnoses			41 (27/66)

Reprinted by permission from Chu, Day: J Fam Pract, 12(4):657–660, 1981.

conferences presented by one of the authors. The conferences included presentation of the initial study results, discussion of the health consequences of smoking, and physician attitudes toward smoking patients and prevention. Following the educational conferences, antismoking and smoking cessation literature was placed throughout the family medicine center and made available to both patients and physicians. One year after the initial study and educational program, a larger follow-up study was done. A total of 505 charts of active patients were randomly selected and reviewed to validate the findings of the initial study and also to determine the possible effectiveness of the educational program in altering physician behavior.

Table 1 summarizes the statistical data from both smoking audits. The percentage of smokers and nonsmokers was comparable in the two studies conducted one year apart. There was a large number of patients (31 percent in 1979 and 21 percent in 1980) whose smoking status could not be determined from the information available on the health history questionnaire or in the remainder of the chart. Although the initial smoking recognition rate by the family physicians was very low (18 percent), there was a dramatic and statistically significant improvement in the follow-up study (51 percent). Table 1 also demonstrates higher recognition rates for smokers with underlying medical conditions that are known to predispose them to higher morbidity and mortality. These associated diagnoses included respiratory and cardiovascular conditions as well as hypertension, diabetes, pregnancy, and use of birth control pills.

The failure to recognize patients who smoke precludes any attempt to counsel or intervene with smoking cessation programs. Family physicians need to explicitly determine and document the smoking habits of all their patients before they can begin to help curb this single most important and preventable cause of illness, disability, death, and high medical costs.

Rose JH: The use of amantadine and influenza vaccine in a type A influenza epidemic in a boarding school. J R Coll Gen Pract 30:619–621, 1980

In the winter of 1977, reports of 'red flu" were circulating. The vaccine given to the school the previous September was known not to contain this virus. Reports from Russia and elsewhere had shown that the cyclic primary amines with a three-dimensional bird-cage structure called the amantadine series had inhibitory properties on influenza A virus. The backing of the local public health laboratory was sought, and the family practitioner committee quickly agreed to pay the cost of a trial of amantadine.

On September 30, 1977, 380 (65.7 percent) boys out of a possible 578 in a West Country public boarding school were given Duphar trivalent vaccine by gun, 0.5 ml. The 31 youngest boys were given 0.25 ml. These boys were subsequently given amantadine. The immunization was voluntary, and many of the older boys avoided the gun either because they feared it or doubted its efficacy. The epidemic started on January 15, 1978, and there was a sudden increase in numbers a week later. On January 22, amantadine, 100 mg, was given to 31 of the younger boys. It was continued, given daily after breakfast, until the school broke up for the half term, for a total of 23 days. On their return ten days later (snow prolonged half term), there were no further cases of influenza, so the drug was not restarted.

The public health laboratory service swabbed 33 boys; 19 viral isolations were made: 15 Texas 1/77 H3N2; four A/USSR 90/77 HN. Table 1 shows the number of boys treated for influenza and the number of those vaccinated. Table 2 shows the number of boys with influenza and whether they were treated with amantadine or not. However the results are analyzed—by severity of symptoms, length of illness, or lack of symptoms—previous immunization seems to have had no protective effects. The 31 boys to whom amantadine was given found it easy to take, and no side effects were noticed, although the boys were unusually quiet for the first few days. None of these boys developed influenza. On several occasions, these boys were seen talking with those in the sickbays, and several of their masters were ill during the epidemic. Several of the boys also had siblings with influenza.

These preliminary findings indicate that it would be beneficial to extend the use of amantadine. Policy was changed the following year when there was a further outbreak of influenza. Amantadine seemed to be largely protective, but the virologic studies reported virus B/E/95/79. Policy was changed in 1980, and a general immunization program was abandoned, as the experience described showed it not to be protective, especially when a new strain such as A/USSR emerges.

Table 1. *Number of Boys with Influenza Compared with Number Immunized (Percentages in Brackets)*

	Immunized	Not Immunized	Totals
Number of boys with influenza	106 (*63.9*)	60 (*36.1*)	166 (*100*)
Number of boys without influenza	274 (*66.5*)	138 (*33.5*)	412 (*100*)
Totals	380 (*65.7*)	198	578

Reprinted by permission from Rose: J. R. Coll Gen Pract, 30:619–621, 1980.

Table 2. *Effect of Treatment with Amantadine*

	Amantadine 100 mg Daily	Without Amantadine	Totals
Number of boys with influenza	0	166	166
Number of boys without influenza	31	381	412
Totals	31	547	578

$\chi^2 = 11.2$ p < 0.001.
Reprinted by permission from Rose: J R Coll Gen Pract, 30:619–621, 1980.

Pieroni RE, Coplin TW, Leeper JD: Tetanus and diphtheria immune status of patients in a family practice. J Fam Pract 11(3):403–406, 1980

Despite their relative infrequency in this country, tetanus and diphtheria are associated with considerable morbidity. It is regrettable that even though relatively safe and effective immunization agents are available, there has been no substantial decrease in the case-fatality ratio of these disorders during this century.

This study was undertaken to help determine the tetanus and diphtheria immune status in outpatients of widely varying ages in a family practice setting. The study was conducted in a double-blind manner. Sera obtained randomly from 37 patients seen at a family practice center were evaluated for protective antibodies against tetanus and diphtheria using in vivo toxin neutralization methods. The patients' ages ranged from 1 to 99 years.

Seventy-four percent and 83 percent of patients were found to have protective antitoxin titers against tetanus and diphtheria, respectively. No significant differences in immune status were detected among different sexes or races.

A large proportion of tetanus cases are found among elderly persons, a population whose immune status has been shown to be inadequate in several studies. Following active immunization in early childhood, combined tetanus and diphtheria toxoids (adult Td) is recommended for those greater than 6 years of age, with booster immunizations at 10-year intervals to sustain immunization. Primary immunization for adults who have never received toxoid consists of three intramuscular injections of Td, with 4 to 6 weeks separating the first and second doses and 6 to 12 months between the second and third doses.

Hansen NH: Rubella prevention in family practice with RA27/3 vaccine. J Fam Pract 11(4):537–542, 1980

In a 1964 rubella epidemic in the United States, more than 20,000 infants were born with one or more effects of congenital rubella—principally cataracts, glaucoma, deafness, cardiac malformations, and central nervous system problems such as mental retardation and cerebral palsy. Despite many millions of doses of vaccine administered since its introduction in 1969, rubella has not yet been satisfactorily controlled.

Key elements for successful elimination of rubella risk in a family practice appear to be the utilization of an ongoing approach to all patients at risk, during any care for which they present, as part of everyday practice; a method offering high compliance levels; a vaccine offering high conversion rates when administered to those susceptible to rubella.

The objectives of this two-practice study are:

1. To review the status of rubella immunization prior to inception of the study.
2. To test rubella HI titer levels of female patients of childbearing age.
3. To administer RA27/3 vaccine (Almevax) to susceptible patients and to test response by repeating rubella HI titers eight weeks after vaccination.
4. To determine the frequency and nature of adverse effects of RA27/3 vaccine.
5. To review the success of this intervention after 18 months and to compare the levels of compliance reached by inviting patient participation within episodes of care with that reached by telephone invitation.

Levels of immunity by age group are displayed in Table 1. An immediate (eight weeks) positive response of 98.3 percent was shown to RA27/3 vaccine. At the 18-month review, 67 (77 percent) of those

Table 1. *Levels of Immunity by Age Group (515 Tested)*

Age (Years)	Titer				% Susceptible
	<1:8	1:8	1:16	>1:16	
12–20	4	27	2	123	19.9
21–30	28	17	4*	219	16.9
31–40	4	5	1	82	9.8
Total	36	49	7	424	16.9 Average

*Two among this group were in high-exposure occupations.
Reprinted by permission from Hansen: J Fam Pract, 11(4): 537–542, 1980.

Table 2. *Frequency and Nature of Adverse Effects*

No reported reaction	37 (64.9%)
Any reported reaction(s)	20 (35.1%)
Sore throat	
1st week	5
2nd week	9
3rd week	1
Total	15 (26.3%)
Mild joint pains	6 (10.5%)
Fever	6 (10.5%)
Lymphadenopathy	5 (8.8%)
Soreness at site of injection	5 (8.8%)
Rash (2nd week)	4 (7.0%)

Reprinted by permission from Hansen: J Fam Pract, 11(4): 537–542, 1980.

deemed suitable for vaccine had received it. Of the 20 (23 percent) not yet given vaccine, only one was a refusal. Seven of the nine patients leaving the practice during the study were informed and agreed to seek vaccination elsewhere. Five of their new physicians were informed, thus assuring that for all nine patients leaving, either the patient or the new physician was notified.

In one patient, possible adverse effects (sore throat and fever) required loss of time from work. The remaining adverse effects were consistently mild (Table 2). Thirty-seven patients (64.9 percent) had no reaction at all.

A suggested protocol, utilizing RA27/3 vaccine in a family practice, is as follows:

1. As a part of well-child care, all 15 to 18-month-olds are to be given combined measles, mumps, and rubella vaccine (preferably including RA27/3 vaccine).
2. When admitted to the practice, all children under the age of 12 years should be reviewed with regard to immunization history and appropriate immunization carried out.
3. When women from ages 12 to 40 years are admitted to the practice, HI titers should be performed and susceptible women immunized under appropriate contraceptive protection.

4. All present female patients of ages 12 to 40 years should be tested for immunity as they present for any care.
5. All susceptible women should have this result placed on their problem list until vaccinated.

For practices utilizing public health facilities for vaccination services, careful patient follow-up for compliance is necessary.

Quality of Care Assessment In Family Practice

COMMENTARY

THE papers and abstracts in this section deal with the assessment of quality of care in a family practice setting. The complexities of the many issues involved in this task are lucidly examined in the opening paper by Donabedian. As he points out, quality of patient care involves both technical and interpersonal components. Many factors relate to the quality of care that results from the patient's encounter with the physician, including expected benefits, risks, costs, effectiveness of communication, and patient compliance.

Further useful background for this subject is provided by the excellent paper by Buck, Fry, and Irvine, which reports the recommendations of a conference sponsored by the Rockefeller Foundation. This conference involved primary care physicians and researchers from Europe and North America in the discussion of what research is needed and what approaches are feasible to set standards of quality in primary care.

This section presents a number of methods for monitoring the process and quality of patient care, including the use of various types of audit, morbidity data, criteria mapping, and tracer techniques. The results and implications of a number of disease- and problem-specific audits are described. Excellent progress is being made in the development and application of practical approaches to this important area. Further development is clearly needed, however, before the ongoing measurement of quality of care is both accepted and valued as an essential part of everyday family practice.

PAPERS

The Quality of Medical Care:
A Concept in Search of a Definition*†

Avedis Donabedian

Patient care has two components: technical and interpersonal. The quality of technical management depends on the balance of its expected benefits and risks. The quality of the interpersonal process consists in conformity to legitimate patient expectations and to social and professional norms. Since this conformity is expected to result in social and personal benefit, a unified definition of quality can be derived by including the benefits and risks of both aspects of care. When the patient's health and welfare are judged by professional criteria, and the cost of care is not considered, one has an "absolutist" definition of quality. By contrast, an "individualized" definition accepts the informed patient's valuation of the consequences of care, and includes the cost to the patient as an unwanted consequence. The "social" definition includes monetary cost even when not borne directly by the patient, may place a different valuation on patients and their interests, and pays attention to the social distribution of the cost and net benefits of care. Thus, the physician who wishes to do the best for each patient

*Reprinted by permission from *The Journal of Family Practice* 9(2):277–284, 1979; presented as The First Ward Darley Lecture, at the School of Medicine, Department of Preventive Medicine and Comprehensive Care, The University of Colorado, Denver, Colorado, March 5, 1979.

†This paper is based on Chapter 1 of Donabedian, A. (1980). Explorations in Quality Assessment and Monitoring, Vol. I: The Definition of Quality and Approaches to its Assessment: Ann Arbor, MI: Health Administration Press.

may be in conflict with what society dictates to be the best for all. The health care professions must resolve this moral dilemma.

I suppose that from time immemorial individuals and societies have been concerned about the quality of the advice and care they have received from those to whom they have looked for guidance and help. But, of late, our confidence in all our "experts" seems to have eroded to an alarming degree, and our demand that the quality of their performance be scrutinized and improved has been, accordingly, loud and insistent. The medical profession, in particular, has felt the consequences of this challenge, not because its performance has been particularly deficient, but because it is of such moment to life and well-being.

But what, one may ask, is this thing called the quality of medical care, in the pursuit of which we are so mightily mobilized? What is it we seek? And if, perchance, we were to encounter it in one place or another, would we recognize that we had found it? This is the question before us today. This is the quest on which we are about to embark.

The Two Components of Care

The search for a definition of quality can usefully begin with what is perhaps the simplest complete module of care: the management by a physician, or any other primary practitioner, of a clearly definable episode of illness in a given patient. It is possible to divide this management into two domains: the technical and the interpersonal. Technical care is the application of the science and technology of medicine, and of the other health sciences, to the management of a personal health problem. Its accompaniment is the management of the social and psychological interaction between client and practitioner. The first of these has been called the science of medicine and the second, its art. But this terminology is not universally accepted, and could be misleading. According to some, the technical management of illness can conjure up behaviors so mysteriously and elegantly appropriate as to merit the admiting appellation of "art." On the other hand, the management of the interpersonal relationship is an "art" mainly by default: because its scientific foundations are relatively weak, and because even the little that is scientifically known is seldom taught. Since technical care is neither completely nor exclusively a science, and interpersonal care is capable of growing, at least partly, into a science, the distinction between science and art can be accepted only as an imperfect representation of the distinction between technical and interpersonal care. The same can be said of the distinction between "care" and "cure," despite the alliterative euphoniousness of this terminology. Technical care is often far from curative; and it is not necessarily less caring than the management of the interpersonal process.

The terminology used is, of course, not as important as the general agreement on the usefulness of the distinction between the two domains of care: technical and interpersonal. However, one should also note that the two domains are interrelated, and that it may be difficult to distinguish the two. It is easy to see how the interpersonal relationship can influence the nature and success of technical management. One could also plausibly suggest that the nature of the technical procedures used and the degree of their success will influence the interpersonal relationship. Finally, in the application of psychotherapeutic techniques the technical and interpersonal elements in management could be virtually inseparable. However, in most cases the distinction can be made, and is not only useful, but of fundamental importance to the definition of quality.

What Constitutes Goodness

So far, I have argued that quality is a property of, and a judgment upon, some definable unit of care; and that care is divisible into at least two parts: technical and interpersonal. It is necessary, next, to say what constitutes quality or goodness in each of these parts. At the very least, the quality of technical care consists in the application of medical science and technology in a manner that maximizes its benefits to health and minimizes its risks. The degree of quality is, therefore, the extent to which the care provided is expected to achieve the most favorable balance of risks and benefits. What constitutes goodness in the interpersonal process is more difficult to summarize. The management of the interpersonal relationship must meet socially defined values and norms that govern the interaction of individuals in general and in particular situations. Partly, these norms are reinforced by the ethical dicta of the health care professions and by the expectations and aspirations of individual patients. It follows that the degree of quality in the management of the interpersonal relationship is the extent of conformity to these values, norms, expectations, and aspirations. But it could be argued that the consequence of this conformity is some form of social and personal good, and the absence of conformity a kind of loss. Moreover, to the extent that the interpersonal process contributes to the failure or success of technical care, it contributes to the balance of benefits and risks that flow from that care. Finally, the benefits and risks, no matter what their nature, must be valued jointly at least by the patient in addition to the practitioner responsible for care. All these postulates lead us to a unifying concept of the quality of care, as that kind of care which is expected to maximize an inclusive measure of patient welfare, taking account of the balance of expected gains and losses that attend the process of care in all its parts. This is a concept fundamental to the values, ethics, and traditions of the health care professions: at the very least to do no harm; usually to do some good; and ideally, to realize the greatest good that is possible to achieve in any given situation.

How simple it all seems to be; and how reassuring to end our initial exploration in this way, at a pleasantly familiar resting place. But the simplicity and plausibility of this unifying concept of quality hides a great complexity beneath the surface. And while we shall not have the time to descend far into these darker depths, it is necessary to give at least an intimation of what perils we may find there.

Benefits, Risk, and Cost: A Unifying Model

Figure 1 shows an attempt to pull together and to further develop several of these thoughts in a somewhat more formal, though still hypothetical, model. In the upper panel of the figure the volume of services is related to several variables. The first of these is benefits to health. The shape of the curve that relates the volume of services and benefits is, of course, unknown. I have assumed that as services are added there is, at first, a rapid increase in benefits and, later, a slowing down so that, toward the end, large additions to the services provided produce very small increases in benefits, or none. If benefits to health are used as the sole criterion of quality, there is no clear-cut level of services which corresponds to optimum care. One must presumably continue to add services until no measurable additional benefits accrue. But that is to proceed without considering the risk inherent to a greater or lesser degree in all health care.

The hypothetical curve relating volume

of services and risk to health, as shown in Figure 1, is roughly the mirror image of the path traced by benefits. The services prescribed and used first have large benefits and small risks. Then, as services are added, each increment has progressively larger risks and smaller benefits. If the postulates inherent in these curves are accepted, it is possible to plot for each additional step in the progression of services the health benefits minus the risks expected at that step assuming, of course, that benefits and risks are measured in the same units. The result is shown in the lower panel of the figure. The curve of "benefits minus risks" rises to a peak and then falls to zero, which is the point at which benefits equal risks. The most important feature of this curve is that it has a maximum point, which clearly identifies optimum technical equality. Of course, the shape of the benefit-minus-risk curve, and the position of its highest point, depend on the shapes of the curves of benefits and risks. These, in turn, are deter-

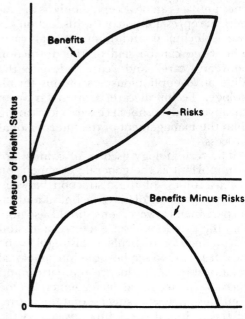

Fig. 1. Hypothetical relationships between the quantity of health services received and the benefits and risks of these services to health.

mined by the condition of the patient, the efficacy of medical science in the care of that condition, and how skillfully medical science is applied. Advances in medical science and technology, by definition, improve the ability to achieve greater benefits, lower risks, or both. However, when improperly or unskillfully applied, scientific innovations could also increase the potential to do harm without corresponding increases in benefits. But at any given state of medical science, the highest skill in its application is evidenced by obtaining the highest possible benefits with the lowest possible risk at any given volume of service. This means that the curve of benefits-minus-risks will attain the highest possible peak, and the strategy of management that, on the average, achieves this result represents the highest level of quality, other things being equal. Anything less is less than perfect quality; but only convention and usage can fix the rough boundaries of what is meant when quality is judged to be "fair" or "poor."

At this point a few clarifying remarks may be in order. In Figure 1 it is assumed that risks do not exceed benefits at any level of service, so that, at worst, health status is expected not to alter. In reality, risks can exceed benefits, so that there is a deterioration in health which is attributable to the care received. That this is poor quality no one would question.

It is also important to emphasize that the peak in the curve of benefits-minus-risks represents the state of medical science as well as the way in which it is applied. This is important because the assessment of the efficacy of the science and technology must be clearly separated from the assessment of the quality of technical management. The latter is a judgment on how well the science and technology are used. Quality, then, is not represented by health status, but by the extent to which improvements in health status that are possible are realized.

It is now time to add to the analysis yet another variable, which is the cost of providing health care services. The upper panel of Figure 2 portrays this new situation showing a steady increase in cost as services are added.

Assume that it is possible to put a money value on the expected benefits and risks to health that correspond to any level of health care services consumed. When this is done, one can plot a curve that shows, at each level of services, the expected monetary value of benefits minus the sum of the monetary value of risks and monetary costs. The lower panel of Figure 2 shows this curve and how it compares to the curve of benefits-minus-risks. The new curve is shifted to the left, it extends below the zero line, and its peak is lower. In effect, a new standard has been established for the quality of technical management. This new standard includes the fundamental postulate that monetary cost is an unwanted consequence of care and, for that reason, can

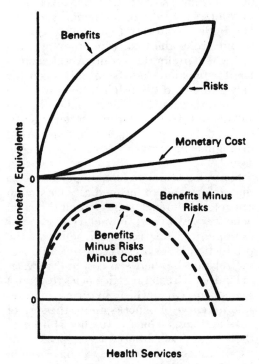

Fig. 2. Hypothetical relationships between the quantity of health services received and the benefits, risks and costs of these services.

be added to the expectations of risk in the assessment of the net benefit of technical management. The construction of the new standard also implies that monetary cost and benefits or risks to health are not incommensurate: that they can be valued in some comparable manner, even if very roughly.

It seems that in recent years several scholars have arrived at essentially similar formulations of the role of monetary cost in the definition of quality. One example is to be found in a manuscript on Quality Assurance of Health Services being prepared by Vuori for the European Office of the World Health Organization. (Vuori VH: Quality assurance of health services, unpublished). In addition to considering the consequences of including or excluding costs in the definition of quality, Vuori raises the question of whether optimal quality is the level of services that maximizes net benefits minus cost or the level that maximizes the ratio of net benefits to cost. He finds it obvious that the consumer would prefer the first, while the "producers" would prefer the second. Another similar formulation has been advanced by Havighurst and Blumstein who emphasize the differences in health care policy that result not only from including monetary costs in the definition of quality, but also from distinguishing private costs from social costs.[1]

Several additional factors pertinent to the performance of the medical care system can enter the model through their effect on benefits, risks, and monetary cost. For example, the degree of efficiency in the production of services of course influences the relationship between cost and services in Figure 2. Greater inefficiencies result in a steeper cost curve which, in turn, would result in a curve of benefits minus the sum of risks and costs which is further shifted to the left, and which has a lower peak. The use of unnecessary services will have a similar effect by lowering benefits and increasing risk relative to any level of monetary cost.

Still another factor, and one that is fundamental to the model, is that of valuation or utility. It is postulated that individuals vary in the manner in which they value the expectations of health benefits, risks, and monetary costs that accompany the receipt of care in any condition. If so, there is another set of curves (not shown in the figures) which represents these subjective valuations, and which could lead to a different specification of the quantity and mix of services that represent the best in technical care. It is, of course, possible that the valuation of benefits, risks, and monetary cost might correspond in such a way as to leave their joint interrelationship unchanged. But this is unlikely. Patients and physicians are likely to vary in their propensity to incur risk in the expectation of a given benefit; and the valuation placed on monetary cost is likely to be more responsive to income than the valuation placed on increments of health status. But all this is subject to empirical exploration.

The Unifying Model and Interpersonal Care

The unifying model was described as if it applied only to defining the quality of technical management. However, as already pointed out, it is possible, at least hypothetically, to conceive of various strategies and styles in the management of the interpersonal process as having expected benefits and risks to one or several aspects of the patient's welfare. There are monetary costs as well, since the practitioner's personal attention requires time, and costly amenities must be added to assure comfort, privacy, convenience, and other features that contribute to the patient's satisfaction. It follows that curves similar to those shown in Figures 1 and 2 could be used to define a standard of the quality of interpersonal care. One argument for keeping this as a separate measure of quality is the difficulty of expressing in a common unit of measurement the multiplicity of expected gains and losses to the many objectives of care in the two forms of management. Important as this problem is, it is not a barrier to conceiving the possibility of one measure or standard of quality that is the final sum of all possible benefits, risks, and monetary costs that result from care. In fact, there is ample evidence in everyday experience that patients are able to assess the various benefits, risks, and costs within a common framework, and to make reasonable exchanges between one seemingly nonmeasurable attribute and another. At the extreme, in acute life threatening illness, many of the niceties of care are gladly relinquished, even though, in retrospect the patient may resent deeply having had to do so. In certain chronic illnesses, where little improvement in physical function can be expected, and the main objective of care is to help the patient to cope with a disability, the elements that enter the management of the interpersonal relationship become very important.

The Balance of Benefits and Risks in the Unifying Model

The balance of benefits and risks in the unifying model of quality is the result of several considerations. The first is the likelihood of occurrence of benefit or harm under any specified situation. The second is the magnitude of benefit or harm, which is the degree of deviation in health and welfare from what is expected in the absence of any health care intervention. Duration of benefit or harm can be seen either as a component of magnitude or as an additional feature. Promptness or delay in the occurrence of benefits or harm, together with duration, make up what might be called the time perspective on benefits and risks. This perspective is important because the valuations placed on benefits and risks can vary depending on whether these are immediate or delayed; and it is likely that individuals differ from each other in their relative preferences for the present as

compared to the future. The clients and practitioners very probably take all of these factors into account, in a very rough and poorly understood way, in the decisions that they make about what to do or not to do. But more rigorous application of the model would require careful study and quantification of these factors.[2]

Some Implications of the Unifying Model

The unifying model asserts that individual expectations and valuations, as well as monetary cost, can enter the definition of the quality of care. I also believe that these are important considerations in the determination of what is the most appropriate care in actual practice. But, in addition to noting that these factors *can* and *do* enter the definition of quality, we need to consider whether they *should*. To define quality is to establish a norm, which means that the definition must be defensible on normative grounds.

Before adopting any given position it would be useful to consider several alternatives. Perhaps the simplest position is to assert that health care professionals should, as experts in the matter, have the prerogative of defining what is meant by "health status," what their intervention can contribute to health, and how that contribution is to be measured. The quality of medical care would be defined as the management that is expected to achieve the best balance of health benefits and risks. It is the responsibility of the practitioner to recommend and carry out such care. All other factors, including monetary cost, as well as the patient's expectations and valuations, are regarded as obstacles or facilitators to the implementation of the standard quality. They do not modify the standard itself. Though seldom explicit, this viewpoint is strongly represented when professional groups construct general formulations of the kind of care that constitutes quality. However, I hesitate to call it the "professional" definition, because I do not believe it represents the full range of professional values and responsibilities. I do not want to call it the "technical" or "scientific" definition because I want to leave room for kinds of intervention or aspects of management that are not now considered to be scientific or technical. Perhaps it should be called the "absolutist" definition, since it has the fewest conditions attached to it. In a similar vein, Vuori uses the term "absolute quality" to describe the standard of quality when "we omit . . . the significance of the economic factors to the persons concerned." (Vuori VH: Quality assurance of health services, unpublished, p. 39.) However, the absolutist definition of quality is still conditional on the nature of the health problem to be managed, and on the state of the science, technology, and "art" of medicine and its allied disciplines.

There is an alternative view. A long and honorable tradition of the health care professions holds that the primary function of medical care is to advance the patient's welfare. If so, it is inevitable that the patient must be involved together with the practitioner in defining the objectives of care and in placing a valuation on the benefits and risks expected as a result of alternative strategies of management. In fact, it can be argued that the practitioner merely provides expert information, while the task of valuation falls on the patient or on those who can, legitimately, act on his behalf. In principle, the patient as the best judge of his own welfare, must direct the physician. In practice, the patient often will ask the health care professional to act on his behalf. In that case the practitioner is expected not to substitute his own valuations for those of the patient, but to act in the best interests of the patient, considering what the practitioner knows or can find out about the patient's circumstances and valuations. Sometimes, the practitioner has good reason to believe that the patient is not in a position to make a proper assessment of the expected risks and benefits. For example, it may be

impossible for the patient to predict how well he can adapt to a seemingly crippling amputation, or to an operation that results in the loss of sexual function. Under these circumstances the patient should be given unbiased information about how other patients have responded to these disabilities and, if possible, arrange for the patient to meet with others who have gone through similar experiences. Since this is time consuming, the practitioner may be tempted to speed things up by "steering" the patient to a preconceived decision. But even such a decision must be, in the practitioner's opinion, the best, in the long run, for the patient. And in all these decisions, whether by the patient or on his behalf, the monetary cost of care and its impact on the patient's welfare would seem to be a legitimate and necessary consideration.

When the judgment of quality takes into account the patient's wishes, expectations, valuations, and means, we may speak of an "individualized" definition of quality, since patients differ considerably with respect to each of these. Patients are also different from one another in type and stage of illness, and also in the demographic and social characteristics that influence the course of illness and its response to treatment. Given all these sources of variation, it is reasonable to ask whether it is possible to formulate specific, but generally applicable, criteria and standards of the quality of care. Many would argue that this is not possible, and would insist that the standard of quality must be established case-by-case.

One important implication of including so many factors in the definition of the quality of care is a possible reduction in the ability to formulate generalizable criteria and standards. The inclusion of monetary cost as a factor in this definition has additional implications of its own. It is necessary to include cost whenever the patient pays at least part of the cost, if the patient's net welfare is the criterion of quality. But including the monetary cost of care is tantamount to saying that the patient's ability to pay influences the standard of quality. This might be ethically acceptable if the benefits of care are enjoyed only by the patient, and the distribution of income itself rests on an ethically justifiable foundation. If it is asserted that there is a right to medical care, even these justifications would be insufficient. Thus, the inclusion of monetary costs as an ingredient in the "individualized" definition of quality, while necessary to that definition, does pose a moral problem for the practitioner who must accept, in the interests of the patient, less than the greatest net benefit to health that medical science can confer. In fact, an analogous moral problem is created by any individual variation in the valuation of benefits and risks that is introduced because of social or economic factors whose distribution in the population could be considered inequitable. Thus the "absolutist" definition of quality seems to us to be morally neutral, whereas the "individualized" definition obviously is not. This may be why the formal pronouncements of medical leaders are couched in terms of the former, even though actual practice probably conforms more to the latter.

It is possible, of course, to virtually remove monetary costs as a factor in the individualized definition of medical care by instituting some form of comprehensive health insurance, together with paid sick leave. The patient can now demand, and the practitioner provide, all the care that makes a net contribution to the patient's health and welfare. But the costs have not simply disappeared. They persist, important as ever, in the social sphere. And since society must, sooner or later, demand that costs be controlled, the practitioner, once again, faces a moral dilemma. His responsibility for, and commitment to, the patient demand that he provide all the care that may do the patient good. And yet his responsibility to society, or his own dependence on social or institutional approval, demand that, because of monetary cost, he should stop somewhat short of the maxi-

mum health benefit attainable for any given individual.

This brings us to a third definition, which is the "social" definition of quality. The factors that enter this definition are the same as those that do so at the individual level, but the quantities could be different. There is also a new criterion. In addition to the aggregate net benefit (or net utility) for an entire population, the social distribution of that benefit within the population becomes very important.

Differences between the social and the individualized definitions of quality arise in different ways. To the extent that monetary costs, for capital investment or for operations of the program, are shifted from individuals to the collectivity, or from one segment of the population to another, monetary cost would have a different impact on the two definitions. Another reason for the difference between the two definitions is that some forms of care are more highly valued at the social level because they benefit not only the individual who uses them, but others also. Elements of care that are introduced as part of planned research, formal education, or informal learning by trial and error, might be a constituent of quality as socially defined, because they are expected to benefit others, including the patient, in the long run, even though they may not contribute to the current care of the patient. Finally, society may place different valuations on the health and welfare of different segments of the population distinguished by sex, occupation, and so on. This may reflect social values, economic considerations, or political influence and power. Thus, social valuations may rest on what is socially expedient rather than socially just, which raises still another ethical problem for the practitioner. It is one thing to ask the practitioner to place a limit on the care of some in the interest of fairness to all. It is quite another thing to require this in order to serve the interest of the economically privileged or the politically influential. There is a general presumption in democratic societies that social valuations represent a superior ethic. This may not always be the case.

Choosing a Definition of Quality

The analysis done so far leads to the conclusion that there are several definitions of quality, or several variants of a single definition; and that each definition or variant may be legitimate in its appropriate context. While this formulation is useful for analysis, it does not help as a guide to public policy or personal action. For example, there is still the question of what definition should be espoused by a health care professional who provides personal health care services for which he is responsible, and by the professional association that legitimizes the practitioner's point of view. I feel that having raised the issue, I am obligated to express an opinion, even if it is tentative.

I am convinced that the balance of health benefits and risks is the essential core of a definition of quality. I am reasonably certain that risks and benefits must be compared primarily as valued by the fully informed patient or his legitimate representative. A good case could also be made for including the avoidance of useless care, which incidentally also lowers cost, as an element in the definition of quality. The efficiency of production, to the extent that it is determined by factors other than practitioner decisions in the management of individual patients, should be excluded from the definition of quality, though it remains as an important consideration in its own right. As to the social valuations placed on health benefits and risks, I believe that these should be excluded if they differ from individual valuations. The reason is to avoid diluting the loyalty of the practitioner to the individual patient. Social valuations that differ from individual valuations should be expressed by resource allocation at the aggregate level, including the institution of special programs, special benefits, and the like. The responsibility of the prac-

titioner would then be to do the best for each patient within the framework of social constraints and facilitations.

The only element in the definition of quality that remains truly problematic is the role of monetary costs as balanced against net benefits to health. I believe that, in real life, we do not have the option of excluding monetary costs from the individualized definition of quality. Their inclusion means that the practitioner does for each patient what the patient has decided his circumstances allow. In doing so, the practitioner has discharged his responsibility to the patient, provided the patient has been helped to tap every available means of paying for care. It is true that this may result in care and the benefits of care being distributed inequitably, or in a less than socially optimal manner. But this problem can be solved only by social action. When this action includes controls over the use of health care services, it is the practitioner's role, as I see it, to act as the patient's advocate, so that the system can be made most responsive to each patient's interests. The consequence is an inevitable tension between the practitioner and the mechanisms of social control, which implies a conflict between the individualized and social definitions of quality.

It seems to me that this conflict between the individualized and social definitions of quality can be resolved if the direct and indirect costs of care are borne by society, and, at the same time, the practitioner is made responsible for the welfare of an entire group of people. An ethically defensible social definition of quality could then be applicable. In this definition, all person-years of life at full function would be equal in value. All persons would have equal access to care, but would contribute to the costs of care in a manner that is equitably related to their ability to pay. Given a specified quantity of resources devoted to medical care, the highest quality of care would be that which yields the highest net utility for the entire population. It is the responsibility of the professional schools to discover and to teach those strategies of care that are most likely to achieve this result. When this happens, the care provided to each individual, using these strategies, would conform to the social standard of quality.

I am not sure that this Utopian solution is fully realizable. Until it is implemented, it seems inevitable that the individual practitioner will be subject to the conflict engendered by the simultaneous application of the three definitions of quality: the absolutist, the individualized, and the social.

Acknowledgments

I wish to thank the Department of Preventive Medicine and Comprehensive Health Care at the University of Colorado for inviting me to present this paper as The First Ward Darley Lecture on March 5, 1979.

In preparing the paper I have benefited from discussions with Professor John Wheeler, my friend and colleague at the School of Public Health of The University of Michigan. However, the paper, as it stands, represents my opinions alone. In particular, it does not in any way speak for the National Center for Health Services Research that has so generously supported the work on which the paper is based, under Grants 1-RO1-HS-02081-01, 5-RO1-HS-02081-02, and 3-RO1-HS-02081-02S1.

REFERENCES

1. Havighurst CG, Blumstein JF: Coping with quality cost trade-offs in medical care: The role of PSROs. Northwestern Univ Law Rev 70(1)15-20, 1975
2. McNeil BJ, Weichselbaüm R, Pauker SG: Fallacy of the five-year survival in lung cancer. N Engl J Med 299:1397, 1978

A Framework for Good Primary Medical Care—The Measurement and Achievement of Quality*

Carol Buck, John Fry, and D. H. Irvine

A conference was initiated by the Royal College of General Practitioners and sponsored by the Rockefeller Foundation at its Study and Conference Centre in Bellagio, Italy. The purpose was to assemble a small group of primary physicians and research workers from Europe and North America to discuss ways of improving the quality of primary care. The conference accepted the following objectives:

1. To define primary care and to discuss its aims,
2. To determine what research is needed in order to set standards of quality for primary care,
3. To suggest methods for implementing improvements in the quality of primary care.

Background

Background papers (Buck, 1974; Fry, 1974; Jefferys, 1974; Lee, 1974) were distributed in advance; the salient points were:

1. In definitions of primary care, emphasis is usually placed on availability, accessibility and continuity, and on the coordinating function. All definitions imply that the role of primary care is of such importance that its quality has an overwhelming influence on the quality of the whole system of medical care.
2. The content of primary care varies from one country to another, with large differences between the developed and developing countries. Measurements of quality must allow for this.
3. Characteristics of the providers also vary throughout the world, and further variations are likely to arise as the result of deliberate experiments in the use of nonphysicians as providers. Such experiments should give a stimulus to the measurement of quality of care. It is unlikely that any 'best' system will ever emerge, given that cultural and economic factors determine what is regarded as best.
4. Two important trends are appearing:
   a. the replacement of the solo physician by a group of physicians and the addition to the group of other health workers who may provide some preventive and counselling services more competently than the physician.
   b. the development of specific postgraduate education for primary physicians.
5. In investigating or controlling the quality of primary care it is helpful to use Donabedian's classification (1966):

Structure of care—the setting, the qualifications of the providers, the administrative arrangements and the policies of the primary care service.

Process of care—the preventive, diagnostic and therapeutic actions taken by the provider of care.

Outcome of care—the change in health status of the receipient of care.

6. Non-medical factors, both personal and environmental, have a strong influence on health and may often be more important than medical care. A

*Reprinted by permission from *Journal of the Royal College of General Practitioners*, 24:599–604, 1974.

by-product of research into the quality of care would be the highlighting of urgent needs to alter non-medical determinants of health.

7. In appraising quality of care, it has been traditional to rely on the examination of structure and process, assuming their relationship to outcome is well understood. In fact, knowledge of the best clinical management of many conditions is deficient and research is needed into process/outcome and structure/outcome relationships before standards of quality can be set.

8. The outcome of preventive and therapeutic actions against chronic diseases is usually not clear for many years, hence the importance of being able to link records that refer to one patient if process and outcome are to be related.

9. In the management of emotional illness and social handicap the conventional medical approach, with its reliance on physical therapies, may have to be extensively modified before an acceptable level of quality can be achieved.

10. Studies of quality that relate to the outcome of primary care must consider the objectives of care. Providers and consumers of care have different implicit objectives, which are not necessarily symmetrical or reciprocal, and no two providers or consumers are likely to have exactly the same range or order of objectives.

11. Resistance to evaluating the quality of primary care exists both among the providers and within governments or other third parties engaged in financing care. Among providers, inertia delays some steps necessary for studies of quality. A reluctance to improve record-keeping is an example. Furthermore, not all providers view with equanimity the prospect of being evaluated by their peers or a central bureaucracy. Among third parties, there is unwillingness to divert scarce funds into studies of quality of care.

12. The implementation of any system for monitoring the quality of primary care must not absorb excessively the time of physicians in reviewing the work of their peers. Thus, acceptable sampling procedures and routine indicators of quality must be developed.

Summary of Conference Discussions

(1) Definition and Content

Two definitions were considered. The first was from the Royal College of General Practitioners (1972):

> The primary care physician is the doctor who will provide first contact care and where possible continuing and terminal care to a defined population of patients. He will make his assessments in physical, psychological and social terms.

The second was from Dr. Alberta Parker (1973):

> The primary level of care is the one where the health care system is entered and basic services received and where all health services are mobilised and co-ordinated. In functional terms, the two definitions differ little. The second one, however, avoids specifying the provider.

The content of primary care differs from one country to another because disease patterns vary and there are differences in the relationship between the primary and other components of the medical care system. Such international variations must be kept in mind, so that standards of quality will be clinically and administratively appropriate for the country in which they are to be applied.

Because it may be easier to set quality standards for some aspects of primary care than for others, the temptation to let ease of measurement take precedence over the importance of what is being measured must be resisted.

There was recurrent discussion of the difference between primary *health* care and primary *medical* care. The former introduces concepts of health promotion, enhancement of social well-being and environmental modification not usually implied in the latter. The degree to which the primary care physician should be held responsible for health care in the fullest sense was arguable, although there was agreement that primary medical care should not be isolated from health care. As a member said, "the primary physician has pastoral responsibilities."

(2) Process and Structure

When members of the conference tried to list specific elements of the structure and process of care, it became clear that the distinction between the two is not firm. Some elements of structure were mentioned which relate to the features of the community in which the consumers of care reside, while others apply to the physical and administrative characteristics of the service in which care is provided. Many of the latter blend imperceptibly into the clinical action usually listed under process.

It may be less important to distinguish between the categories of structure and process than to specify all the potentially important elements of both which need to be investigated in relation to outcome.

(3) Outcome of Care

Since the ultimate criterion of quality must be in terms of what happens to the patient, the specification and measurement of outcome is vital to the control and improvement of quality. In one group discussion eight elements of outcome were listed:

a. Prevention of disease or control of the disease process,
b. Improvement or preservation of the patient's level of function in his family, at work and in his social activities,
c. Relief of the patient's symptoms, distress and anxiety, and avoidance of iatrogenic symptoms,
d. Prevention of premature death,
e. Minimising the cost of the illness to the patient and his family,
f. Giving the patient satisfaction with his care,
g. Relieving or at least clarifying the patient's interpersonal problems,
h. Preserving the human integrity of the patient from an ethical point of view.

It was recognised that another group might have produced a different list and also that there could be argument about the relative importance of the items. If consumers were to make such a list it might be very different.

Providers, consumers and third party financers of care should be invited to specify the outcomes they consider important. Consumers of care can affect outcome by the manner in which they seek or comply with care, and this in turn will be influenced by their perception of a desirable outcome.

(4) Research to Establish Standards of Quality

Each member was asked to list up to ten health problems commonly encountered in primary care in developed countries and for which optimum standards of management cannot at present be set. The following clinical conditions were the most frequently listed:

a. Hypertension
b. Acute otitis media
c. Acute back pain
d. Acute bronchitis with asthma
e. Acute urinary infections
f. Angina of effort
g. Acute sore throat
h. Low haemoglobin
i. Depression

The list indicates the difficulty of controlling the quality of primary care when standards for such common conditions cannot be set. The best clinical management must be determined by scientifically acceptable methods, such as the traditional randomised control trial. It was suggested that because of the urgency of the need to set quality standards, controlled trials should be supplemented by applying multivariate statistical techniques (appendix) to uncontrolled situations in order to choose the optimum from among competing methods of management.

Randomised controlled trials and the multivariate analysis of data from uncontrolled situations can be applied to the analysis of structure as well as process. If there are many uncertainties about the optimum process of clinical management, there are equally urgent uncertainties about the influence on outcome of many structural variables of which the following were given particular importance:

1. The composition of the primary care team,
2. The number of patients cared for,
3. The training of the primary physician,
4. The participation of the primary physician in hospital care,
5. The provision of instructions for self-care to patients
6. The use of the problem-oriented record.

It was agreed that there is a place for both national and international research projects. International comparative studies of outcome would be particularly valuable in determining the importance of structure because differences in some structural variables are much greater between nations than within any single nation.

The difficulty of allowing for other than structural differences in such comparative studies was recognised but not regarded as insoluble. To expedite studies of this sort it was suggested that potential research collaborators be asked to provide detailed information about the cultural, economic and structural characteristics of the community and the clinical setting in which they provide primary care. It would then be possible to choose the most appropriate participants for specific studies and to identify the research issues which can be attacked in this way.

At both national and international levels, collaborative research must be encouraged because it is difficult for a single investigator to acquire the volume of data or the range of structure and process variation necessary to reach definitive conclusions. The research literature is of little help because it describes completed research rather than studies being contemplated.

Would-be investigators with similar interests often remain unaware of each other's existence. Thus, a means of communication is necessary because conferences alone cannot meet the need. It was agreed that an international mechanism for fostering collaborative research in primary care must be established.

(5) Implementation of Quality Control in Primary Care

When standards of quality have been set by studies of the relationships between structure, process and outcome, feasible methods for monitoring quality must be developed. A sampling approach is indicated since it would be impracticable to review all aspects of care for which standards might exist.

The idea of using indicator (or tracer) conditions is attractive. These would be health problems for which optimum management has been established and which are common enough in primary care to make quality of care given to them important.

Two difficulties were discussed. First, that indicator or tracer conditions which have so far been proposed refer to the management of diagnosed conditions. Yet primary care deals in the first instance with undifferentiated symptoms rather than with clear-cut diagnostic entities. To take a specific example, primary care needs standards that begin with the management of fever, irritability and earache in a child rather than with the care of streptococcal otitis media.

The second difficulty is that a set of indicator conditions might be put into use which missed completely the fact that very often the symptoms brought to the primary physician do not represent the patient's underlying problem. For example, a physician might provide exemplary management of repeated visits for minor sore throat of a child and yet fail to appreciate that the mother brought the child so often to the physician because she was trying to achieve a discussion of her own near-suicidal depression.

If the list of indicator conditions being used to monitor quality did not include the appraisal of "token" visits, his failure to understand the situation would be missed. Although this is an example of one of the most subtle aspects of the primary physician's function, it is extremely important because it is one of the functions that distinguishes him from other providers of care.

Some impatience was expressed with delaying the implementation of quality control while the research needed to identify optimal levels of structure and process is awaited. It was therefore suggested that some interim procedures for monitoring quality should be adopted. Two approaches were put forward:

1. To use health problems for which there is already acceptable evidence of a relationship between process and outcome. It was not feasible to review the documentation permitting the preparation of a list of such interim indicators of quality. However, this is a potentially useful approach, as long as it is not allowed to institutionalise a meagre and inadequate list which might forestall research needed to create better indicators of quality.
2. To adopt the approach hospitals have taken toward the appraisal of quality, whereby such "critical incidents" as deaths and surgical interventions are regularly reviewed, by, for example, re-

viewing all deaths, complications of illness, and iatrogenic health problems. Although useful as an interim measure, such an approach tends to emphasize poor outcomes of an acute and dramatic nature, thereby deflecting attention from less vivid but equally undesirable consequences of poor primary care.

In implementing quality control the motivation of the primary care physician was discussed. Monitoring of quality should become an integral part of the physician's continuing education. Thereby the intellectual and emotional participation of the physician in setting and maintaining quality standards could be secured, in contrast to a grudgingly passive acceptance of standards that might result from a purely bureaucratic process of control.

Because of marked differences among countries in the role of professional associations, universities and third parties in peer review and cost control, and in the organisation of continuing education, the manner in which the control of quality is implemented must be tailored to the circumstances of each country.

Recommendations of the Conference

1. That consideration be given to the establishment of an international committee to further the study of primary care in national systems of medical and health care.

   The committee should be provided with secretarial and library staff. It would be asked to arrange for reviews and abstracts of published literature and for information on research work in progress. It would establish communication with similar groups in health systems and circulate information to interested groups and individuals. This committee would help research in primary care and in identifying problem areas.

   It would convene international task

forces to examine specific problems and to stimulate research. The conference suggested that in the first instance the Royal College of General Practitioners should be invited to set up such a secretariat, provided that finance is obtained.

2. That international organisations be asked to consider sponsoring and encouraging more research into specific clinical problems in primary medical care. These international organisations should be asked to carry out a review of the present position and of further actions necessary on research methods and techniques in primary care.

J. Bush Appendix

The discussion on multivariate procedures was summarised: to assess statistically the quality of primary medical care, the structure/process/outcome paradigm can be transformed to a regression format. The dependent (outcome) variable may be a disease specific indicator, a general health index, or a measure less directly related to health, such as patient satisfaction. The advantages and disadvantages of multivariate analyses over the significance tests more commonly used must be considered; and the form of regression depends upon the form of the dependent variable. Thus, these methods provide techniques for data analysis to assess quality in ongoing practice situations.

A health status index was suggested as an overall outcome variable suitable to test the influence of most known factors, medical and non-medical, on the health status of a defined population. The index is constructed of multiple factors including symptoms, mobility, disability, performance, and social activity that have been scored with measured social values. Both the index and the statistical analysis could be adapted to analysing the outcomes from the diffuse non-specific complaints peculiar to primary care. Short and long-term follow-up studies are needed to allow for prognostic factors. The hope was expressed that a general index incorporating social values could help to resolve the need for a consensus outcome measure.

REFERENCES

Buck, C. (1974). The measurement and improvement of quality in primary health care. Typescript
Donabedian, A. (1966). Millbank Memorial Fund Quarterly, 44, Part 2, No. 3. 166-206
Fry, J. (1974). Primary medical care. Typescript
Jefferys, M. (1974). The quality of primary medical care: outcomes of care for the patient. Typescript
Lee, P. R. (1974). The process of primary medical care. Typescript
Parker, A. (1973). The Dimensions of Primary Care—Blueprints for Change. Presented to Sun Valley Forum. Sun Valley, Idaho
Royal College of General Practitioners (1972). The Future General Practitioner. London: British Medical Association

Medical Audit in General Practice*

P. Curtis

As an educational experience a good system of medical audit is worth any number of postgraduate courses—MCWHINNEY (1972).

Increasing interest is being shown in the standards of medical care in general practice. The method of measuring these standards, known as medical audit, is discussed in relation to general practice in Great Britain.

Introduction

The family doctor is a manager as well as a clinician and uses a wide range of hospital, social, and governmental services. He is instrumental in spending substantial sums of money. It is, therefore, hardly surprising that increasing interest is being shown in the evaluation of quality and costs in primary care (Capstick, 1974).

The evaluation of costs is known as financial audit while the assessment of quality of medical care is called medical audit (*British Medical Journal*, 1974).

Quality of care has been measured by workload studies, prescribing patterns, morbidity, patient satisfaction, referral and consultation rates (Forsyth and Logan, 1962; Cartwright, 1967; Seiler, 1967; Korsch, Gozzi and Francis, 1968; Stolley and Lasagna, 1969; Drury and Kuenssberg, 1970; Pinsent, 1972; Honigsbaum, 1972). This is called external audit (Figure 1) and consists of the assessments of the results of treatment as well as the environmental and functional aspects of the medical system providing care for the patient.

Another method of measurement is to look at the mechanism for determining care, the medical record. This is internal

*Reprinted by permission from *Journal of the Royal College of General Practitioners*, 24:607–611, 1974.

medical audit, which takes a more private look at the way the doctor deals with his patient. Of course, if the record is illegible or incomplete then the pathways of the patient's care reside in the doctor's memory. The doctor's standards or competence cannot then be measured, but this does not necessarily mean that they are bad.

A structured record with a defined collection of demographic, physical, and physiological data (database) is more easily assessed and so hospital records are usually easier to review than those in general practice.

The problem orientated medical record (POMR) lends itself well to medical audit (Weed, 1969; Bjorn and Cross, 1970) precisely because of the defined components of the database, the problem list, and progress notes (*Journal of the Royal College of General Practitioners*, 1973). The POMR is now widely known in Britain and descriptions of its use in general practice have already been published (Metcalfe, 1973; Tait and Stevens, 1973; McIntyre, 1973).

Techniques of Audit

The object of reviewing a record is to examine its adequacy and the methods used by the doctor in diagnosis and management of the patient. Subsequently judgments are made on the doctor's ability to provide a reasonable standard of care. Who makes these judgements? Who sets the standards? Who defines the diagnosis? These questions have not been answered.

The Americans have had to respond to them. The Congressional Legislature (1972) has set up Professional Standards

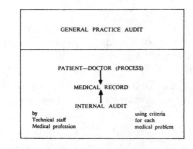

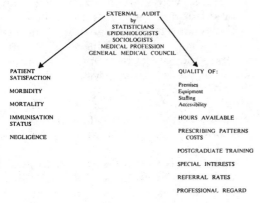

Fig. 1.

Review Organisations (PSRO) which are to assess, by law, the care given to patients under governmental health programmes (Medicare and Medicaid) in hospitals and private practice.

A record can be audited in two ways (Brook and Appel, 1973). Firstly a technical assessment is made. This can be performed by non-medical personnel who check the adequacy of demographic data and completeness of the record. This follows specific guidelines. For instance, one could specify that an adequate record in general practice must contain the name, address, date of birth, sex, marital state, and occupation of the patient. Any secretary or clerk could perform this task. This is known as an *explicit* judgment which is based on strict criteria.

Secondly, a physician can give his subjective opinion about the record. He might think it was neat or that the doctor under scrutiny was probably doing a good job. This is a personal opinion relating to the auditor's attitude and experience and is an *implicit* judgment.

Selecting records for audit can be accomplished in a variety of ways (Lembcke, 1967; Brook, 1972) including random sampling and following tracer diseases such as hypertension and myocardial infarction (Rubin, 1973; Kessner *et al.*, 1973). Will it be possible to measure the quality of care in general practice? It is unlikely that this will occur in the near future. Firstly, there is no tradition of reviewing the general practitioner's work in Britain and there would be strong resistance to it. In general, medical audit is very threatening to physicians and is best taught to those with unformed medical habits—the medical students (Peterson, 1973).

Secondly, there is no convincing proof yet that the end results of care are improved by measuring professional competence (Fessel and Van Brunt, 1972; Marson *et al.*, 1972; Brook and Appel, 1973). Thirdly, the long-term aspects of disease and the problems of diagnosis in general practice make it difficult to set standards and criteria of care.

One can illustrate some of the problems which become apparent when an audit of, for instance, tonsillitis is undertaken in general practice. Let us assume that the general practitioner has written in his notes: "Tonsillitis—Rx Penicillin V." Does this tell us that he has performed adequately? What are the criteria for good care in such a case? They could be:

1. Adequate history of sore throat,
2. Evidence of examination by the doctor,
3. Throat swab sent to the laboratory,
4. Description of drug and dose given.

If so, the doctor under audit has failed to provide adequate care. Yet many an excellent doctor writes just such a note during a busy surgery. Perhaps if he had more time and training he might fulfil the above criteria.

More time means the introduction of paramedical personnel to take on many of the traditional tasks of the general practitioner. These tasks include the treatment of minor trauma and trivial disorders as well as the surveillance of chronic diseases. This trend is well established in the United States with the growing physician-assistant and family nurse-practitioner programmes.

The primary care physicians who use paramedical staff in this way therefore have more time to devote to accurate record keeping, patient management decisions, medical audit, and education. Many followers of Balint (1964) would argue that this trend represents a retreat by the doctor from patient contact with a consequent reduction in his effectiveness "as a drug".

Problems of Audit

Table 1 shows a simple record audit sheet in which section 1 (basic data) presents no auditing problems except that it is unlikely that many of our general-practice records would be thus regarded as adequate. Dawes (1972) in a survey of eight practices showed that ten per cent of the files examined had no age recorded, 99 per cent had no indication of marital status, while 60 per cent had no occupational status.

In section 2 (problems) the main difficulty arises in the definition of a problem. The patient, his doctor, and the auditor may have differing views about the definition of, for instance, obesity. When does it become a problem in the records? Perhaps when the patient's weight is 20 per cent greater than the expected level. Maybe the patient just feels overweight or looks obese to the observing general practitioner. Can these differing view points be audited?

Finally, in section 3 (plans) how can one suitably deal with the problems of obesity. Should one prescribe appetite suppressants, weight reduction, psychotherapy, antidepressants, hypnotherapy, exercise, or group therapy? Unless there is a consensus of opinion on what is adequate therapy for this condition, accurate auditing is not possible.

It is obvious that the only way to audit records effectively is to define, fairly rigidly, the criteria of the diagnosis and treatment of each disease. Naturally as medical opinion changes these criteria will have to be altered on a regular basis. Unfortunately the content of general practice includes often indefinable symptoms as well as problems which have social, environ-

Table 1. *Simple N.H.S. Record Audit*

	Yes	No
Basic Data		
(1) Were the following obtained and recorded?		
a. Demographic data		
b. Past medical history		
c. Family history		
d. History of previous medication		
e. Menstrual history for females		
f. Present complaint		
Problems		
(2) a. Were all the problems recognised from the basic data and history?		
b. Are new problems added to the list when necessary?		
Plans		
(3) a. Were all the problems acted upon?		
b. Were all the problems acted upon suitably?		

mental, and psychological components. These are difficult to audit.

Dollery (1971) has proposed a statutory body, independent from the Department of Health and Social Security, which would undertake external audit in hospitals and general practice. For this to be effective there would have to be a great improvement in the collection of data in all areas of the National Health Service.

An internal audit could possibly be set up in this country through the network of postgraduate centres with both financial and educational incentivies for the participants (Capstick 1974). This might involve random sampling of hospital and general-practice records with discussion, at a monthly meeting, of the problems raised by the audit. This should have an educational result rather than a punitive one. Alternatively, this task could be taken on by the general-practitioner committees.

The prospect of auditing the care of patients using the present National Health Service record would daunt most doctors. A redesigned record would offer some chance to examine the methods of care used by general practitioners (Royal College of General Practitioners, 1973). It seems likely that the process of medical audit will occur soon in Great Britain where medical services use a significant proportion of the national budget. The Government may well decide to start quality control for the taxpayers' money long before general practice begins to look at its own standards.

REFERENCES

Balint, M. (1964). The Doctor, His Patient and the Illness. Second edition. London: Pitman Medical

Bjorn, J. C. & Cross, H. D. (1970). The Problem-Oriented Private Practice of Medicine. Chicago: Modern Hospital Press

Brook, R. H. (1972). A Study of Methodologic Problems Associated with the Assessment of Quality of Care. ScD. Thesis, Johns Hopkins University. National Centre for Health Sciences Research and Development

Brook, R. H. & Appel, F. A. (1973). New England Journal of Medicine, 288, 1323-1329

Capstick, L. (1974). British Medical Journal, 1, 278-279

Cartwright, A. (1967). Patients and their Doctors; A Study of General Practice. London: Routledge & Kegan Paul

Dawes, K. S. (1972). British Medical Journal, 3, 219-223

Dollery, C. T. (1971). The quality of health care, p. 5-32. In Challenges for Change, (ed. G. McLachlan). London: Oxford University Press

Drury, M. & Kuenssberg, E. V. (1970). British Medical Journal, 4, 42-44

Fessel, W. J. & Van Brunt, E. E. (1972). New England Journal of Medicine, 286, 134-138

Forsyth, G. & Logan R. F. L. (1962). Studies in Medical Care, p. 66-68. In Towards a Measure of Medical Care. Nuffield Provincial Hospital Trust. London: Oxford University Press

Honigsbaum, F. (1972). Journal of the Royal College of General Practitioners, 22, 429-451

Journal of the Royal College of General Practitioners (1973). Editorial, 23, 301-302

Kessner, D. M., Kalk, C. E., & Singer, J. (1973). New England Journal of Medicine, 288, 189-194

Korsch, B. M., Gozzi, E. K. & Francis, V. (1968). Paediatrics, 42, 855-871

Lembcke, P. A. (1967). Journal of the American Medical Association, 199, 543-550

McIntyre, N. (1973). British Medical Journal, 2, 598-600

McWhinney, I. R. (1972). British Medical Journal, 2, 277-279

Marson, W. S., Morell, D. C., Watkins, C. J. Zander, L. (1973). Journal of the Royal College of General Practitioners, 23, 23-31

Metcalfe, D. H. H. (1973). Practice team, 22, 11-13

Peterson, P. (1973). Journal of the American Medical Association, 224, 884-885

Pinsent, R. J. F. H. (1972). Update, 5, 599-600

Rubin, L. (1973). Group Practice, 22, 7

Sanazaro, P. J. (1974). Brtish Medical Journal, 1, 271-274

Seiler, E. R. (1967). Journal of the Royal College of General Practitioners, 13, 197-204

Stolley, P. D., & Lasagna, L. (1969). Journal of Chronic Diseases, 22, 395-405

Tait, I. & Stevens, J. (1973). Journal of the Royal College of General Practitioners, 23, 311-315

Weed, I. L. (1969). Medical Records, Medical Education and Patient Care. Cleveland: Case Western Reserve University

Peer Review of a Small Group Practice*

Theodore J. Phillips, Amos P. Bratrude, and Francis C. Wood, Jr.

How does one group of physicians go about rating the medical care given by another? Variously described as "peer review," "medical audit," or "patient care appraisal," attempts to answer this question have recently received much emphasis. Such assessments usually serve either a disciplinary or an educational purpose, and the two do not mix well. Disciplinary assessments are generally intended to improve patient care by limiting costs or restricting physician privileges. The assessors are not obliged to provide constructive feedback or opportunity for reform to the person or institution under investigation. Educational appraisals, however, aim at helping physicians identify the subjects in which they need additional training or a better conceived program of patient care. Such an educational appraisal is reported here with 1-year follow-up documenting the results.

The methodology for peer review is still being developed. Early approaches as pioneered by Brown concentrated on hospitalized patients and medical record review.[1] Such assessments are now becoming common in hospitals throughout the country and are beginning to be accepted by their medical staffs.

Taking peer review out into the community is new. Hamaty has reported a West Virginia project to evaluate office practices for individual physicians.[2] This article will describe a pilot project to assess a small group practice. The report includes results of a follow-up one year later to measure the

*Reprinted by permission from *The Journal of Family Practice*, 7(1):28-33, May 1974.

usefulness of the initial assessment for the physicians requesting it.

Origin of Study

Those who organized the Washington/Alaska Regional Medical Program (W/ARMP) in the late 1960's particularly emphasized continuing education. This generated immediate interest among the region's rural practitioners. When asked to describe their educational needs, however, many physicians replied that they could not identify these until someone audited their current level of practice. Although a method had yet to be developed, one physician persisted in request for an audit. By November, 1970, a Department of Family Medicine had been formed at the University of Washington Medical School, and its chairman agreed to undertake the requested audit on behalf of the W/ARMP as the coordinator of an evaluating team.

The clinic under review is located in a town of 6,500 persons and provides all available immediate care for the townspeople and the surrounding villagers who constitute a total population of 8,000 in an isolated rural area of the Pacific Northwest. One group of physicians (three when the study began in January, 1971, and four upon follow-up 15 months later)† runs the

†In 1971 the group consisted of: Family Physician—15 years' practice following internship, Family Physician —7 months' practice following internship; General Surgeon—6 years' practice and Board Certified. In 1972 another Family Physician had been added with 9 months' practice following an internship

clinic with access to the community's recently built 25-bed hospital.

Methods

General Preparations

After exchanging ideas of specific information desired from the audit, the coordinator and the requesting physicians agreed upon the following goals.

1. *Education:* To help the clinic physicians identify the subjects in which they could benefit from further study.
2. *Audit methodology:* To develop an evaluation procedure for wider application.
3. *Curriculum development:* To collect information on the functioning of a primary care clinic which would assist in development of family physician curriculum in the School of Medicine.

The team coordinator was already familiar with the clinic's locale through 6 years of practice in the same region before he entered academic medicine. For a second team member he called on a W/ARMP organizer who is a full-time family physician with (at that time) 11 years of experience in a remote town similar to the one where the clinic is located. The clinic physicians had been asked to submit a list of five diseases whose management the reviewers could inspect in the records for an in-depth appraisal of patient care. The reviewers selected two of the five, diabetes and urinary infection, as index diseases. The coordinator then invited an internist-endocrinologist with many years of experience in academic medicine (and a particular interest in diabetes) as the third member. The team thus included one physician familiar with the clinic's geographic locale, one familiar with the type of practice, and one an expert on one of the index diseases. Prior to their audit, the team reviewed literature on practice audit and patient care appraisal.[2–7]

The clinic physicians were asked to submit their criteria for the optimum management of diabetes and urinary infection in both office and hospital so that the reviewers could compare ideal against actual performance. One reviewer organized the criteria into checklist form which was adapted by a medical record librarian for use in abstracting information from records of patients with the index diseases. The librarian then spent one day at the clinic abstracting office and hospital records assembled for her by the staff, as well as making notes on the quality of record keeping.

All arrangements for the initial visit were made by letter and telephone. The three team members did not meet together until actual departure for their visit to the clinic. Once there they were able to complete the investigation in 2½ days.

Specific Assessment Methods

ASSESSING PATIENT CARE ON SITE. Using the clinic physicians' criteria, the evaluators examined abstracted records of all patients hospitalized in 1970 with urinary infection (14) or diabetes (8). As a second method of patient care assessment, the team also reviewed a sample of 20 hospital records (all patients in hospital at time of the visit) and 30 clinic records (pulled at random from the files).

Donabedian has stressed that the ultimate measure of patient care is the final outcome at the end of therapy.[3] Fessel has shown that the course of care noted in a patient's record may have no relation to his outcome later.[4] As an index of outcome, the assessors thus looked for notes on the patient's condition during the year following treatment for any particular problem.

As a third assessment method, the reviewers observed clinic physicians at work, on hospital rounds, in the emergency room, at the clinic, answering phone calls at home, at a lunch meeting with community members and at the mental health clinic.

While reviewing the records and making direct observations, the team asked these questions about medical care:

a. Was it rational and based on current medical knowledge?
b. Did it emphasize prevention?
c. Did it make use of intelligent cooperation between patient and physician?
d. Did it treat the individual as a whole?
e. Did it maintain a close and continuing personal relationship between the physician and the patient?
f. Was it coordinated with social work and other allied professions?
g. Did it coordinate all types of medical services? [(a) through (g) adapted from Lee and Jones, 1933][5]
h. Was the care rendered easily available and acceptable to the patients?
i. Was it documented? [(h) and (i) adapted from Esseltyne, 1958][6]
j. Was the care provided comprehensive in the sense of approaching all four stages of disease as defined by James?[7]
   —Stage 1: the foundations of disease
   —Stage 2: presymptomatic disease
   —Stage 3: symptomatic disease
   —Stage 4: chronic disease
k. Do the medical records help achieve efficiency and continuity of patient care?
l. How is the follow-up of patient problems carried out?
m. How do physicians and other clinic personnel share time and tasks?

ASSESSING PRACTICE MANAGEMENT. The team inspected physical facilities, including both hospital and clinic. Clinic management was checked with an eye to appointment scheduling, the system for recording charges, fees, billings, collections, circulation pattern of patient charts, supportive services and their quality and level of use, and personnel policies. The reviewers also examined hospital medical staff practices, the routine for clinical rounds, communica-

tions between physicians and with the other members of the hospital staff, hospital-staff relations and laboratory usage.

ASSESSING THE FUNCTION OF THE CLINIC TEAM. Throughout their observations the reviewers tried to evaluate the manner in which the physicians and other clinic and hospital staff members worked together, what facilitated good functioning and what stood in the way of continuous improvement.

ASSESSING PATIENT SATISFACTION. Noting that earlier reviews of physician performance had not tried to assess patient satisfaction as an index of care, the reviewers decided to take advantage of the clinic's iso-

Table 1. *Community Medical Survey*

M F _____ S M W D _____ Age _____

Occupation _____

Husband's Occupation _____

1. How long have you lived here? _____
   Came from? _____
2. Do you have a family doctor? _____
3. When did you last see him? _____
4. Do you have a medical problem now? _____
5. Are you under care now? _____
6. Do you have a good hospital here? _____
7. What do you do for problems your family doctor can't handle? _____
8. Is it hard to talk to, or see the doctor? _____
9. How long do you wait in the office? _____
10. Can you get care on weekends—nights—etc.? _____
11. Is the medical care you get in this area good? _____
12. Have there been any changes in health–medical care in the past year? _____

lated setting for a community survey. After discussion with faculty from the University of Washington School of Public Health, a simple questionnaire was designed (Table 1) to learn on what occasions community residents used the clinic and what they thought of the level of care. This was done to assess the feasibility of such a survey only. There was no attempt at developing statistically significant data.

Radio and newspapers ran announcements of the auditors' forthcoming visit. During the visit one team member interviewed 16 community residents (9 men and 7 women) ranging in age between 18 and 72 years. They were surveyed away from the hospital and clinic setting and asked 11 questions, many of which were open-ended to elicit a discussion of health care rather than a listing of statistics.

FOLLOW-UP ASSESSMENT. The reviewers summarized their findings in a list of 22 specific recommendations (Table 2).

One year later the team returned for two and one-half days to learn the effects of their suggestions. The same method was followed once again to assess patient care, practice management, functioning of the clinic team and community attitudes. The assessors studied patient care through the same two index diseases, this time reviewing the records of 19 patients hospitalized with urinary infection and 11 with diabetes. At the request of the clinic physicians, they also reviewed against criteria the clinicians had submitted earlier the management of 11 patients hospitalized for alcoholism. Reviewers also examined the records of 18 patients hospitalized at the time of the follow-up visit and a random sample of clinic records.

The follow-up community survey this time included 14 persons between the ages 14 and 67, eight of them male and six female. The interviewer used the same questionnaire as in the first survey but added the question: "Have there been any changes in the health-medical care here in the past year?"

Table 2.

Summary of Recommendations—1971	Implemented by 1972?
1. Continue as group of general family doctors	No
2. Each member of group could pursue an area of special interest for benefit of the entire group	Yes
3. Each member should work at developing proficiency in all areas of family practice	Yes
4. Each member should undertake regular short-term postgraduate study in his area of interest	Yes
5. Establish a regular group conference for educational purposes	Yes
6. Establish a regular staff conference to discuss clinic operation and policy—including office personnel	Yes
7. Establish a system of communication with the itinerant public health nurse	Yes
8. When seeing a patient with whom he is not familiar, each physician should review more regularly the past and family histories previously recorded	Yes
9. Make clinic records more specific in outlining plans for patient management	Yes
10. Regularly record the interpretation of electrocardiograms	Yes
11. Consider a more frequent interval for patient appointments	Yes
12. Consider more regular use of short, return follow-up visits	Yes
13. Consider a duplicate or numbered charge slip for tighter money control in the office	No
14. Consider use of a standard relative value fee schedule	No
15. Modify office routine so that patients are not asked to carry clinical records from examining room to business office	Yes
16. Become more familiar with services now available through the hospital laboratory	Yes

(*continued*)

Table 2—*Continued*

Summary of Recommendations—1971	Implemented by 1972?
17. Consider removing physical therapy unit from the office	Yes
18. Tighten up scheduling and starting time for surgery	No
19. Include nurse in physician rounds at hospital	No
20. Consider improved communication with physicians at Naval base nearby	Yes
21. Consider planning for extended care facility or nursing home in community	Yes
22. Repeat audit in one year	Yes

Findings

ASSESSMENT OF PATIENT CARE. The reviewers noted a distinct improvement in the diagnosis and treatment of urinary infection patients between the first and second visits. As Table 3 shows, improvement in the handling of this disease was a matter of bringing performance, as documented in patients' records, up to well defined criteria.

In the case of diabetes, however, after examining the 1971 report the clinic physicians revised their criteria. The 1971 criteria, for example, had recommended oral hypoglycemic drugs for almost all newly discovered diabetics, and these in fact were being used in seven out of the eight cases reviewed. The 1972 criteria called for these drugs only in special instances, and only four of the 11 cases reviewed were on such drugs. Another change in criteria was a deemphasis on maintaining perfect control of the patient's blood sugar in favor of assessing his status according to weight, symptoms and urine sugar. This change in criteria between the first and second visits meant that comparison of performance was not really as helpful as in the case of urinary infections.

The reviewers examined 30 randomly selected clinic records in 1971 and a comparable number in 1972. After their first visit they had recommended that, at the time of a patient visit, the physician review that patient's past and family history in the record, especially when unfamiliar with the patient. They also suggested that plans for diagnosis and treatment be outlined more specifically so that one doctor could easily take over a case from another. By 1972 the clinicians were dictating approximately half their records. Both recommendations had been implemented in the dictated records but not in others. The recording of interpretations on the electrocardiogram was also suggested to help one team member pick up from another. This was being carried out in 1972.

Hospital records were in excellent condition in both 1971 and 1972. They indicated close physician follow up and an efficient record keeping system. The hospital maintained a good disease and operations index. Inclusion of more detailed plans in hospital discharge summaries was the one recommended change in 1971, and a 1972 check showed that this was being done.

Observation of physicians and staff in action, along with record review, led to other suggestions for improvement in patient care. To give follow-up care to patients returning to remote villages, the reviewers had recommended equipping the travelling public health nurse with the hospital patient's discharge summaries. Since then the hospital has installed a radio-phone, and the doctor on call has regularly held evening radio contacts with the villages. The clinic also sends instructions and suggestions to the public health nurse in writing and by radio.

Unfamiliarity with the capabilities of a new technician who served both hospital and clinic appeared responsible for the clinician's underutilization of the laboratory. Reviewers recommended that they rely more heavily on the sophisticated lab testing available. Follow-up revealed that

Table 3.

Criterion	Performance 1971	Percent	Performance 1972	Percent
Urinary Tract Infection in Hospitalized Patients				
Careful Physical Exam (e.g.: including careful genital-pelvic and rectal exam)	4/14	28.6	16/19	84.2
Blood Pressure	13/14	92.9	18/19	94.7
Urinalysis	14/14	100.0	19/19	100.0
Urine Culture	11/14	78.6	17/19	89.5
Radiologic Study	3/14 received studies, but criteria and records too vague to tell how many more were included	21.4	5/5 both needed and received studies according to more precisely defined criteria	100.0
Treatment: 10 days of antibiotics and a follow-up urine culture.	Information unavailable to assessors		Length of treatment known in 18/19 (94.7%). The clinic did follow-up cultures for 11/19. (Of the 8 others, 3 were transferred to other towns for care, 3 failed to return for appointments, 1 signed out of the hospital. Record was in doubt for only 1 case.)	

while hospital patient volume remained the same, utilization of laboratory services rose markedly.

Exploring the possibility of establishing a nursing home or extended care facility for patients who did not need acute hospital care was also recommended. A year later the hospital administrator reported specific plans underway for such a service.

ASSESSMENT OF PRACTICE MANAGEMENT. The clinic had been sandwiching drop-in visits between formal appointments scheduled at 30 minute intervals. Reviewers suggested that the clinic accept scheduled patients every 15 to 20 minutes, in order to dispel the community belief that appointments were difficult to obtain except for acute problems, discourage a reliance on drop-ins, and encourage physiians to re-

quest that the patient return for follow-up care. Since then the clinic has scheduled appointments at more frequent intervals. Followup visits have been requested of patients more frequently than before.

Formerly patients carried their records from the examining room to the business office. The reviewers criticized this practice and observed that it might pressure the physician to write shorter, less complete comments on the chart than he would were the patient not waiting to carry it off. This practice has since been discontinued.

For more stringent fiscal control the reviewers suggested duplicating the charge slip to protect against loss by the patient or inefficiency or dishonesty by a business office employee. No change had been made one year later.

In billing patients the clinic had not been

keeping strictly to its fee schedule, which the reviewers thought could be more flexible and more rationally thought out. They recommended consideration of the relative value fee schedule. This has since been used in charging for surgery and hospital care, but has not been routinely followed for office visits. In a group practice, the reviewers said, much better agreement should be possible on charges for specific services.

Business practices in the office were still judged as weak on the follow-up visit. A further suggestion was made that the business manager be sent to survey other offices and methods or that a professional team come in to evaluate and improve current practices. The reviewers noted that for either measure to be effective, the physicians would have to show a greater desire for change.

To avoid wasting time and lowering hospital staff morale, it was suggested that physicians try to arrive on time for scheduled surgeries. The situation appeared to have remained the same during the following year.

ASSESSMENT OF CLINIC PERSONNEL AS A TEAM. In 1971 reviewers observing clinic physicians found that they neither thought of themselves nor functioned as much as a team as might be expected. Rather than remaining generalists they seemed to be heading toward reorganization as a group of specialists in separate disciplines. The evaluators proposed that each member instead develop his proficiency in all areas of family practice since the clinic's position as an isolated medical unit in a rural community makes the physicians dependent upon each other professionally. The reviewers also recommended that each physician pursue an area of special interest from which he could share his knowledge with the others in the group.

One year later observers saw that the group had moved even further toward some speciality organization, but this appeared to be working well. At the same time the members had begun sharing special knowledge to a greater extent. Although one member of the group is surgically trained and does nearly all the surgery, he was assisting the newest member to develop some emergency surgical skills. The suggestion that clinicians attend short-term courses and post-graduate study programs was acted upon by all three members during the intervening year. Each clinician had improved family practice proficiency as well, so that each adequately covered for the others in the broad range of medical practice. The exception was one member who did not practice obstetrics.

Staff conferences were strongly recommended by the reviewers in several instances. A regular weekly morning conference at the hospital for all physicians was suggested for its educational value. Its institution appears responsible for one of the most striking changes between the two visits—the consistency and standardization of practice developed. For example, the revised criteria for management of diabetes which were submitted for the follow up review indicated there had been combined effort by the physicians as a group. Review of records of patients with diabetes indicated general adherence to these criteria. In addition, informal conversation revealed that each physician was much more knowledgeable about his associates' patients and management routines than had been true at the time of the first visit.

A regular conference for other clinic personnel was also suggested and has been held once and sometimes twice a month. Although the physicians call these meetings "frustrating," they have increased communication and permitted discussion of policy decisions.

Having a nurse accompany the physician when he makes hospital rounds was highly encouraged by the reviewers so that the nurse could record and implement any instructions given to the patient and so that she could provide added information about him. A check one year later showed that this was sometimes done when the nurse was not involved in care elsewhere.

ASSESSMENT OF PATIENT SATISFACTION. The follow-up community survey produced very similar responses in 1971 and 1972. Those questioned knew where to get health care, how to go about it, and felt that access to the clinic was easy. Most of them did not specify a particular physician as their family doctor. Four of the sixteen reported a practice of going outside the area of medical care in the first survey in 1971 while none of the fourteen in the second survey did. The first survey included several store-owners who may have been better able to pay for such trips than the working people who constituted almost all those questioned in the follow-up interview.

The follow-up survey was also intended to ascertain whether the original survey had been valid and whether the public had noted any changes in health care delivery. Not even the addition of a fourth physician to the practice was noted by those asked in 1972 about any significant change in health care during the past 15 months. They described the last major improvement in medical care as the building and opening of the hospital which had occurred several years earlier.

Discussion

The peer review reported here was not strictly disease-oriented and clinical, but it had broader goals. It included hospital as well as office practice and touched upon practice management, staff communications and community satisfaction.

The follow-up visit demonstrated that such an audit can produce measurable results. Physician performance measured against self-determined criteria for at least one index disease showed significant improvement. For the other index disease the first review led to re-evaluation of management. Implementation of 17 of 22 recommendations from the review committee provided another measure of change upon follow up one year later. Five situations showed no change where the reviewers had

suggested some change might be indicated. Two of these concerned business practices, one involved surgery schedules and one involved the inclusion of nurses on hospital rounds. The lack of implementation of the other recommendation (retreat from specialization), suggested to the reviewers that their specific advice may not have been appropriate in the first place.

Implementation of two recommendations, staff rounds and communications with surrounding villages, far exceeded the reviewers' expectations. Stimulation of interest in continued self-evaluation was another observable result, shown by increased sophistication of the criteria submitted for index disease handling and by the request that a third index disease be examined during the follow-up visit. Clinic physicians have also reported a project to develop additional criteria for their own examination of performance in managing other illnesses.[8]

The project appears to have satisfied its initial purposes. With respect to education, all three physicians present during the initial audit have since attended post-graduate courses in subjects recommended by the evaluation team. As for the development of family physician curricula, the study not only provided descriptive information about the functioning of a small, private, primary care clinic, but also stressed the importance of teaching students and residents how to perform well as a team. The project convinced the reviewers that considerable learning and conscious effort is required for four physicians to work together successfully. In training students for clinical practice, medical schools have emphasized acquisition of information and skills but have often neglected attitudes and understanding necessary for such learning. During the audit it became apparent that the clinic physicians did not succeed as well as possible with group problem-solving. On such issues as specialization versus general competence for all, the clinic's role in the community, and the event of the group's responsibility for health care beyond the clinic's doors, the members had difficulty resolving problems together.

The project also succeeded in developing a workable evaluation procedure which can be conducted in less than three days on site and with limited disruption of the practice. Further refinement of this approach could undoubtedly be achieved. Reviewers might use more sophisticated measures of patient care outcome such as those suggested by Williamson.[9] They could put more time and effort into defining acceptable patient care criteria in the way Hamaty describes. Expert consultants in practice management could be added to the team. A sampling system with greater statistical reliability could be used for the community survey. A pollster skilled in assessing community opinion and attitudes could be hired to administer a pre-tested and sophisticated questionnaire. On the other hand, the most comprehensive evaluation might not be the optimal one.

An important value of the audit method presented here, however, is that it represents true peer review through which both the reviewed and the reviewers have much to gain. An unexpected result of this project was that the reviewers have looked at their own practices and educational responsibilities from a new perspective and have instituted such changes as using cultures more often in treatment of urinary infection and emphasizing the teaching of attitudes and understanding. In this sense the method could be useful to geographic or professional medical groups, such as state medical societies, or to local specialty organizations as a tool for continuing education. It seems particularly adaptable for isolated and rural practice where physicians from one town could be evaluated by their peers in another similar community.

Acknowledgments

The research of this paper was supported by the Washington/Alaska Regional Medical Program and, in part, by the Department of Health, Education and Welfare—PHS—Health Professions Special Project, Grant No. 1 D08-PEOO393-01.

Thanks are due to Mrs. Annie Demming, medical record librarian of Palmer, Alaska, for her considerable assistance in this project. Dr. Robert Day, Chairman, Department of Health Services, University of Washington School of Public Health and Community Medicine offered valuable advice in planning for the community survey. Mrs. Vivian Bowden provided assistance in tabulating and reporting data.

REFERENCES

1. Brown Clement R Jr, Uhl Henry SM. Mandatory continuing education, sense or nonsense? Journal of the American Medical Association 213, No. 10, September 7, 1970, 1660–1667
2. From West Virginia: the doctor's office becomes his classroom. Patient Care, May 30, 1971, pp. 39–43
3. Donabedian A. Evaluating the quality of medical care. Milbank Memorial Fund Quarterly 44 (3): 166–203, Part 2, 1966
4. Fessel WJ, Van Brunt EE. Assessing quality of care from the medical record. The New England Journal of Medicine 286, No. 3, January 20, 1972, pp. 134–138
5. Lee RI, Jones LW. Fundamentals of Good Care, Publications of the Committee on the Cost of Medical Care, No. 22; Chicago, University of Chicago Press, 1933
6. Esseltyne Calwell D. Principles of Physician Remuneration, papers and proceedings of the National Conference on Labor Health Services: Washington D.C., June 16–17, 1958, Washington, D.C.: American Labor Health Association, 1958, p. 122
7. James George. The general practitioner of the future. New England Journal of Medicine, June 11, 1964, p. 1286
8. Johnson Bob. Horizons in medical evaluation. Alaska Medicine 14, No. 4, October 1972, pp. 112–114
9. Williamson John W. Evaluating quality of patient care. Journal of the American Medical Association 218, No. 4, October 25, 1971, pp. 564–569

Assessment of Quality of Care by Profiles of Physicians' Morbidity Data*

Jack Froom

A process model for the assessment of quality of care in the ambulatory setting by diagnostic profiles of participating physicians is presented. This model allows comparison of the individual physician's morbidity profile with those of his peers in family practice and other primary care disciplines. Deviations from peer group profiles set the stage for education focused on accepted criteria for diagnosis and management of specific clinical problems. Initial experience indicates that physicians will participate in the project and can benefit from the experience. It is anticipated that further experience with the method described will demonstrate that it is a valid technique to evaluate quality of care and that changes in physician behavior can be demonstrated following educational experiences based on deviant morbidity profiles.

In recent years, there has been increasing interest in peer review and the assessment of quality of care in the United States. In 1972, the United States Congress enacted Public Law 92-603 which mandated the creation of physician groups called Professional Standard Review Organizations (PSRO). The function of these organizations is to provide peer review concerning the suitability and quality of care rendered

*Reprinted by permission from *The Journal of Family Practice*, 3(3):301–303, 1976. This paper was presented at the Sixth World Conference on General Practice-Family Medicine held by the World Organization of National Colleges, Academies and Academic Associations of General Practitioners-Family Physicans (WONCA) in Mexico City, Mexico, November 6, 1975.

to patients insured under Medicare, Medicaid, and Title V of the Social Security Amendments. Although the law relates primarily to hospitalized patients, it is likely that ambulatory care will come under scrutiny in the near future.

Donabedian[1] has described three parameters by which quality of care may be assessed:

1. Structure—which includes a measurement of health facilities available;
2. Process—which includes management of health and illness; and
3. Outcome—which includes what eventually happens to the patient.

   Although evaluations of outcome are the most desirable, they are the most difficult to perform. Outcome measurements often require extended periods of observation. In addition, there is a lack of precise information about the natural history of diseases. This makes it difficult to relate medical interventions to health outcomes.

There have been a number of attempts to assess quality of care by process management. Assessment by chart review in offices of internists led Kroeger and coworkers to conclude that only 67 percent of physicians kept records which were adequate for review purposes based on legibility and completeness.[2] Other measurements of the medical record[3,4] show similar problems of incomplete data recording. Some groups have defined specific criteria for the diagnosis and management of a group of health conditions[3,5] and suggest that quality assessment may be made by comparision of actual performance with these selected criteria. The use of preselected specific criteria may be a poor method because the selected criteria tend to become unduly rigid.

This paper presents an attempt to assess quality of care in the ambulatory setting. *Process* is measured rather than outcome, although the potential for outcome measurement is created. This study was undertaken with acceptance of the following assumptions:

1. Process measurements can produce evidence of quality of care.
2. The diagnoses that a physician makes are an important parameter of process measurement.
3. Individual physicians' performance in diagnoses should be compared to that of peer groups rather than against idealized standards.
4. Participation should be voluntary.
5. Feedback to participating physicians should have no adverse consequences, such as loss of income or prestige. Reviews of insurance claims often carry such penalties.

The project had the following goals:

1. To define local standards of medical care within three groups of primary care physicians, (a) family physicians, (b) internists, and (c) pediatricians, by analysis of morbidity data.
2. To identify deviations from the standards among participating physicians by comparison of their morbidity profiles with those of their peer groups.
3. To educate physicians about currently accepted diagnostic criteria and therapy for those conditions identified in which they were deviant from their peer groups.
4. To document changes in physician behavior by continuous monitoring of morbidity data and comparison with data generated prior to the educational experience.

This is a preliminary report which describes the method and some of the early results. All of the goals described above have not yet been implemented.

Method

Enrollment of participating physicians began in January 1972. Currently there are 56 family physicians and general practitioners (including family medicine residents) in 11 practices recording data on 60,000 patients. In addition, there are ten internists in seven practices with 25,000 patients and five pediatricians in two practices with 15,000 patients. The diagnostic and demographic data are recorded both manually and on computer tape allowing retrieval of diagnostic data by either method. Each participating practice has the following systems installed:

1. *Age/Sex Register*—The Age/Sex Register has been described elsewhere,[6] but briefly it is a file of 3 × 5 cards which are color-coded for sex and contain the following information: name, age, date of birth, area of residence by census tract, marital status, and physician. Cards are filed by color and by date of birth. Active patients are defined as those patients who have had a physician encounter within the preceding two years.

2. *A Classification of Diseases*—An ideal classification of health problems for use in primary care has not been available and the hospital classifications currently in use have not been found suitable for recording health problems in the ambulatory setting.[7] In 1972, the best available classification appeared to be the Metcalfe modification of the Royal College of General Practitioners Classification of Diseases. This classification was adopted and used in all practices. In November 1974, the International Classification of Health Problems for Primary Care (ICHPPC) was approved by the World Organization of National Colleges and Academies of Family Medicine-

General Practice. This classification had been tested for one year in multiple sites in nine countries and will be introduced into our participating practices at a later date.

3. *The Diagnostic Index—E-Book*-The Diagnostic Index—E-Book was devised by Eimerl and also has been described elsewhere.[8,9] This index is a manual method for recording morbidity data by diagnostic groupings. Diagnostic data are also recorded on daily work sheets, keypunched, and stored on magnetic tape. The diagnostic data are linked to the patient's master file already on computer tape.

Periodic computer printouts which describe individual physicians' morbidity experience compared with that of their peer groups are distributed to participating physicians. These physicians are also encouraged to use data recorded in their manual systems for self-audit and for outreach to their patient population.[10]

Results

It was first necessary to analyze the age-sex composition of each practice and to compare these figures with the total of the peer group practices. Table 1 compares the age-sex distribution of Dr. S.' practice (a family physician) with all family medicine patients in the study. It illustrates that corrections for frequency of those health problems that are age related will be necessary because Dr. S.' patient population is somewhat older than that of his peer group.

Table 2 illustrates the type of report that was periodically sent to all participating physicians. This table compares the frequency of diagnoses of the most common communicable disease problems diagnosed by that physician (N.L.) with the peer group (family physicians), with the total population, and with the other primary care specialties. Similar tables are prepared for each of the 22 sections of the modified RCGP classification used in the study. These reports permit each physician to

Table 1. *Age-Sex Analysis of Patient Population*

Age in Years	All Family Doctors		Dr. S.	
	No.	% of Total	No.	% of Total
Males				
0–4	2,957	4.9	19	0.4
5–9	3,533	5.9	63	1.3
10–14	3,341	5.6	139	3.0
15–24	5,244	8.8	617	13.4
25–34	3,810	6.4	338	7.3
35–44	2,777	4.6	188	4.1
45–54	2,356	3.9	354	7.7
55–64	1,790	3.0	306	6.7
65+	1,629	2.7	192	4.2
Total	27,437	46.2	2,216	48.1
Females				
0–4	2,824	4.7	17	0.4
5–9	3,311	5.6	49	1.1
10–14	2,981	5.0	152	3.3
15–24	6,789	11.4	650	14.1
25–34	5,445	9.2	314	6.8
35–44	3,433	5.8	223	4.8
45–54	2,928	4.9	441	9.6
55–64	1,986	3.3	299	6.5
65+	2,285	3.8	243	5.3
Total	31,982	53.8	2,388	51.9
Total	59,419		4,604	

compare his practice with those of his peers and with other specialty groups.

Another goal was to identify those physicians whose diagnostic frequencies deviated most from those of the peer group. We were more interested in examining the most frequent health problems rather than the rare ones. For example, Table 3 illustrates the marked variation in the frequency of the diagnosis of depression among some of the family physicians and family medicine residents in our group.

Discussion

Our initial experience demonstrates that many physicians will participate in a morbidity recording project for an ex-

Table 2. *Comparative Morbidity Report for Common Problems by Category*

Category 1. Communicable Diseases

RCGP No.	Description	Frequency of Diagnoses Number	Cases/1,000
	Family Physicians (Practice population 63,933)		
025	Warts, viral	674	10.5
005	Intestinal infections	447	6.9
021	Dermatophytosis	286	4.4
017	Infectious mononucleosis	165	2.6
027	Other virus infection	163	2.5
	Doctor N.L. Practice No. 7 Family Physician (Practice population 3,275)		
021	Dermatophytosis	38	11.6
025	Warts, viral	36	11.0
023	Epidemic winter vomiting	12	3.7
006	Scarlet fever	11	3.4
017	Infectious mononucleosis	11	3.4
	Total Population (Practice population 89,353)		
005	Intestinal infections	1,250	14.0
025	Warts, viral	1,023	11.5
027	Other virus infection	632	7.1
021	Dermatophytosis	371	4.2
031	Pyrexia without rash	353	4.0
	Pediatricians (Practice population 13,380)		
005	Intestinal infections	747	55.8
027	Other virus infection	457	34.2
025	Warts, viral	343	25.6
015	Mumps	202	15.1
031	Pyrexia without rash	201	15.0
	Internists (Practice population 12,040)		
005	Intestinal infections	56	4.7
016	Infectious hepatitis	39	3.2
014	Herpes zoster	33	2.7
017	Infectious mononucleosis	19	1.6
027	Other virus infection	12	1.0

Table 3. *Comparative Morbidity Report for Depression*

Category 5. Mental Illness		Diagnosis 134. Depression	
Physicians	*Patient Population*	*No. Cases this Diagnosis*	*Cases/1,000*
All physicians	89,353	1,762	19.7
Family physicians	63,933	1,311	20.1
Internists	12,040	449	37.3
Pediatricians	13,380	2	0
Family Physicians			
J.C.	2,804	191	68.1
S.H.	547	13	23.7
G.G.	501	11	22.0
T.G.	3,420	67	19.7
D.N.	573	11	19.2
L.Z.	2,359	39	16.5
N.L.	3,032	44	14.5
T.K.	3,340	46	13.8
T.Ke.	3,739	42	11.2
G.L.	1,684	14	8.3
J.A.	790	6	7.6
L.S.	4,624	17	3.6
R.P.	1,422	5	3.5
V.G.	2,776	7	2.5
J.W.	3,029	1	0.3

tended period of time. Some of our group have been recording diagnostic data for almost three years. There has been only one physician who dropped out of this study for reasons other than moving from the area. The demonstration of diagnostic frequency deviance from the peer group has, in general, been of interest to the physicians rather than threatening to them. Visits to the offices of the physicians for audit of charts of cohorts of those patients with diagnoses in which these physicians had deviant frequencies is planned as the next step. Continued monitoring of diagnostic frequencies will demonstrate whether this educational experience has had any effect on the physicians' subsequent diagnostic behavior.

We believe that some of the recent antagonism demonstrated by physicians to peer review and to the assessment of quality of care can be reduced if physicians are compared with their peer group's performance rather than to a set of arbitrarily defined standards. Assessment of quality of care will have the greatest chance of improving care if physicians voluntarily participate in the project and if they can be educated about their actual performance with their own patient populations.

REFERENCES

1. Donabedian A: Evaluating the quality of medical care. Milbank Memorial Fund Quarterly 44(pt 2):166–206, 1966
2. Kroeger HH, Altman I, Clark DA, et al: The office practice of internists. 1. The feasibility of evaluating quality of care. JAMA 193:371–376, 1965
3. Brook RH: Quality of Care Assessment. A Comparison of Five Methods of Peer Review. Rockville, Maryland, National Center for Health

Services Research and Development. DHEW Pub HRA-74-3100, 1973

4. Fitzpatrick TB, Riedel DC, and Payne BC: Character and effectiveness of hospital use. In McNervey WJ (ed): Hospital and Medical Economics. Chicago, Chicago Hospital Research and Educational Trust, 1962, pp. 361-592

5. Taylor FC, Payne BC, Mann FC, et al: The Use of Hospital Utilization Review Manual. Criteria and Record Abstracts for Medical Review in a Hospital Committee Setting. Ann Arbor, Michigan, Center for Research in Utilization of Scientific Knowledge, Institute for Social Research, University of Michigan, 1970

6. Farley ES Jr, Treat DF, Baker CF, et al: An integrated system for the recording and retrieval of medical data in a primary care setting: Part I. The age-sex register. J Fam Pract 1(1):45-46, 1974

7. Westbury RC, Tarrant M: Classification of diseases in general practice: A comparative study. Can Med Assoc J. 101:603-608, 1969

8. Eimerl TS, Laidlow AJ: A Handbook for Research in General Practice. Edinburgh and London, E & S Livingstone Ltd, 1969

9. Froom J: An integrated system for the recording and retrieval of medical data in a primary care setting. Part 3. The diagnostic index-E-book. J. Fam Pract 1(2):45-48, 1974

10. Henk M. Froom J: Outreach by primary care physicians. JAMA 233:256-259, 1975

Application of the Tracer Technique in Studying Quality of Care*

Stephen R. Smith

Assessment of the quality of care provided within an active family practice was attempted by evaluation of the physicians' management of a tracer illness—in this case, hypertension. The prevalence in adults was nine percent. The discrepancy between this and higher rates described in the literature appeared to be due to population differences. Management of hypertension by participating physicians complied with a minimal care plan designed by the Institute of Medicine in 78 percent of the cases. The tracer technique for assessing quality of care appears to be a promising method which can be adapted to active community practices with a minimal allocation of time, money and other resources. By requiring a review of the practice against contemporary standards, the tracer technique also enhances the quality of care through self-teaching and evaluation.

Quality of health care is a subject presently under intensive investigation. While there is little debate in regard to the right of the patient to receive "quality" care, there is much controversy regarding the definition of "quality." Third party payers are interested in the cost of quality, the government is involved in setting standards, and community groups are demanding access and accountability as integral parts of "quality" care.

In addition to the problem of defining quality, there is also the problem of objectively measuring quality. In order to measure anything, standards must be available for comparison. Unfortunately, such standards are rare in medicine. Although many "authorities" are quite willing to express opinions on subjects within their expertise, these opinions often are based on data subject to differing interpretations; consequently, no single standard can be defined. This is partly due to the sparcity of carefully collected data on the natural history of diseases and the impact of modern treatments on the outcomes. In the end, these should determine the acceptability of any particular assessment.

The impact of multiple variables on the course of illness is seldom completely understood. Nevertheless, the health profession is required to deal with these illnesses in the most effective way possible, based on the present fund of knowledge. Just as treatment of these illnesses is not postponed until more definitive information is available, neither can evaluation of how well the health profession deals with the problems be postponed any longer. It is clear that any judgment of "quality" is not absolute, but merely reflects the currently accepted standards which must be reviewed periodically and updated.

Since the process of evaluation requires one to review the current opinion on the natural history, epidemiology, diagnosis, and management of certain diseases, it becomes a learning and teaching process as well. The process through which quality is evaluated is as important as the conclusions attained. In order to adequately evaluate their own practice, physicians must review the latest literature, debate and re-evaluate their data base in regard to what constitutes a minimum work-up, and survey their practice in regard to record-keeping, history-taking, physical examinations, laboratory procedures, and prescribing patterns. Having done this, these physicians will be more

*Reprinted by permission from *The Journal of Family Practice*, 4(3):505–510, 1977. Originally reprinted from *The Journal of Family Practice*, 1(3/4), 1974.

aware of their own practice, better informed and up-to-date, and better able to provide the best possible care to their patients. This is a goal that any method of evaluation should seek to achieve.

This paper outlines a procedure for assessing quality of care using a tracer technique as carried out in the group practice of the Family Medicine Program at the University of Rochester. The entire study was conducted by one physician in this group without outside funding or use of sophisticated techniques, equipment or consultants. The project attempted to demonstrate that this method is a practical technique which practicing physicians may use without a large commitment of time, money or other resources.

The Tracer Technique

The tracer technique assumes that careful evaluation of the manner in which physicians diagnose and manage a few selected disease entities will be representative of the practice as a whole. Thus, if a pertinent family history is consistently recorded in the charts of patients with three or four diagnostic entities, it can be assumed that a pertinent family history is obtained on patients with other diagnostic entities not specifically studied.

A recent article by Kessner et al[1] reviewed a modification of the tracer method developed by the Institute of Medicine of the National Academy of Sciences and its theoretical applicability to active community practices. This study employed the framework described by Kessner and applied it to an actual practice. In order to select those illnesses that would provide the most meaningful information, certain guidelines were followed.

First, there must be general agreement on a standard minimum treatment plan. Although the treatment of streptococcal pharyngitis is fairly well defined and agreed upon, the treatment of acne is not. Thus, there must be some generally accepted consensus on the management of the disease. By management, one includes not only specific treatment, but also measures for prevention, diagnosis, and rehabilitation.

Secondly, the tracer disease must be amenable to easy and objective diagnosis that can be made by the average physician without use of sophisticated equipment or techniques not readily available. The disease must be one in which its natural history will be affected by appropriate therapy. It would not be very useful to evaluate different modes of treatment for physiologic bowlegs, since in mild cases this resolves without specific therapy. The disease selected should also be one that has sufficient prevalence so that it is commonly encountered. At the same time, it should be a type of condition that requires the active intervention of the health profession. Alcoholic hangover is highly prevalent, but the nature of the illness does not warrant intensive evaluation regarding quality of care.

Finally, the effects of nonmedical factors on the tracer should be understood. Such variables as economic conditions, religious and cultural behavior patterns and environmental factors, for example, should at least be identified and their role in the evolution of the disease taken into account.

Methods

Benign hypertension was chosen as the tracer illness for this study. Recent studies indicate that early and vigorous treatment of hypertension can substantially reduce the morbidity and mortality associated with this disease.[2-4] Hypertension is a common problem in the general office practice. Its diagnosis is easily made and can be specifically defined.

Several aspects in the total management of hypertension were investigated. First, an attempt was made to evaluate how well the entity was diagnosed in the population at risk. This was done by comparing the popu-

I. Screening
   A. *Method.* The systolic pressure is recorded at the onset of the first Korotkoff sound, and the diastolic at the final disappearance of the second or the change if the sound persists.
   B. *Criteria.* An individual patient is judged in need of evaluation for elevated blood pressure if the mean of three or more systolic or diastolic pressures exceeds the age-specific criteria specified below:

Males and Females	Systolic	Diastolic
		(mmHg)
18–44 years	140	90
45–64 years	150	95
65 or older	160	95

II. Evaluation
   In the evaluation of elevated blood pressure, the history and physical-examination data listed below should be obtained early in the evaluation.
   A. *History.* (1) Personal and social history; (2) family history of high blood pressure, coronary-artery disease, or stroke; (3) previous diagnosis of high blood pressure (females, toxemia of pregnancy or pre-eclampsia) and time of first occurrence; (4) previous treatment for high blood pressure (when started and when stopped, and drugs used); (5) chest pain, pressure, or tightness; location, length of symptoms, frequency of symptoms, effect of deep breathing, description of feeling (crushing, smothering, strangling), symptom temporarily curtails activity, and pain radiates into left shoulder, arm, or jaw and is accompanied by nausea, shortness of breath or fast or fluttering heart beat; (6) feet swell; (7) shortness of breath; (8) patient awakens wheezing or feeling smothered or choked; (9) patient sleeps on two or more pillows; (10) prior history of kidney trouble, nephrosis or nephritis; (11) history of kidney infection; and (12) prior x-ray examination of kidneys.
   B. *Physical Examination.* (1) Weight and height; (2) blood pressure—supine and upright; (3) funduscopic; (4) heart—abnormal sounds or rhythm; (5) neck—thyroid and neck veins; (6) abdomen—standard description, including abdominal bruit; and (7) extremities, peripheral pulses and edema.

   C. *Laboratory.* (1) Urinalysis; (2) hematocrit or hemoglobin; and (3) blood urea nitrogen or serum creatinine.
   D. *Other Tests.* (1) Electrocardiogram; if the patient is less than 30 years of age or if diastolic pressure is 130 mm of mercury or greater; and (2) rapid-sequence intravenous pyelogram.

III. Diagnosis
   A. *Essential Hypertension.* As described in above under I-B Criteria provided there is no evidence of secondary hypertension.
   B. *Secondary Hypertension.* Hypertension secondary to renal, adrenal, thyroid, or primary vascular disease.

IV. Management
   All drugs are prescribed in acceptable dosages adjusted to the individual patient, contraindications are observed, and patients are monitored for common side effects according to information detailed in AMA Drug Evaluations 1971 (first edition). Fixed-dosage combinations should not be used for initial therapy.
   A. *Mild Essential Hypertension* (*Diastolic Pressure of 115 mm of Mercury*). (1) Initial treatment with thiazides alone in a diuretic dose; (2) if pressure is not reduced by 10 mm of mercury or to lowest level that patient can tolerate without symptoms of hypotension in two to four weeks, alpha-methyldopa, reserpine of hydralazine is added to thiazide.
   B. *Moderate Essential Hypertension* (*Diastolic Pressure of 115 to 130 mm of Mercury*). (1) Initial treatment with thiazide and alpha-methyldopa, reserpine, or hydralazine; (2) if no response after two to four weeks, change to thiazide-reserpine-hydralazine or thiazide-guanethidine combination.
   C. *Severe Essential Hypertension* (*Diastolic Pressure of 130 mm of Mercury or Keith-Wagener Grade III or IV Funduscopic Changes*). Refer to specialist or hospitalize (or both).
   D. *Secondary Hypertension.* Treat, or refer for treatment of, primary condition.
   E. *Undetermined Etiology or No Response to Treatment.* Hypertension of undetermined cause or not responding to treatment regimens above requires further evaluation, to include: (1) determination of serum sodium and potassium; and, if not previously performed, (2) rapid-sequence intravenous pyelography.

Fig. 1. A Minimal-Care Plan for Hypertension. Developed by Kessner and Kalk for the National Academy of Sciences. Reprinted with permission of the authors and publishers from A Strategy for Evaluating Health Sciences, DM Kessner and CE Kalk, National Academy of Sciences and the New England Journal of Medicine, January 25, 1973.

lation distribution of the practice to the population of the community. Once assured that the practice population was a representative one, the prevalence of the illness diagnosed among the practice population was then compared to the prevalence as reported from the literature.

Next, the actual management of the disease was considered. The Institute of Medicine had recently outlined a minimum standard of care for hypertension.[1] This included history, physical exam, laboratory studies and treatment. The protocol is outlined in Figure 1.

Ten percent of the charts in which hypertension had been diagnosed and coded were reviewed. The charts were selected at random. Historical data were noted as positive, negative, or not recorded. Physical exam data were considered to have been performed if there was an explicit note so stating or if the appropriate box had been checked on the physical exam checklist in the chart. Most charts were problem-oriented in the fashion after Weed, and this study was conducted using the techniques outlined by Metcalfe.[5]

Results

The population distribution of the Family Medicine Group closely paralleled that of the general community of Monroe County as delineated in Table 1. The practice population also shared a similar socioeconomic distribution to that of the general population. Thus, it appeared that all specific age or sex groups were adequately represented.

In the total practice population of 6866, there were 453 cases of hypertension diagnosed and coded in the diagnostic index. When the population over the age of 15 is considered, the prevalence of hypertension in the Family Medicine Group is nine percent. The overall rate is twice as high in females as males.

To reconfirm this prevalence rate, 100 randomly selected charts from the total practice population were reviewed. In only

Table 1. *Comparison of Populations: Family Medicine Group and Monroe County*

	Family Medicine	Monroe
Men		
0–14	13.6	14.8
15–44	21.2	20.0
45–64	6.7	9.6
65+	2.6	3.9
Total	44.5	48.2
Women		
0–14	12.0	14.1
15–44	30.7	21.2
45–64	8.4	10.6
65+	4.4	5.8
Total	55.5	51.8
Socioeconomic Status*		
Class I (highest)	19.2	12.0
II	26.1	28.4
III	36.9	40.2
IV	13.9	13.0
V (lowest)	3.9	6.4

*Determined by the technique of Wagenfeld and Willie, (1962) for use in Syracuse and Onondaga County, New York. The unit of analysis is the census tract and the data are based on the 1960 census. The socioeconomic areas are delineated on the basis of a five-part Composite Index. Unpublished communication, available on request from the author.

one chart was the blood pressure greater than the age-specific criteria for hypertension and the diagnosis not made. Similarly, in the 45 charts of hypertensive patients that were reviewed, two were eventually found not to be hypertensive. One of the two patients was obese and had the blood pressure measured using a standard-sized cuff; when a large cuff was used, the patient was normotensive. The other patient was diagnosed as hypertensive based on one recording of the blood pressure and subsequent readings were normal.

Thus it appears that the prevalence figure of nine percent is a valid one for the Family Medicine Group's adult population. This prevalence rate is contrasted to that reported by other sources. The United States Health Survey[6] reported a prevalence of roughly 20 percent, the Framing-

Table 2. *Chart Review Work Sheet for Hypertension with Cumulative Results*

	Positive	Negative	Not Recorded
I. History			
1. Personal and social history	19	22	4
2. Family history (HBP, ASHD, DVA)	32	9	4
3. Previous diagnosis HBP	34	5	6
4. Previous treatment HBP	21	6	18
5. Chest pain, description	12	18	16
6. Ankle swelling	10	15	20
7. Shortness of breath	18	13	14
8. PND	3	18	24
9. Orthopnea	7	14	24
10. History of renal disease	13	29	3
11. History of UTIs	10	31	4
12. History of IVPs	3	9	33

	Performed	Not Performed
II. Physical Exam		
1. Height and weight	42	3
2. BP upright	15	—
supine	13	—
unspecified	36	—
3. Funduscopic	44	1
4. Cardiac	45	0
5. Neck and JVs	45	0
6. Abdominal exam and bruits	42	3
7. Extremities, pulses and edema	43	2
III. Laboratory		
1. Urinalysis	44	1
2. Hct or Hgb	43	2
3. BUN or creatinine	41	4
4. EKG (30 y.o. or less, BP 130+)	39	0
5. IVP	18	27

	Correct	Incorrect
IV. Diagnosis		
1. Essential	39	1
2. Secondary	1	0

	Satisfactory	Unsatisfactory
V. Management		
1. Mild (DBP 115 or less)	30	7
2. Moderate (116–130)	4	1
3. Severe (DBP 131 or more)	0	0
4. Secondary	1	0
5. Undetermined (Na, K, IVP)	1	3

ham Study[4] 18 percent, and the Baltimore study,[7] 25 percent. The rate of diagnosis of hypertension among these family medicine patients was therefore less than half that of large screening studies.

In the work-up of hypertension, the data prescribed by the minimal care plan as shown in Table 2 were obtained in the large majority of cases. The social, personal, family, and past medical history of hypertension and kidney disease were obtained from over 90 percent of the patients. It is interesting to note a positive family history in 73 percent of the patients. Other history items such as previous treatment and specific symptoms were recorded less often. A prior history of renal x-rays was recorded only 26 percent of the time.

In the physical exam, the appropriate examinations were conducted in over 95 percent of the cases. However, the determination of both supine and upright blood pressures were recorded in only 29 percent of the patients; the rest were unspecified, which in most cases probably was sitting.

Laboratory procedures were also uniformly obtained except for IVPs. All patients with a diastolic blood pressure of 130 mmHg or greater, or who were less than 30 years old, received an EKG. There were many patients, however, who had EKGs taken without these criteria, apparently for other reasons. IVPs were not obtained on six out of every ten hypertensive patients.

The diagnosis was correctly made and/or appropriate studies undertaken in 91 percent of the cases. One case of essential hypertension was diagnosed when actually no hypertension existed. In three cases a definitive diagnosis was not made nor were appropriate studies undertaken to determine the etiology.

In regard to treatment, 35 cases (78 percent) were treated in a satisfactory manner as outlined by the Institute of Medicine. In the ten cases that were not treated satisfactorily, six were not treated at all, two not treated aggressively enough and two treated incorrectly. Of the latter two patients, one was treated with phenobarbital and the other was treated with a diuretic even though he was not actually hypertensive. Of the six who were not treated at all, four never returned for follow-up after the diagnosis was made, so that therapy could not be initiated. The etiology of the hypertension was not adequately determined in three of the ten cases.

The total amount of time spent in preparing the protocol, retrieving and reviewing the charts, recording and analyzing the data amounted to approximately 24 hours. No costs were incurred outside the theoretical cost of 24 hours labor and the cost of materials which was subsumed in the office overhead and estimated at less than five dollars. While this study was conducted entirely and solely by a physician, a large part of this type of review could be adequately performed by someone other than a physician working from a detailed protocol.

Comment

This study, based only on one tracer disease, cannot be considered an adequate assessment of the quality of care provided by the Family Medicine Group of Rochester. The study of hypertension does not adequately investigate how the group provides preventive or rehabilitative services. Ideally, this study should be coupled with that of two or three other entities which would focus on other aspects of the health-care delivery system.

It did, however, raise some interesting points. The discrepancy between the prevalence rates is particularly interesting. The 1959 study by the Society of Actuaries[8] did not use the same age-specific criteria as employed in this study. When their stricter criteria are applied (i.e., diastolic pressure greater than 92 mm Hg to the age of 50, then greater than 97 mm Hg), the prevalence is four percent as compared to 25 percent when 87 mm Hg and 92 mm Hg are used. The present study uses 90 and 95 mm Hg and the prevalence falls in between. In the Baltimore study, when 140/90 is used for those up to 50 years old, 160/95 for those over 50, and three screening levels are required for diagnosis, the prevalence is still 23 percent. However, 42 percent of their population were 50 years old or more, whereas only 19 percent of the Family Medicine population is over 50. The population of the United States over 50 years old is approximately 26 percent. Not only are there population differences in regard to age, but other factors, such as race, socioeconomic status, self-selection factors and location, are also unequal between the two groups. The study in Baltimore is that of a large urban population, compared to the small urban, suburban, and rural mixture seen in the Family Medicine Group population. Thus it appears that population differences could contribute to the variation in prevalence shown in Table 3.

Two variables influenced the frequency and regularity with which data were recorded: the person responsible for recording the data and the presence of a checklist. The nurse usually recorded the patient's family, social, personal, and past medical history. The physician usually asked about the present illness, symptoms, and other disease-specific data. Where the nurse was responsible, the data were recorded about 90 percent of the time. Where the doctor was responsible, the data were recorded about 55 percent of the time. It was impossible to determine if the questions were never asked, or if they were asked and the answer simply not recorded. Where a checklist was available, as in the physical exam, the data were recorded over 90 percent of the time. It was assumed that the examiner was competent and thorough. Thus, if "Abdomen" was checked as normal, it was assumed that the examiner had listened for renal bruits and heard none.

It is noteworthy that in only one case out of 45, or about two percent, was hypertension due to a secondary cause, as far as could be ascertained using the Institute's criteria. Of the cases of essential hypertension, 86 percent were mild, 12 percent were moderate and none were severe. The one case of secondary hypertension was treated properly by the family physician without referral. This study would indicate that hypertension is a widespread disease which can be readily diagnosed and properly treated by the family physician in almost all cases.

The use of the tracer technique appears to be a promising quality assessment method which can be utilized in family practice with a minimal allocation of time, money and other resources. By requiring a review of the practice against contemporary health-care standards, the tracer technique also enhances the quality of care through self-teaching and evaluation.

Table 3. *Prevalence of Hypertension Rochester, New York and Baltimore, Maryland*

Family Medicine	
Age	Prevalence (%)
29	2.8
36–49	15.9
50+	18.4

The Baltimore Study	
Age	Prevalence (%)
35	1.4
36–49	15.4
50+	43.1

REFERENCES

1. Kessner, DM, Kalk CE, Singer J: Assessing health quality—the case for tracers. N Engl J Med 288:189–194, 1973.
2. Veterans Administration Cooperative Study Group on Antihypertensive Agents: Effects of treatment on morbidity in hypertension. I. Results in patients with diastolic blood pressure averaging 115 through 129 mm Hg. JAMA 202:1028-1034, 1967

3. Veterans Administration Cooperative Study Group on Antihypertensive Agents: Effects of treatment on morbidity in hypertension. II. Results in patients with diastolic blood pressure averaging 90 through 114 mm Hg. JAMA 213:1143-1152, 1970

4. McKee PA, Castelli WP, McNamara PM, et al: Natural history of congestive heart failure: The Framingham study. N Engl J Med 285:1441-1445, 1971

5. Metcalfe DHH: Knowing what goes on, or, cohort review in primary care. Del Med J 44(9):252-256, 1972

6. US Department of Health, Education, and Welfare National Health Survey: Hypertension and hypertensive heart disease in adults. United States, 1960-1962. National Center for Health Statistics, US Public Health Service Publication No. 1000, Series 11, No. 13, Washington, DC, Superintendent of Documents, 1966

7. Chronic Illness in the United States. Chronic Illness in a Large City, June 1949-June 1956. Vol. IV. The Baltimore Study, Cambridge, Massachusetts, 1957

8. Society of Actuaries: Build and Blood Pressure Study, vol. 1. Chicago, Society of Actuaries, 1959

Physician Preference for Criteria Mapping in Medical Care Evaluation*

Sheldon Greenfield, Sherrie H. Kaplan, George A. Goldberg, Mary Ann Nadler, and Rosalyn Deigh-Hewertson

This study was designed to determine which of three quality assessment methods most validly identifies deficient care. Process criteria were developed to assess outpatient care for urinary tract infection using each of three methods: a limited "list" of seven criteria, an extensive "list" of 40 criteria, and a criteria map (CM) which uses branching logic to identify applicable criteria according to the specific needs of each case. Defining deficiency as compliance with less than 60 percent of criteria, the extensive list found all 66 cases deficient; the limit list, 27 (41.0 percent); and the CM system, 15 (22.7 percent). After excluding the extensive list because of its nondiscrimination, 23 discrepancies in rating remained between the limited list and the CM. Ten physicians unaware of the results reviewed all 23 cases. In 12 of these 23 cases, at least seven of the ten physicians preferred the rating of one method over another; the CM assessment was preferred in 11 of the 12 cases (P < .01). Criteria maps, providing a patient-specific approach, offer a more valid assessment of medical care than either the extensive or limited list.

Comparisons of medical audit scores with measures of outcomes of care[1-3] have often failed to demonstrate positive associations between medical process and patient outcome. In such studies, the scores from measures of patient outcome have usually exceeded those for medical process. This relatively consistent finding suggests a sys-

*Reprinted by permission from *The Journal of Family Practice*, 6(5):1079-1086, 1978.

tematic difficulty with the "measurement" of process. As recently suggested by Brook,[4] one of the possible factors contributing to the process/outcome measurement disparity is the inherent inability of a list of process criteria to reflect the patient-specific medical decisions/actions which are most relevant to that patient's outcomes. The logical processes of the physician, who sequentially collects preliminary patient data, identifies positive findings, and takes specific actions based on those findings, are excluded from evaluations which rely on a criteria list.

The authors have developed a method called Criteria Mapping[5] which, by tracking physician logic for a given problem or diagnosis, limits the actual number of criteria applied to a given patient's case to those criteria which are relevant to that case. Criteria constructed in this way have greater potential for identifying those specific medical processes that will lead to discrete patient outcomes. Results using this method have been shown to correlate with discrete outcomes for at least one problem—chest pain as evaluated in an Emergency Department.[6]

This paper reports the findings of the first in a series of studies undertaken to compare representative explicit criteria lists with criteria mapping, to determine which method more accurately measures medical process. In this study, physician judgment is used as the standard of reference in the analysis of three process assessment methods. Quality-of-care assessment methods are designed to identify cases which would be considered by physicians to be inadequately managed. A method which more closely conforms to these physician judgments of adequacy can be considered of greater utility than one which shows less conformity with physician judgment.

Methods

Setting and Problem Selection

A family practice training unit affiliated with the University of California, Los Angeles (UCLA) served as the site for the study and supplied patients' records for evaluation. Urinary tract infection (UTI) in adult females was chosen because of the frequency of occurrence in this setting, the relatively important role of primary care in the control of acute morbidity, and the po-

tential for prevention of chronic renal disease.

The Process of Assessment Methods

Three evaluation methods were chosen for comparison: two criteria lists—one an extensive, comprehensive list, the other a more abbreviated list—and a criteria map. These three methods were selected as representative of the types of process assessment measures currently in use. The first method, an extensive list containing 40 items applicable to each case, was generated by the American Society of Internal Medicine.[7] A portion of this list appears in Table 1. It is clear from inspection that this

Table 1. *Long List Criteria for Quality of Care*[7] *First Section**

Acute Urinary Tract Infection in the Female

	A. History (specific reference to vesical dysfunction):
Score: _____	1. Frequency of urination
_____	a. Day
_____	b. Night
_____	2. Obstructive symptoms
_____	3. Pain
_____	a. Nature
_____	b. Location
_____	c. Radiation
_____	4. Hematuria
_____	5. Pattern of incontinence
_____	6. Chronology of symptomatology
_____	7. Previous urologic disease
_____	8. Previous urologic treatment
_____	9. Previous urologic instrumentation
_____	10. Obstetrical history
_____	11. Gynecologic history
_____	12. Medication initiated for this illness prior to contacting physician
_____	13. Duration of symptoms before contacting physician
_____	14. Previous evaluation of genitourinary system
_____	15. Temperature
_____	16. Chills
_____	17. History of recent sexual contact
_____	18. History of other recent infection

---

*A total of 22 additional criteria for the physical examination, laboratory, therapy, and follow-up examination constitute the remainder of this list.

Table 2. *Abbreviated List (Complete)*

1. Mention of presence or absence of any one or all of the following:
   a. dysuria
   b. frequency
   c. urgency
2. Urinalysis showing
   ≥10 white blood cells per high power field
3. Urinalysis showing
   ≤10 epithelial cells per high power field
4. Appropriate antibacterial agent to include *only one* of the following:
   a. sulfonamide
   b. ampicillin
   c. tetracycline
   d. nitrofurantoin
   e. trimethoprim-sulfa
5. Antibacterial agent given at least 10 days
6. Repeat urinalysis requested
7. Repeat urinalysis obtained 10 to 14 days after therapy is initiated

list includes items for evaluation of the most complex cases of urinary tract infection. The more economical "abbreviated list" (Table 2) contained only items applicable to *all* cases. This list was developed by the family practice unit medical staff using the California Medical Association's Patient Care Audit method, and is representative of an abbreviated list which has limited ability to evaluate complex cases.

The third method, a criteria map, was initially developed by members of the Department of Medicine at UCLA and was subsequently modified by the family practice unit. Because of the branching, patient-specific format of these criteria (as shown schematically in Figure 1), the actual items applicable to each case varied. The map contained a total of 97 items, but an average of five criteria applied to any given case. For example, different criteria would apply if the patient had vaginal symptoms, or was pregnant, or had a previous history of urinary tract infection, or was diabetic. In these cases, a more in-depth evaluation is required and is accounted for in the criteria map. However, for uncomplicated urinary tract infection—which accounts for the

majority of adult female patients with UTI presenting at a family practice unit—only a few criteria apply (Figure 2). In addition, many "options" for diagnosis and treatment are provided in the criteria map (accounting for many of the total 97 items), such as alternative confirmation of the diagnosis by "any of bacteriuria, pyuria, or a positive urine culture." These options allow for accepted variations in clinical "styles" (eg, choice of range of antibiotics, diagnostic techniques) not accounted for by a criteria list. If any of these findings are present, the subsequent criteria for treatment and follow-up apply. If none of these findings are present, the abstractor need not proceed to that section of the map

SCHEMATIC REPRESENTATION OF PART OF
URINARY TRACT INFECTION CRITERIA MAP

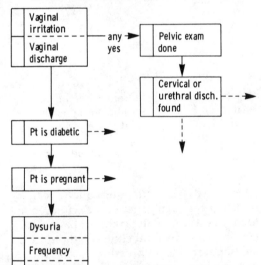

Fig. 1. Boxes to the left of each item are provided for coding. Positive responses to an item lead to the next item on the right. Negative responses or "missing" information are directed down to the next vertical item. The abstractor looks only for the items to which he/she is directed by the arrows. Here, if neither vaginal irritation nor vaginal discharge were reported in the record, the abstractor follows the arrow down and does not seek information concerning the performance of pelvic examination or the discovery of cervical or urethral discharge.

URINARY TRACT INFECTION CRITERIA MAP:
UNCOMPLICATED INFECTION AND ACUTE PYELONEPHRITIS

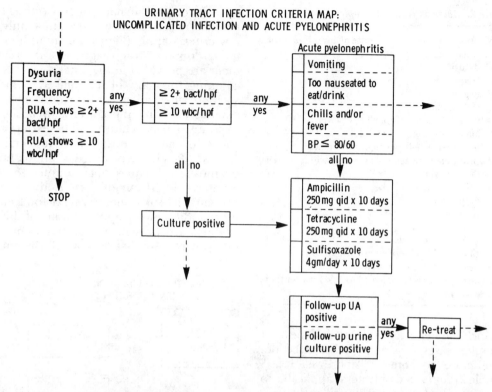

Fig. 2. Boxes to the left of each item are provided for coding. Positive responses to an item lead to the next item on the right. Negative responses or "missing" information are directed down to the next vertical item. "STOPs" are placed after items for which subsequent items would exceed the limits of the criteria map. The abstractor looks only for the items to which he/she is directed by the arrows. Therefore, for any individual case, only a fraction of the available criteria is applied.

which deals with the subsequent (conditional) criteria. In general, the criteria map identified various subgroups of patients according to individual clinical findings (eg, chills, fever, blood pressure ≤ 80/60 mm Hg, positive urine cultures). Subsequent criteria are then applied only to patients with the relevant predisposing clinical findings.

When development of the three criteria sets was complete, the content of each was reviewed by the principal investigator to ensure that the standards (not the criteria themselves) required by each set were comparable (eg, positive urinalysis meant ≥ 10 white blood cells/high power field for all methods).

Using each of the three methods described above, the charts of 66 patients presenting to the family practice unit with either symptoms of urinary tract infection or a positive routine urinalysis were abstracted. For the purpose of this study, an individual patient score was computed for each case, using each of the criteria sets. Those cases failing to meet an arbitrary level of 60 percent of the required criteria were rated "inadequate." (This very liberal limit was chosen to allow for reasonable variation in care based on the underlying assumption that many of the criteria commonly designated for urinary tract infection are of uncertain clinical value.)[8] If, for example, a case complied with 75 percent of the California Medical Association (CMA) criteria, 50 percent of the criteria-map criteria, and 40 percent of the American Society of Internal Medicine (ASIM) criteria, it would receive, respectively, "Adequate," "Inadequate," and "Inadequate" ratings.

When discrepancies in ratings between the methods occurred, an external estimate of the quality of care was used to indicate which method more accurately reflected the quality of care. It was decided not to use the outcomes of care for this usually self-limited disease, since outcomes such as symptomatic relief may be unrelated to good care for urinary tract infection (that is, they are likely to correlate poorly with process). In addition, poor outcomes, such as persistent positive culture, are infrequent, and a prohibitively large sample size would have been needed to obtain a sufficient number of negative outcomes to show a significant correlation between processes and outcomes.[8,9] Lastly, while patient outcome is clearly one form of validation of medical process, and is currently the focus of considerable attention, it has limited feasibility as a method for validation of patient care audits. For these reasons, it was decided to validate the methods of medical process assessment by using physicians' independent evaluations of the adequacy or inadequacy of process.

Ten UCLA primary care physicians of varying ages and both sexes—six internists and four family physicians (none of whom was involved in the criteria development)—were presented with an abstract of each case with conflicting method assessments. Essentially all the information in these short ambulatory care notes was put into the abstract; abstracts were used to avoid the effect of poor handwriting and recognition of signatures. In addition, conflicting judgments regarding the adequacy of the care for that case and the corresponding reasons for the judgment rendered by each method were provided. An example of the abstract presented to the physicians is shown in Figure 3. Each physician was asked to read each case abstract and the accompanying evaluations by each method, and to decide which method most appropriately evaluated the care. The methods were labeled only "A," "B," or "C" in order to prevent easy identification. In addition, to reduce the effects of preexisting bias toward any of the methods, the physicians were not shown any of the criteria sets in advance of completing the case reviews.

Fig. 3. Case #213—Medical Record Abstract.

___ Patient complains of pain over bladder and burning on urination.

___ No costovertebral angle tenderness, but suprapubic tenderness.

___ Urinalysis shows 2–3 red blood cells per high power field; 40–55 white blood cells per high power field with few clumps; moderate bacteria; many epithelial cells.

___ Patient was treated with Azo Gantrisin for 10 days.

___ Urine culture from this visit shows 25,000 E coli per cc.

___ No follow-up urinalysis or culture requested.

Method A: Adequate	**Method B:** Inadequate
___ Urinalysis positive	___ No follow-up urinalysis ordered or done
___ Patient was treated with appropriate antibiotic	___ Urinalysis shows epithelial cells
___ Negative culture and no previous history of UTI; therefore, no follow-up necessary	
Agree ___	Agree ___

Table 3. *Charts Judged Inadequate by Each Method*

	Total Number Charts	Number Inadequate	% Inadequate
Long list	66	66	100.0
Abbreviated list	66	27	41.0
Criteria map	66	15	22.7

Results

As illustrated in Table 3, of the total of 66 charts abstracted, using the standard of ≥ 60 percent as the requirement for adequate care, the long list judged all cases as having received inadequate care. The abbreviated (limited or "short") list found 41 percent of the cases to be inadequate, while the criteria map showed 22.7 percent (15 out of the 66) to be inadequate.

Because the long list failed to discriminate even minimally between adequate and inadequate care (ie, all charts were found to be inadequate), further comparisons were made only between the abbreviated list and the criteria map review results.

To determine whether using an "adequate" cutoff point of 60 percent could have been responsible for the differences in ratings by these methods, the data were reviewed for rank order correlations of method scores. No correlation between rank orders of the two methods was found, indicating that the differences found (22.7 percent vs 41 percent) were not artifacts of scaling. In addition, the data were analyzed using 50 percent and 75 percent adequacy cutoffs; use of these levels did not change the results significantly.

The review procedure is summarized in Figure 4. There were 23 cases in which the two methods, mapping and the abbreviated list, gave opposite ratings as to the adequacy of care. These 23 cases were then subjected to physician review. The results of the physician review of these 23 cases are presented in Table 4. In a total of 12 cases, physicians showed a definite preference for one method over the other, as evidenced by a high degree of concordance, ie, at least seven physicians agreeing with the rating of one method over the other for any case. Of these 12 cases, method A (criteria mapping) was chosen 11 times. In only one instance of definitve physician preference was method B (the abbreviated list) chosen over method A. If the two methods were equally likely to be preferred, the chance of seeing a preference this extreme is less than 1 in 100 (P < .01), by a test of proportions.

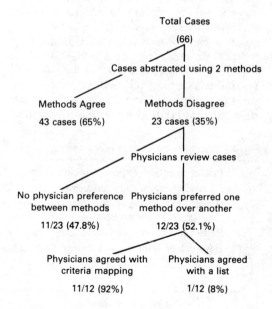

Fig. 4. Review procedure. The methods disagreed in a substantial percentage of cases (35 percent). When physicians perferred one method's decision over the other, they nearly always agreed with the criteria mapping decision. Thus, criteria mapping comes closer to judging quality of care in the same way as physicians would judge it.

Table 4. *Method Choice in Cases with High Concordance (≥7/10 Physicians)*

	Cases with High Concordance
Method A	11
Method B	1
Total	12
Total Cases	23

Examination of these 11 "highly preferred" cases revealed that 8 of the 11 either had complications or unusual presentations, all of which could be explained or included in the various branches of the criteria map, but could not be captured by the list. Five had unusual presentations such as lower abdominal pain, dyspareunia, nocturia, etc. Two had a history of urinary tract infection requiring more investigation and follow-up than a list could fully encompass, and one had a persistent infection which was documented by a positive culture and required follow-up. Criteria map assessment of the case illustrated in Figure 3 did not include follow-up urinalysis since the intitial culture was negative.

For the remaining 11 cases of the 23, the physicians made no definitive choice between either of the methods. Review of these records revealed straightforward, uncomplicated cases in which physician choice would be expected to vary according to individual preference for specific criteria. In these cases, additional qualifying clinical information usually provided by a criteria map would not contribute to the adequate/inadequate decision.

To determine whether the choice of method was affected by the individual physician's tendency to judge cases consistently as adequate or inadequate, the physicians' choice of method was analyzed by method rating (adequate or inadequate) for each case. Physicians were just as likely to choose the criteria map assessment (method A) for a case which had been rated adequate as for one which had been rated inadequate. Similarly, physicians chose the

list method as often when it judged a case adequate as when it judged it inadequate. The criteria mapping method was preferred over the list method regardless of rating.

Discussion

This study was concerned primarily with the relative accuracy with which a method could assess the quality of care rendered. Additionally, there was interest in determining whether a method could, by increased accuracy of evaluation, reduce the need for physician review of cases.

Consequently, attention was focused on the 23 discrepant judgments (35 percent). In those 11 cases (47.8 percent of the 23) for which the physician choice was discernible—that is, those cases where there was clear consensus—the explanation for that choice (as indicated by participating physicians) was that the method chosen (ie, criterian mapping) more completely explained the clinical details of the case. That is, when the cases were more complex, criteria mapping provided a more valid assessment of the care. Where the cases were relatively more simple and straightforward, there was no basis for either system to provide a more discriminating evaluation, and therefore physicians had no strong preference for either method.

The choice of method was not based on whether the method resulted in an adequate or inadequate rating; preference for criteria mapping was consistent regardless of the rating this method rendered. Subjective opinions or implicit judgments about quality of care in the absence of objective evaluations have proven to be unreliable in the past.[10] One factor which may have contributed to the variability of these judgments is that each physician-judge in an implicit review may apply his or her own unique standards of care to the evaluation effort. In an attempt to control this problem, physicians in this study were specifically asked to choose between two conflicting ratings and accompanying explanations in reviewing the data in the case abstract. Therefore, the physician judgment required was to determine the relative completeness and validity of each assessment, rather than independently to rate the case.

Because of the poor correlation between process and outcomes for urinary tract infection,[8] outcomes were not used as validation. Instead, this approach—that of using physician judgment—attempted to approximate the "real life" circumstances under which quality-of-care evaluations are performed. That is, it is usual practice for physicians to review the questionable cases identified by a quality-of-care evaluation.

The inherent inability of a criteria list to account for the progressive logic of the medical care process can account for the relatively low scores obtained from applying either list to the care documented. The physician, in caring for the individual patient, collects certain data and takes action (either management or collection of further information) on the basis of the data collected. The medical care process is conditional—not all things are done for all patients with the same disease or complaint. The single explicit list, intended for application to all cases of a specific disease or diagnosis, fails to account for this conditionality. Thus, routine cases requiring only a few criteria fail to comply with extensive lists of criteria designed to account for very complicated cases; similarly, more abbreviated lists designed to apply a limited number of criteria to all cases fail to provide a meaningful evaluation of the more complicated cases. It is not surprising, then, that low performance scores are frequently found when lists are used to evaluate medical care. However, the criteria map applies only relevant criteria, in sequential fashion, to an individual case, so these criteria are more patient-specific than disease-specific. It would be expected that when these conditional, decision-oriented criteria are used to measure care, a more valid assessment of care results.

The choice of urinary tract infection for a comparison of these two methods put the criteria mapping method at a considerable disadvantage. The strength of criteria mapping lies in the measurement of care of those diagnoses which have multiple divergent subgroups of patients, more complicated cases, or more options for diagnosis and treatment. Since the majority of cases of urinary tract infection in women are relatively straightforward, little conditionality is required and therefore, with respect to ability to assess care, relatively little difference would be expected between the criteria map and a list. A comparative assessment of almost any other problem (with the exception of the most self-limited conditions such as upper respiratory tract infections) would be expected to show even greater differences between evaluations of the methods. Nevertheless, the fact that the criteria mapping method was consistently preferred in the assessment of this problem suggests that even for simple problems, medical practice varies sufficiently to require flexibility in the evaluation of care.

Although criteria mapping may appear to be more involved, it is neither more complicated nor more extensive than a criteria list. It is only as complex as the individual case requires. Indeed, for patients with uncomplicated urinary tract infections, this method provides more flexibility: most of the branching criteria will never be abstracted, and the map will consequently require fewer criteria than even the abbreviated list. For more complex cases, the criteria map may require as much information as an extensive criteria list. However, unlike the list method, the map method would require additional information *only* for the relatively few cases which warrant a complete analysis.

Criteria mapping, which balances economy of criteria and allows for case complexity, seeks to make sense of evaluation of medical care by tracking physician logic. If quality-of-care evaluation is to provide meaningful results, it is essential to reflect the medical decision process accurately. Extensive criteria lists, even those modified by weighting techniques, may have the effect of increasing the cost of health care without contributing to the health of patients.[2] On the other hand, abbreviated lists may not provide enough of the essential information to permit a valid evaluation of medical care, and as a result many records may require subsequent (and costly) physician review.

Current trends in quality-of-care assessment reflect increased awareness of the need to incorporate the idea of logic or conditionality into assessment measures. Some studies have accounted for conditionality by subcategorizing patients into basic/inclusive subgroups (ie, diabetics, individuals over 40 years of age, males/females, etc).[11] Criteria mapping has attempted to incorporate both broad subgroupings of patients *and* clinical variations in patient presentations in the formulation of a method capable of accurate and efficient medical care evaluation.

It may be concluded that even for an uncomplicated, rather standard outpatient problem with minimal recording, the criteria mapping approach is as feasible, and more discriminating, than either a simple or a complex list. It corresponds better with the actual process of medical care, offers an alternative to the more rigid and less satisfying list, and shows potential for ultimately narrowing the gap between process and outcome measures.

Acknowledgment

Supported by Grant No. HS 01320, from the Center for Health Services Research and Development, United States, Public Health Service. The authors wish to thank Dr. Shan Cretin, Dr. Robert H. Brook, Ms. Linda Worthman, and Ms. Nancy Solomon for careful review of the manuscript. We are also grateful to Dr. Charles E. Lewis for continuing support and advice.

Author's Update

In recent continuing research on the use of criteria mapping to evaluate physician performance, we designed a study to validate this approach.* If criteria mapping measures the quality of care accurately, scores resulting from using a criteria map to review charts should show a relation to patient outcome. In other words, if the care is good and the criteria map scores indicate that it is good, the patient should have good outcomes; if the care is inadequate, and criteria mapping scores indicate that it is inadequate, the outcome should be poor. In this study of patients with chest pain, we demonstrated a correlation between medical process measured by criteria mapping and patient outcome. Several groups around the country are currently developing criteria maps in which they are using a scoring (weighting) system developed by us as part of this research. Continuing work on this approach continues to indicate its value as a measure of physician performance.

REFERENCES

1. Nobrega FT, Morrow GW Jr, Smoldt RK, et al: Quality assessment in hypertension: Analysis of process and outcome methods. N Engl J Med 296:145, 1977
2. Brook RH, Appel FA: Quality-of-care assessment: Choosing a method for peer review. N Engl J Med 288:1323, 1973
3. Romm FJ, Hulka BS, Mayo F: Correlates of outcomes in patients with congestive heart failure. Med Care 14:765, 1976
4. Brook RH: Quality—Can we measure it? N Engl J Med 296:170, 1977
5. Greenfield S, Lewis CE, Kaplan SH, et al: Peer review by criteria mapping: Criteria for diabetes mellitus. Ann Intern Med 83:761, 1975

*Greenfield S, Cretin S, Worthman L, et al. Comparison of a Criteria Map to a Criteria List in Quality-of-Care Assessment for Patients with Chest Pain: The Relation of Each to Outcome. Med Care, 19:3, 1981

6. Greenfield S, Nadler MA, Morgan MT, et al: The clinical investigation and management of chest pain in an emergency department: Quality assessment by criteria mapping. Med Care 15:898, 1977

7. Hare RL, Barnoon S: Medical care appraisal and quality assurance in the office practice of internal medicine. American Society of Internal Medicine, National Center for Health Services Research and Development, US Department of Health, Education, and Welfare, HSM 110-70-420, 1973

8. Lindsay MI, Hermans PE, Nobrega FT, et al: Quality of care assessment: Part I: Outpatient management of acute bacterial cystitis as the model. Mayo Clin Proc 51:307, 1976

9. Brook RH, Davies-Avery AD, Greenfield S, et al: Assessing the quality of medical care using outcome measures: An overview of the method. Med Care 15(Suppl):1, 1977

10. Richardson FM: Peer review of medical care. Med Care 10:29, 1972

11. Jacobs CM, Jacobs ND: The PEP Primer: The JCAH Performance Evaluation Procedure for Auditing and Improving Physician Care. Chicago, Quality Review Center, Joint Commission on Accreditation of Hospitals, 1974

A Review of the General Practitioner Obstetric Service in Colchester 1970-1979*

J. D. Owen

I report here on an audit of the work of a general practitioner maternity unit situated in the same building as a consultant obstetric unit. Between 1970 and 1979, 10,588 patients were admitted under the care of general practitioner obstetricians. The perinatal mortality rate averaged 6.9. I show in the report how an audit of such a unit can be carried out, and demonstrate that general practitioner obstetricians still have a valid and useful place in a district obstetric service.

Introduction

In 1963 the Staff Committee of the Colchester general practitioner maternity unit initiated a form of audit. It is based on a punch card system designed to record the basic details of every patient admitted to the general practitioner unit. The findings from the audit are circulated to all interested parties as an annual report. The present paper is based on figures extracted from these reports.

Method

The information recorded on the punch card includes age and parity, past obstetric history, major abnormalities in pregnancy, type of labour, complications if any, and finally, details of the baby and the duration of the patient's stay in hospital. In the early years practitioners took turns to do the punch card summaries but, with several

*Reprinted by permission from *Journal of the Royal College of General Practitioners*, 31:92-96, 1981.

people being involved, discrepancies inevitably appeared owing to differing interpretations of the available data. Since 1971 a retired senior midwife has undertaken the task of making the punch card record, and the analysis is now consistent from year to year.

Results

Table 1 shows the number of patients booked, admitted, delivered and transferred in the Colchester general practitioner maternity unit between 1970 and 1979.

The discrepancy between bookings and admissions to the general practitioner unit is accounted for partly by miscarriages and removals from the district, but chiefly by referrals during pregnancy to the consultant antenatal clinics. The delivery figures for the consultant unit are included for comparison, but it should be remembered that this unit serves the whole of north-east Essex and not only Colchester.

The number of admissions is made up of patients delivered in the general practitioner unit plus the number physically transferred, but the transfer rate is arrived at by adding to these transferred cases those patients delivered by the obstetric registrar in the general practitioner unit.

Perinatal Mortality

The most important measurement in an obstetric audit is perinatal mortality. When our audit began in 1963 the perinatal mortality rate per 1,000 admissions was

243

Table 1. *Bookings, Admissions, Deliveries and Transfers, Colchester General Practitioner Unit (1970–1979).*

	1970	1971	1972	1973	1974	1975	1976	1977	1978	1979
Bookings	1512	1549	1496	1529	1409	1386	1470	1499	1429	1506
Admissions	1094	1154	1084	1108	937	1006	940	998	1077	1155
Deliveries	1018	1058	1006	1010	894	952	875	926	1000	1039
Transfers	76	96	78	98	43	54	65	72	77	116
Consultant unit deliveries	1187	1330	1370	1443	1554	1480	1580	1556	1732	1771

22.4. The rate for 1979 was 6.9 per 1,000. Comparisons with the perinatal mortality rate for England and Wales and with that for north-east Essex are shown in Figure 1. The average perinatal mortality rate for the general practitioner unit during the period 1970 to 1979 was 6.9; the apparently large fluctuations (Figure 1) are due to the small number of deaths.

Every case of perinatal mortality which occurs in the area is studied in detail by the North-East Essex Perinatal Mortality Survey (Owen, 1977), and this survey is continuing. However, analysis of the cause of perinatal loss, using the Aberdeen clinicopathological classification (Baird and Thomson, 1969), fails to reveal a clear pattern. For instance, none of the four "mature, cause uncertain" losses in 1979 was considered to have had an avoidable factor.

Table 2 classifies the perinatal deaths among admissions to the Colchester general practitioner unit between 1970 and 1979. This includes those transferred to the specialist unit.

The percentage of babies dying from malformation in the whole north-east Essex area during the period 1970 to 1979 was only 20 percent of the total loss. The fact that 40 percent of the general practitioner unit deaths were made up of malformations suggests that high-risk groups are being properly referred to consultant antenatal clinics before admission to the general practitioner unit. The "mature, uncertain" group is made up mainly of unpredictable intrapartum accidents, and the "premature, uncertain" deaths are made up of un-

explained intrauterine deaths and the loss of small preterm babies.

Accurate record keeping and adhering to rules about blood tests are additional indicators of obstetric efficiency. In 1966, 10 percent of antenatal record cards were inadequate, but in the last five years this figure has never been higher than half of one percent. The cases concerned are usually late or unbooked cases who have not attended for any antenatal care.

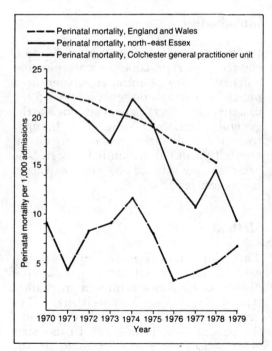

Fig. 1. Perinatal mortality rates per 1,000 births, England and Wales, Colchester general practitioner unit, north-east Essex (1970–1979).

Table 2. *Perinatal Deaths, Colchester General Practitioner Unit (1970–1979)**

	1970	1971	1972	1973	1974	1975	1976	1977	1978	1979	Total
Malformation	2	3	3	5	4	3	1	2	3	3	29
Mechanical	0	1	1	0	1	1	0	0	0	1	5
Premature, uncertain	4	1	1	2	2	3	1	1	2	0	17
Mature, uncertain	2	0	3	3	4	1	1	1	0	4	19
Pre-eclampsia	1	0	0	0	0	0	0	0	0	0	1
Antepartum haemorrhage	0	0	1	0	0	0	0	0	0	0	1
Serological	1	0	0	0	0	0	0	0	0	0	1
Total	10	5	9	10	11	8	3	4	5	8	73
Perinatal loss/ 1000 cases admitted	9.0	4.3	8.3	9.0	11.7	8.0	3.2	4.0	4.6	6.9	6.9

*Figures include cases transferred to the specialist unit.

Transfers to Consultant Unit

About 30 general practitioners use the Colchester general practitioner unit. Each will have his or her own criteria for transferring a patient to specialist care. In 1966 the transfer rate was 2.3 percent. In the last eight years the rate has varied between 6.7 percent in 1974 and 11.4 percent in 1979, the mean transfer rate being 8.4 percent.

Since 1970, it has been possible to analyse, in some detail, patient transfers in relation to age and parity, and type of problem. Table 3 shows the percentage of each age and parity group transferred and clearly confirms that the elderly primigravida is most likely to come to transfer, although after 1972, when the criteria for admission had been altered to exclude primigravidae over 35, the percentage of this group transferred fell considerably. The mean transfer rate for primigravidae aged between 19 and 29 is 12.4 percent and that for the elderly primigravidae is 29.6 percent. This compares with 4.1 percent and 3.0 percent respectively for gravida 2 to 4. Between 1976 and 1978 the transfer rate was lower for the older age group than

Table 3. *Age and Parity of Patients Transferred to the Consultant Unit (1970–1979)*

	Percentage Transferred									
	1970	1971	1972	1973	1974	1975	1976	1977	1978	1979
Primigravida										
Age <19	5.1	5.6	11.7	6.5	2.3	—	6.8	12.2	14.0	8.0
19–29	14.1	8.8	15.0	14.1	7.6	7.4	12.5	13.3	13.2	17.5
30–39	33.0	33.0	50.0	8.3	13.3	20.0	5.8	9.0	9.0	42.8
Gravida 2–4										
Age <19	—	—	—	—	25.0	33.0	—	—	—	—
19–29	3.3	2.7	4.9	8.8	1.9	3.0	4.3	4.6	3.4	8.2
30–39	2.9	4.3	2.9	2.2	2.2	3.7	6.4	4.0	6.0	4.0
Mean transfer rate	6.9	8.3	7.2	8.6	4.6	5.3	6.9	7.2	7.1	10.0
Including registrar deliveries	6.9	8.3	7.2	10.5	7.1	6.7	7.6	9.0	8.0	11.4

for the 19 to 29 age group. However, very small numbers of older primigravidae are involved—only 21 were admitted in 1976, 22 in 1977 and 21 in 1979, compared with 320, 293 and 341 of the 19 to 29 age group. These figures suggest that great care is generally exercised in booking older women into the general practitioner unit.

Figure 2 illustrates the pattern of the major causes of transfer from the general practitioner unit to specialist care, and includes those cases in which the obstetric reg-

istrars helped with the forceps delivery when there was delay in the second stage.

Transfers due to failure to establish labour after ARM or after spontaneous rupture decreased dramatically after 1975. It was at this time that the use of IV Syntocinon in the unit became an accepted procedure. There are now two electronic i.v. infusion counters available, but their use is subject to there being adequate nursing staff and the practitioner who instigates the procedure being available throughout the labour.

The routine use of IV Syntocinon does not, however, seem to have reduced the numbers transferred because of prolonged labour. In the last two years IV Syntocinon has been used in approximately 10 percent of all cases, yet transfers due to prolonged labour still represented 29.5 percent of the cases transferred in 1979. Included in this group are cases variously classified in the punch card audit as high head at term, persistent occipito-posterior, cervical dystocia, uterine dysfunction, and disproportion. There are usually elements of all five factors in prolonged labour. The high heads and disproportions should be screened out before the onset of labour, but persistent occipito-posterior and uterine dysfunction are not so predictable.

There was a steady decline in the number of cases of pre-eclampsia transferred (PET) until 1979, when the figure reached 10 percent. It had begun to look as though all cases of PET were being screened out and referred to specialist antenatal care, but in 1979 there were 14 cases admitted who showed toxaemia of sufficient severity to warrant immediate transfer to the specialist unit.

Delay in the second stage of labour is the second most common cause of transfer to specialist care, representing 17.4 percent of the total number of transferred cases for the period 1970 to 1979. Approximately four fifths of this category (123 out of 158) were delivered by an obstetric registrar in the delivery suite of the general practitioner unit.

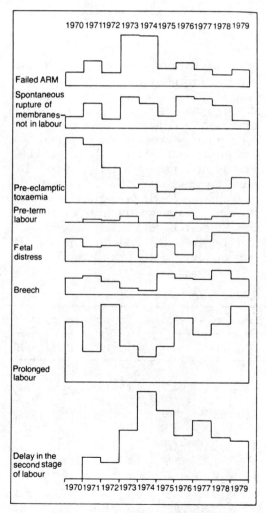

Fig. 2. Reasons for transfer to specialist care as a percentage of total transfers (1970–1979).

Table 4. *Forceps Deliveries by Obstetrics Registrars; Transfers Due to Prolonged Labour and Delay in the Second Stage (1973–1979)*

	Transfers Due to Prolonged Labour (Percentage of All Transfers)	Transfers Due to Delay in Second Stage (Percentage of All Transfers)	Forceps Deliveries by Obstetrics Registrars (Percentage of All Forceps Deliveries in General Practitioner Unit)
1973	15.0	20.0	29.3
1974	10.4	35.8	36.3
1975	14.7	27.9	24.2
1976	27.7	18.0	21.9
1977	20.0	24.4	25.0
1978	24.1	17.2	16.9
1979	29.5	15.1	20.2

Since 1974 the percentage of cases of prolonged labour has increased, whilst there has been a drop in the incidence of delay in the second stage. There has also been a reduction in the percentage of forceps deliveries carried out by registrars in the general practitioner unit. As Table 4 suggests, it is possible to infer from these developments that there is now earlier referral in those cases that are liable to end in forceps delivery and earlier diagnosis of poor progress in labour.

Further reasons for transfer include antepartum haemorrhage, prolapsed cord, patients referred for induction, malpresentations such as brow, a meningomyelocele, and several cases of retained placenta, but the numbers involved in each problem are too small to show graphically.

Procedures

Table 5 enumerates various procedures that are carried out. It shows that there was increased use of amniotomy in the mid-decade, usually by forewater rupture, but that latterly the ARM rate has been falling. The forceps rate, even allowing for forceps deliveries by registrars, remains fairly constant over the 10 years, and compares with that shown in figures published for other general practitioner units (Richmond, 1977; Marsh, 1977).

Episiotomy is performed more commonly in primigravidae than in multigravidae. However, second degree tears are more common in the latter group. This suggests that midwives perhaps hope to get away without stitches more often than they ought in multigravidae. The audit has been able to distinguish between episiotomy and second degree tears only for the last 3 years.

Intravenous Syntocinon is used in two ways: either in conjunction with ARM, or when labour is not becoming established after spontaneous rupture of the membranes or is just being sluggish. These cases are classified in the audit as uterine dysfunction. Table 6 shows that Syntocinon is used with ARM as often with multigravid as with primigravid patients, but that its use because of uterine dysfunction occurs twice as often in primigravid patients.

Discussion

The Colchester general practitioner obstetric unit is independent of the consultant unit, although it shares the same building. Relations between general practitioners and consultants are excellent, and there is no interference on the part of the consultants. Changes in policy have evolved gradually by a process of discussion. Some changes are initiated by general practitioners and some by the consultants, but the

Table 5. *Procedures (Numbers; Percentages of Deliveries on Admissions)(1970–1979)*

	1970	1971	1972	1973	1974	1975	1976	1977	1978	1979
Artificial rupture of membranes										
Number	87	109	167	157	138	166	103	127	136	121
Percentage of deliveries	(8.5)	(10.3)	(16.6)	(15.5)	(15.4)	(17.4)	(11.7)	(13.7)	(13.6)	(11.6)
Syntocinon infusion										
Number	51	39	73	52	73	86	102	137	181	169
Percentage of deliveries	(5.0)	(3.6)	(7.2)	(5.1)	(8.1)	(9.0)	(11.6)	(14.8)	(18.1)	(16.2)
*Episiotomy**										
Number								492	492	460
Percentage of deliveries			566	630	613	616	604	(53.0)	(49.2)	(44.3)
*Second degree perineal tears**										
Number								223	218	204
Percentage of deliveries								(24.0)	(21.8)	(19.7)
Forceps deliveries										
General practitioners	44	54	75	53	42	43	32	54	49	63
Registrars	—	6	4	22	24	14	9	18	10	16
Total	44	60	79	75	66	57	41	72	59	79
Percentage of admissions	(4.8)	(5.2)	(7.3)	(6.8)	(7.0)	(5.7)	(4.3)	(7.2)	(5.5)	(6.8)

*Episiotomy and second degree perineal tears were recorded separately only after 1977 and not at all before 1972.

'cog-wheel' system ensures full and open discussion before any changes are implemented.

The result is a dynamic general practitioner unit in which practitioners can offer their patients a personal service during the period of childbirth, and so strengthen the doctor-patient relationship. Knowing that her own doctor will attend her labour is often a great comfort to the expectant woman. The unit attempts to reinforce this feeling.

Table 6. *Use of IV Syntocinon in Induction and Stimulation of Labour (1975–1979)*

	Primigravidae		Multigravidae	
	Induction	Uterine Dysfunction	Induction	Uterine Dysfunction
1975	32	16	30	8
1976	32	27	32	11
1977	49	29	45	14
1978	49	52	55	25
1979	54	43	50	22

The pace of labour in the general practitioner unit is much gentler than in the specialist unit. There is no place for the Cardiff pump, although, as has been shown, extensive use is made of IV Syntocinon to maintain the impetus of labour. In the labour ward some of the ideas put forward by Leboyer (1975) are used—theatre lights are dimmed, and the infant is delivered direct onto the mother's abdominal wall. The body contact gives pleasure and enhances mother/baby bonding.

Labour and delivery in a general practitioner unit should encompass the best elements of a home confinement, namely continuity of care by the family doctor and a peaceful, unhurried approach by the nursing staff provided within the security of a well-equipped hospital environment. With the co-operation of our consultant colleagues we can offer our patients the best of both worlds. Because the specialist unit is nearby, everyone is confident that if a situation develops which a general practitioner cannot control, help is readily available. The importance of specialist assistance being close by is illustrated by the number of patients whose babies are delivered in the general practitioner unit by specialist registrars. However, a transfer rate of less than nine percent for the 10 years covered by this survey does not suggest that their help is misused. The survey also shows that in delivering 1,000 or more patients each year, the general practitioner obstetricians make a significant contribution in terms of manpower which the consultant service would be hardpressed to replace.

It is important to record these observations now because in September 1978 work started on an extension to the Colchester Maternity Hospital which includes a delivery suite in which general practitioners and consultants will work side by side. It is almost inevitable that some independence will be lost, at least in as much as it may prove difficult for patients to remain specifically under the care of their general practitioner.

REFERENCES

Baird, D. & Thomson, A. M. (1969). The survey of perinatal deaths reclassified by special clinico-pathological assessment. In Perinatal Problems. Eds. Butler, N. R. & Alberman, E. D. Edinburgh: E. & S. Livingstone

James, D. K. (1977). Patients transferred in labour from general practitioner maternity units. Journal of the Royal College of General Practitioners, 27, 414–418

Leboyer, F. (1975). Birth Without Violence. Translated from the French. London: Wildwood House

Marsh, G. N. (1977). Obstetric audit in general practice. British Medical Journal, 2, 1004–1006

Owen, J. D. (1977). North-East Essex perinatal mortality survey—1971-1975. British Journal of Obstetrics and Gynaecology, 84, 412–418

Richmond, G. A. (1977). An analysis of 3,199 patients booked for delivery in general practitioner obstetric units. Journal of the Royal College of General Practitioners, 27, 406–413

Audit of Obstetrical Care and Outcome in Family Medicine, Obstetrics, and General Practice*

William R. Phillips, Gregory A. Rice, and Richard H. Layton

To compare obstetrical practices and outcome, hospital charts were audited of 50 patients cared for by each of three physician groups: family medicine residents (FM), private obstetrician-gynecologists (OB), and private general practitioners (GP). The FM patient group was at highest perinatal risk on the basis of maternal age, marital status, socioeconomic status, and obstetrical history. FM patients had fewest total inductions, elective inductions, early surgical rupture of membranes, and augmented labors after conduction anesthesia. Mean duration of total labor and all stages of labor were equal for the three groups except FM multiparas, who had shorter total labors than GP multiparas. FM patients had the least anesthesia, the least analgesia, and the fewest conduction anesthetic blocks. Rates were equal among the three groups for cesarean section, episiotomy, and use of forceps. FM mothers had equal rates of perinatal complications and FM infants had equal Apgar scores compared to the other groups. These data differ from previously published studies. Documentation of quality and character of FM obstetrical care with the resulting favorable comparison to that of obstetricians and general practitioners has important implications for the fields of family medicine and maternal-child health care.

The practice of family medicine includes comprehensive care of family, mother, and newborn infant in continuity through the natural process of pregnancy and child-

*Reprinted by permission from *The Journal of Family Practice*, 6(6):1209-1216, 1978.

birth. Understanding of current trends in the development of the field of family medicine and in the evolution of its role in maternal-infant health-care services requires objective information on the quality and character of obstetric care provided by the family physician. The present study attempts to document the nature of obstetrical care in one family medicine program in an inner-city urban hospital setting, and thereby stimulate discussion and study of the role of obstetrics in family practice and the complementary role of family medicine in obstetrical care.

Method

The hospital records of 150 obstetric patients admitted to Providence Medical Center, Seattle, January through December of 1976, were reviewed from three groups: 50 of the 79 patients delivered by family medicine residents, 50 of the 413 patients delivered by private obstetrician-gynecologists, and 50 of the 88 patients delivered by private general practitioners. Using hospital medical record indexes, all obstetrical patients delivered during the study period were grouped according to specialty of attending physician and 50 patients were randomly selected from each group for inclusion in the study.

The 15 family medicine (FM) residents all worked at Providence Family Medical Center, a family practice residency training program which supplies comprehensive care including prenatal, obstetrical, and pediatric care to families in Seattle's inner-city community. Residents deliver the patients they follow for prenatal care, and deliveries are attended by family medicine faculty physicians or selected private general practice staff physicians. The five obstetrician-gynecologists (OB) were male and all except one were certified by the American Board of Obstetricians-Gynecologists. The seven general practitioners (GP) included two females and none were certified by the American Board of Family Practice. All private physicians in both groups had at least 20 years of practice experience.

Data were abstracted from each patient record to document the patient's demographic profile, selected process factors to assess obstetrical care, and measures of maternal and infant outcome. Comparisons were made between the three physician groups to document the obstetrical care they provided and to evaluate the resulting outcome. With N = 50 for each patient group, results reported in number of patients can be doubled to conveniently find group percentages.

Results

Patient Population

The demographic profile of patients from the three physician groups is shown in Table 1. Family medicine patients were significantly younger (median age 20 years) than either OB patients (median age 27 years) or GP patients (median age 25 years). Significantly larger proportions of the FM patients were never married and on public assistance than in either the OB or the GP groups. More FM patients were primiparas than in the OB group.

Labor

No differences were found between the three patient groups in the number of weeks gestation at delivery or in mean admission hematocrit level (37 percent for all three groups).

Induction of labor was performed signif-

Table 1. *Demographic Data*

	Family Medicine	Obstetrics	General Practice	Difference	
				FM-OB	FM-GP
Maternal Age (Years)					
Mean ± standard deviation	21.4 ± 4.0	28.6 ± 6.1	25.7 ± 5.9	$t = 6.91$ $P < 0.001$	$t = 4.21$ $P < 0.001$
Marital Status (Number)					
Never married	29	4	9	$\chi^2 = 17.42$	
Married ever	21	46	41	df = 2	
				$P < 0.001$	
Financial Status (Number)					
Public assistance	39	8	13	$\chi^2 = 30$	
Private insurance	11	42	37	df = 2	
				$P < 0.001$	
Parity (Number)					
Primipara	30	13	24	$\chi^2 = 12.03$	
Multipara	20	37	26	df = 2	
				$P < 0.005$	

Table 2. *Characteristics of Labor*

				Difference	
Number of Patients	**Family Medicine**	**Obstetrics**	**General Practice**	*FM-OB*	*FM-GP*
Induction of Labor					
Spontaneous labor	47	36	37	$\chi^2 = 9.25$	
Induced labor	3	14	13	df = 2	
Induced with indication	3	3	4	P < 0.01	
Induced without indication	0	10	9	P = 0.036*	P = 0.062*
Rupture of Membranes					
Spontaneous rupture	35	32	34	NS†	NS†
Surgical rupture	15	18	16		
Early surgical	1	7	6	P = 0.037*	P = 0.05*
Late surgical	14	11	10		
Augmentation of Labor					
After conduction anesthesia	1	6	5	P = 0.033*	P = 0.197*
Other indication	3	0	2		

*Fisher-Yates Exact Test for Fourfold Tables.[1]
†χ^2, df = 2, α = 0.05.

icantly less frequently in FM patients than in either OB or GP patients (Table 2). Premature rupture of membranes was the indication for all FM inductions while the OB group had significantly more inductions without any stated indication; a similar difference of borderline significance existed between FM and GP patients. There were no differences between the groups in proportion of patients with spontaneous rupture of membranes. Among those patients with surgical rupture of membranes, how-

Table 3. *Length of Labor*

				Difference*	
Mean ± Standard Deviation	**Family Medicine**	**Obstretrics**	**General Practice**	*FM-OB*	*FM-GP*
Total Labor (Hours)					
All patients	9.5 ± 6.9	7.1 ± 4.1	10.7 ± 7.9	NS	NS
Primiparas	13.0 ± 7.0	8.1 ± 4.7	13.0 ± 8.4	NS	NS
Multiparas	5.0 ± 3.1	6.8 ± 3.7	8.8 ± 6.9	NS	P < 0.02
Stage I (Hours)					
Primiparas	11.9 ± 6.7	7.4 ± 4.7	11.9 ± 8.1	NS	NS
Multiparas	4.6 ± 3.1	6.2 ± 14.3	7.9 ± 6.7	NS	NS
Stage II (Minutes)					
Primiparas	60.4 ± 36.7	36.9 ± 20.0	63.1 ± 27.6	NS	NS
Multiparas	20.9 ± 10.0	27.2 ± 15.7	24.1 ± 13.4	NS	NS
Stage III (Minutes)					
All patients	4.6 ± 3.7	3.8 ± 3.3	3.6 ± 2.0	NS	NS

*t-test, α = 0.05.

Table 4. *Anesthesia*

Number of Patients	Family Medicine	Obstetrics	General Practice	Difference*
Conduction Anesthesia				
Caudal block	1	25	24	P < 0.001
Spinal block	25	19	20	N.S.
Total conduction	26	44	44	P < 0.001
Pudendal, local or none	24	4	3	P < 0.001
General anesthesia	0	2	3	†

*χ^2, df = 2, α = 0.05.
†QNS for significance test.

ever, significantly fewer patients in the FM group than either the OB or the GP group had early surgical rupture of membranes (rupture at cervical dilation less than 4 cm and station less than zero).

Although no significant group differences were found in total frequency of oxitoxin augmentation of labor, significantly more OB patients than FM patients required augmentation for arrest of labor after conduction anesthesia. Comparison of mean duration of total labor or of each stage of labor (Table 3) failed to reveal any differences between patient groups, even when compared within primipara and multipara categories. The one exception was significantly shorter mean duration of total labor among multiparas in the FM group than the GP group.

Anesthesia

Significantly more FM patients had no anesthesia or only local or pudendal block anesthesia than either OB or GP patients (Table 4). Significantly fewer FM patients had conduction anesthesia than did OB or GP patients, the difference being due to fewer caudal blocks performed in the FM group with no difference in the rate of spinal blocks between the three groups. No FM patient had general anesthesia.

Analgesia

Significantly more FM patients received no analgesic than did the other two patient groups (Table 5). Among those patients

Table 5. *Analgesia*

	Family Medicine	Obstetrics	General Practice	Difference	
Number of Patients				χ^2 = 10.94	
Receiving no analgesic	13	8	1	df = 2	
Receiving any analgesia	37	42	49	P < .01	
Doses of Analgesic				FM-OB*	FM-GP*
(Mean ± Standard Deviation)					
All patients	1.9 ± 1.8	1.8 ± 1.4	2.5 ± 1.4	NS	P < 0.05
Patients receiving any analgesic	2.6 ± 1.6	2.2 ± 1.3	2.5 ± 1.4	NS	NS

*t-test, α = 0.05.

Table 6. *Delivery*

Number of Patients	Family Medicine	Obstetrics	General Practice	Difference*
Cesarean Section	5	6	3	NS
Fetal Position				FM-GP
Occiput anterior	44	40	35	$\chi^2 = 5.77$
Occiput posterior	4	8	13	df = 1
Breech	2	2	2	P < 0.025
Forceps				
Low forceps	21	26	28	NS
Mid forceps	1	4	4	
Episiotomy	43	46	41	NS

*χ^2, df = 2, α = 0.05.

who received any analgesic there was no difference between the three patient groups in the number of medication doses given. Among total patient groups, however, FM patients were given significantly fewer doses of analgesic than were GP patients.

Delivery

Between the three patient groups there were no differences in frequency of cesarean section or episiotomy (Table 6). The FM group had lower frequency of use of low, mid, and total forceps, but these differences failed to achieve statistical significance. The FM group had significantly

fewer cases of persistant posterior fetal position than the GP group.

Maternal Complications

The frequency of all complications—hemorrhage, fever, preecclampsia, hypotension, spinal headache—was equal for the FM and OB groups and lower than for the GP group, but the difference was not statistically significant (Table 7).

No difference was found in the frequency of all perineal lacerations between the three groups. Among patients with lacerations, however, the FM group had more fourth degree lacerations than the OB or GP groups. These fourth degree lacera-

Table 7. *Maternal Complications*

Number of Patients	Family Medicine	Obstetrics	General Practice	Difference	
Lacerations				FM-OB	FM-GP
Fourth degree	9	1	1	P = 0.04*	P = 0.0005*
Third degree	1	3	9		
Second degree					
Complications					
Any complication	7	6	14	NS†	NS†
No complication	43	44	36		

*Fisher-Yates Exact Test for Fourfold Tables.[1]
†χ^2, df = 1, α = 0.05.

Table 8. *Infant Outcome*

	Family Medicine	Obstetrics	General Practice	Difference
Apgar Score				
1-Minute Score:				
Mean	8.67	8.34	8.39	NS*
Range	4–10	2–10	0–10	
5-Minute Score:				
Mean	9.65	9.50	9.38	NS*
Range	8–10	4–10	0–10	
Infant Weight				
Mean	7 lb 8 oz	7 lb 3 oz	6 lb 14 oz	NS†
Range	4 lb 10 oz	4 lb 3 oz	3 lb 5 oz	
	10 lb 5 oz	9 lb 10 oz	9 lb 6 oz	

*Mann-Whitney U, $\alpha = 0.05$.
†t-test, $\alpha = 0.05$.

tions in the FM group were significantly associated with primipara births ($\chi^2 = 4.69$, df $= 1$, P < 0.05) and with the use of forceps ($\chi^2 = 5.08$, df $= 1$, P < 0.025) but not associated with infant birth weight, fetal position, or type of anesthesia. Length of postpartum hospital stay was equal for all three patient groups with a mean stay of 3.4 days.

Infant Outcome

Apgar scores at one minute and five minutes were highest for the FM patients, but the differences between the groups were not statistically significant (Table 8). No significant differences were found between groups in infant birth weight. One fetal death occurred in the GP group. Roughly half of each patient group chose to breast feed their infants.

Discussion

The points documented by this audit, of similarities and differences in the obstetrical care provided by family medicine residents, private obstetrician-gynecologists, and private general practitioners, illustrate the quality and character of the family

medicine approach to patient care in continuity through pregnancy and childbirth.

In each area examined, process and outcome measures documented the obstetrical care provided by family medicine residents to compare favorably to that of private OB and GP physicians despite the fact that the family medicine patient population was at significantly higher perinatal risk on the basis of age, marital status, socioeconomic class, and obstetrical history. Compared to their OB and GP colleagues, FM residents attained a record of equal length of labor, equal infant Apgar scores, equal rates of maternal complications, and equal lengths of postpartum hospital stay.

The features of FM obstetrical care that stood in contrast to the care provided by obstetrician-gynecologists and general practitioners characterized FM care as a more "natural" birth process. Family medicine patients were less frequently subjected to elective induction of labor, early surgical rupture of membranes, or oxytoxin augmentation of labor after anesthetic block. They received less analgesia and less anesthesia. Despite this relative lack of intervention, patients had no longer total labors and no increase in incidence of prolonged labor in any stage. In fact, FM residents tended to deliver multiparous women in shorter total time than did the general practitioners. The greater use of conduction anesthesia in the OB and GP patient groups was perhaps responsible for their higher incidence of persistent posterior fetal position.

Although there was no difference in rates of episiotomies and lacerations, the finding that a higher proportion of fourth-degree lacerations occurred in family medicine resident deliveries with the use of low forceps, suggests increased training and experience in this procedure may further improve resident skill.

This study was limited in size and scope and thereby in the generalizations that can be made from these observed associations. Larger studies are currently underway to further assess the suggestive findings and investigate larger patient populations and other patient care settings.

The audit previously published by Ely, Ueland, and Gordon of the University of Washington[3] comparing FM obstetrical care to that of a university obstetrics-gynecology department provides interesting confirmations and contrasts to the data presented here. Both studies found essentially no differences between the FM group and the comparison physician groups in incidence of prolonged second stage of labor or Apgar scores. Both studies documented less use of conduction anesthesia.

Unlike the present study, however, with its description of a high-risk patient population under the care of the FM residents, the University of Washington study compared a high-risk referral OB patient group to a relatively low-risk middle class FM patient population. Within this favorable patient population the University of Washington FM residents achieved a shorter length of postpartum hospital stay than their obstetrician-gynecologist counterparts, but they also recorded significantly longer first stages of labor in nulliparas and significantly higher incidence of maternal complications. In the present study FM physicians equaled the record of both the obstetrician-gynecologists and the general practitioners on these measures.

Caetano's study of birth certificates[4] suggests general physicians may diagnose and report complications of pregnancy and childbirth more accurately than obstetricians. That factor may operate equally in both the present study and that reported from the University of Washington, relatively inflating the complication rates for both groups of FM residents in comparison to the OB physician groups.

The documentation provided by this audit and similar studies provides a basis for the evaluation of the role of obstetrics in a comprehensive family practice and the role of family medicine in maternal-infant health care. Such evaluation comes at a time critical to the continuing growth and formulation of family medicine as a discipline organizing medical knowledge and health-care services, and critical to the development of policy and patterns of the nation's obstetrical care services.

Obstetrics is an integral part of family medicine. Mehl, Bruce, and Renner[5] compared family practices similar except in their inclusion or exclusion of obstetrics. They showed that including obstetrical care in a family medicine practice was associated with improved physician satisfaction with the practice, increased proportion of care provided in continuity and to entire families, larger numbers of pediatric patients, and increases in practice time devoted to problems in the areas of gynecology, orthopedics, minor surgery, and psychosocial problems, especially as treated in the context of the family.

The American Academy of Family Physicians (AAFP) has included prenatal and obstetrical care in the core curriculum for competency-based training in family practice residency training programs.[6] University departments of family medicine and of obstetrics and gynecology have seriously examined their roles in providing physician education in obstetrics.[7] Planning by a joint committee of the AAFP and American College of Obstetrics and Gynecology (ACOG) for achievement of these core training requirements has established family medicine as the training ground for the other "primary care" specialties and supported the qualification of appropriately trained family physicians to take major responsibility for surgical complications of obstetrics.[6,8] The related AAFP/ACOG policy that hospital privileges for such responsibilities should be based on documented training and proven competence rather than arbitrary speciality divisions provides a strong foundation for guarantee of the family physician's role in continuing patient care in the arena of competing specialists.[9]

Consideration of the role family medicine can best play in the evolution of maternal-infant health-care services must take into account these objective assessments of quality and character of family medicine obstetric care. The countercurrents of the continuing debate,[10] such as pressure towards regionalization of obstetric and neonatal care, increased physician specialization, growth of interest in family-centered maternity care, and alternative approaches to childbirth, act in concert to pull family medicine towards the center balance point of the controversy. That point can add another solid cornerstone to the foundation of family medicine as it stands amid the patients, practitioners, and politics of American health care.

REFERENCES

1. Yates F: Contingency tables involving small numbers and the χ^2 test, JR Statist Soc (suppl) 1:217, 1934
2. Mann HB, Whitney DR. On a test of whether one of two random variables is stochastically larger than the other. Math Statist 18:50, 1947
3. Ely JW, Ueland K. Gordon MJ: An audit of obstetrical care in a university family medicine department and an obstetrics-gynecology department. J Fam Pract 3:397, 1976
4. Caetano DF: The relationship of medical specialization (obstetricians and general practitioners) to complications of pregnancy and delivery, birth injury, and malformation. Obstet Gynecol 132:221, 1975
5. Mehl LE, Bruce C, Renner JH: Importance of obstetrics in a comprehensive family practice. J Fam Pract 3:385, 1976
6. Layton RH: The future of obstetrics and gynecology training for family physicians. Wash Acad Fam Physicians J 4:13, 1977
7. Geyman JP: Obstetrics and family practice: Conflict in medical education? Some approaches to problem areas. J Reprod Med 12:59, 1974
8. Stern TL: A landmark in interspecialty cooperation. J Fam Pract 5:523, 1977
9. Hansen DV, Sundwall DN, Kane RL: Hospital privileges for family physicians. J Fam Pract 5:805, 1977
10. Candib L: Obstetrics in family practice: A personal and political perspective. J Fam Pract 3:391, 1976

A Multidisciplinary Audit of Diabetes Mellitus*

Theodore G. Aldhizer, Margaret M. Solle, and Raymond O. Bohrer

A multidisciplinary audit evaluating the quality of care of patients with a primary diagnosis of diabetes mellitus was performed at St. Mary's Hospital in Grand Rapids, Michigan. The audit served to evaluate the treatment and care of diabetic patients, in both the inpatient and ambulatory care settings, and also to identify interaction problems involving patient care among physicians, nurses, dieticians, and social workers.

Analysis of the data indicated that each discipline rendered adequate patient care. As other published audits have also indicated,[1-3] this multidisciplinary audit revealed that documentation of services is frequently lacking and that communication between the involved disciplines was less than desirable. The audit disclosed a need to educate the hospital staff (medical and nursing) as to the role and function of the Social Services Department.

As a result of this audit, definite measures have been instituted in each participating department in an attempt to further upgrade the quality of medical care and improve interdepartmental communication and cooperation.

The focus of a multidisciplinary audit is to evaluate the quality of "total" patient care. Each discipline analyzes its own performance and its interrelation with other disciplines.

Utilizing the audit system,[4] quality of care is objectively reviewed by formulating valid criteria which reflect the acceptable standards of patient care. The actual care rendered, as documented in the patients' medical records, is compared with the criteria. Variations from criteria indicate potential problems that prevent achievement of the expected or predicted patient outcome. Corrective actions are recommended, implemented, and evaluated to determine effectiveness of that action in relation to overall patient care.

Since approximately 1970, medical audits and multidisciplinary audits have been a tool used in acute care hospitals to survey patterns of care and patient outcome. A survey of literature published also indicated increasing interest in the use of medical audits in ambulatory care as well as inpatient settings.[1,2,5] As the interest in audit has increased, it has become obvious that the problems encountered in ambulatory care audit are frequently greater than those in an inpatient audit. According to Christofell and Loewenthal, these problems include less well-defined diagnoses, various stages of disease severity, and nonuniformity and weakness of individual record keeping.[6]

This audit on diabetes mellitus employed the multidisciplinary approach to assess the quality of multiple component care. The audit included care given in both inpatient and outpatient settings and involved social services, dietary, nursing, and family medicine departments in both settings, as well as the internal medicine department as part of the inpatient aspect of the audit. A literature search revealed no previous combined inpatient and outpatient multidisciplinary audit.

St. Mary's Hospital in Grand Rapids, Michigan, is a Catholic hospital owned and operated by the Sisters of Mercy Corporation and serves a population of approximately 550,000. From July 1976 to June 1977 (the time frame from which the sample of cases was drawn for this audit), the

*Reprinted from *The Journal of Family Practice*, 8(5): 947–951, 1979.

hospital's bed capacity was 375. The medical staff consisted of 398 physicians, 33 of whom were family physicians, and 32 internal medicine specialists. In addition, there were 9 dieticians, 266 nurses, and 5 social workers.

The Family Health Center is part of St. Mary's Hospital (with approximately 24,220 patients, 6,960 families at the time of the audit) and serves as the model ambulatory teaching area for the Family Practice Residency in Grand Rapids. The Family Health Center is organized and operated on the basis of the "team concept" developed at Beth Israel Hospital in Boston. Within the center are 18 family practice residents (who during 1976 and 1977 were assuming total patient care with full preceptor assistance), a full-time dietician, 4 registered nurses, 3 health assistants, and a part-time psychosocial worker (from July 1976 to June 1977 a full-time psychosocial worker was present).

The topic of diabetes mellitus was chosen for this multidisciplinary audit because of the chronicity of the disease process and its noted prevalence. Additionally, a diabetic patient requires multidisciplinary involvement in the inpatient and outpatient care and management of his/her disease.

In using the multidisciplinary approach to this audit, various departments were provided the opportunity to participate jointly in evaluating their services to this patient group in the context of the overall care. The objective of the audit was twofold: first, to evaluate the treatment and care of diabetic patients on the basis of established criteria and, secondly, to identify interaction problems involving patient care among the physicians and the nursing, dietary, and social services departments.

Methods

Patients were chosen from the time frame of July 1976 to June 1977. A total of 181 inpatients with diabetes mellitus (primary diagnosis) were reported for that period. A representative sample of 80 patients was randomly selected for the audit. These patients were selected by medical record number, using the H-ICDA code numbers of 250.0, 250.1, and 250.2. Only patients with the primary diagnosis of diabetes mellitus were included in the audit.

The selected sample represented a proportionate number of physicians from the family practice and internal medicine departments. From this sample, 20 Family Health Center patients were identified and chosen for the outpatient record review, some from each of the practicing residents and physicians at the Family Health Center. Diabetes mellitus was diagnosed in 368 patients at the Family Health Center from its inception in 1973 to July 1977.

The following steps were followed to accomplish the audit study:

1. A total of 18 criteria were drawn up by departments involved in the audit: 8 medical criteria, 4 dietary criteria, 2 social service criteria, and 4 nursing criteria. These criteria were organized to reflect prehospitalization, inhospital, and post-hospitalization patient care.

2. A joint meeting was held with representatives from the medical staff, and the nursing, social services, and dietary departments of both the hospital and the Family Health Center. At this meeting all the criteria were reviewed and established. Table 1 illustrates a sample of the format used in defining the elements and instructions of and exceptions to the criteria. Exceptions clarified incidences in which the criteria would not realistically apply. Detailed instructions for each criterion were provided as a guide to assure standard data retrieval and accurate analysis of the compiled data.

3. Medical record review was performed by a registered record administrator (RRA) who was knowledgeable in the audit process as well as the deciphering of medical record content. Separate worksheets listing criteria for each discipline involved in the audit were pre-

pared. Based on the predetermined instructions for each criterion provided by the discipline, the worksheet was used to indicate which criteria the medical record did or did not meet. Compliance with criteria was based on strict adherence of actual documentation within the record to the specified criteria instructions.

4. Records found to be in variation of the criteria were reviewed independently by each department.

Table 1. *Examples of Audit Criteria*

Criteria (Standard, 100%)	Instructions and Definitions for Data Retrieval	Exceptions
Prehospitalization (Family Health Center)		
Medical 1. Method of screening timely and appropriate	Tests done by next scheduled visit to include: fasting blood glucose, 2-hr postprandial blood glucose, random blood glucose, or 3 or 5-hr glucose tolerance test	1. If patient (Pt) is a known diabetic, past records reviewed and review documented in chart.
Nursing 2. Patient education documented: A. Observe films B. Review materials C. Attend diabetic classes	Patient progress notes reflect documentation by nurse or resident at the time the diagnosis is documented in the record	2. A. Pt. hospitalized within 48 hours B. Pt refused C. Family member or significant other person educated
Inhospital (At time of discharge)		
Medical 1. Blood glucose less than 180 mg/100 ml and urine free of ketones	Fasting, 11 AM, 4 PM, or 4 hr postprandial blood glucose within 24 hours of discharge	1. A. Pt expired B. Hemo/peritoneal dialysis (Pt on dextrose)
Social Services 2. Documentation of social services intervention for patients requiring post-hospitalization continued care	Needs or plans documented by social worker via discharge notes or progress notes. Continuing care defined as post-acute medical, nursing, rehabilitative, supervisory	2. A. Pt refused B. MD defers or cancels Social Services referral C. Social Services not indicated D. Lack of appropriate resources for care in the community
Posthospitalization (Family Health Center)		
Dietary 1. Dietician's documentation of appropriate information for patients upon follow-up visits after hospitalization	Progress notes. Dietician documents: 1. Patient's recollection of diet (how it compares to discharge diet) 2. Any special problems with diet 3. Assessment of patient's understanding 4. Plan for patient's continued nutritional care	1. A. Pt refused B. Scheduled appointment not kept C. Physician did not refer patient for continued nutritional care

5. Variations revealing discrepancies were further analyzed by each department to determine causes of problems and potential corrective actions.
6. A joint meeting was held with the above-specified representatives to review all audit findings and to analyze areas of interaction concerning jointly held concerns.
7. Actions of the audit were implemented with plans for follow-up evaluations.
8. Audit findings were reported to the medical staff, involved departments, Administration, Executive Committee, and Governing Board.

Results

Table 2 displays the percentages of records that did not comply with each of the 18 established criteria. These percentages are based on the total sample number of records with the exception of social services criteria, in which percentages are based on the number of cases in which intervention by social services was indicated, and not the total number of cases in the audit. Indications were based on criteria established by the department.

The audit did serve to evaluate the treatment and care of diabetic patients in both inpatient and outpatient settings from a multidisciplinary treatment approach. Physicians, for example, analyzed their performance by reviewing the findings of the audit. The data substantiated that all patients who were hospitalized with diabetes mellitus required hospitalization. Evaluation of patient outcome revealed that 58 of the 80 patient records met the screening criteria, showing a blood glucose level of less than 180 mg/100 ml with urine free of ketones at the time of discharge. Upon physician review of the remaining 22 patients' medical records, all but one were considered justified variations. Examples of justified variations were as follows: a patient transferred to extended care facility with complication of the disease which made "ideal" control impossible at the time of transfer, and an elderly brittle diabetic with blood glucose values stable, but not considered acceptable at time of discharge.

The outcome of the eight medical criteria revealed a mean adherence of 97 percent. The most significant finding, relating to the lower compliance for prehospitalization treatment criteria, was that the current protocol used at the Family Health Center by residents required revision and updating.

Nursing service's mean adherence to their four criteria was 63 percent, with major discrepancies identified in pre, post and inhospital care. Specifically, all of these variances to the criteria were related to patient education and documentation of the education given diabetic patients.

Dietary's mean adherence to its four criteria was 50 percent. Dietary variances were attributable to the lack of documentation of patient education. It is significant that criterion #3 (Table 2, Hospitalization) in retrospect proved to have been inappropriate, since during the time frame of the audit, a dietician's signature confirming diet orders had not been a departmental requirement.

The mean adherence to the social service criteria was 22 percent. The reasons contributing to this low compliance were multiple, including lack of physician awareness of social services' role and function and lack of referrals from nursing service. In some instances, social services involvement was not appropriately documented.

Discussion

As a result of the audit, definite steps have been instituted in each department to upgrade the quality of medical care and interdepartmental communication. Specific examples include revision of the Diabetes Mellitus Protocol used by Family Health Center physicians; initiation of a diabetic teaching program for hospital nursing staff; formulation of a comprehensive protocol for Family Health Center nurses; con-

Table 2. *Percentage of Discrepancies Based on Medical Record Documentation*

Criteria	Discrepancies %
Prehospitalization	
1. Screening for diabetes mellitus (DM) to be done for elements listed (these elements included 15 conditions, in combination or alone, which indicated need for screening)	5
2. Method of screening appropriate and timely	5
3. Interpretation of results appropriate	0
4. Treatment of American Diabetic Association (ADA) diet and insulin or oral agents	15
5. Dietician instruction of patient and follow-up for ADA diet and appropriate documents in patient record	40
6. Documentation of patient education by means of films, written materials, and diabetic classes upon diagnosis of DM, by nursing	35
Hospitalization	
Admission	
1. Uncontrolled DM or complicating or precipitating illness or complications of therapy or disease (to justify admission)	0
2. Appropriate referral of DM patients to social services for physical, social, and psychological problems	76
3. Confirmation of diet orders by dietician within 24 hours of time diet order was written	99
Discharge	
4. Blood glucose less than 180 mg/100 ml and urine free of ketones	1
5. Length of stay (maximum of 7 days)	1
6. Alive	0
7. Documentation of social service intervention for patients requiring continued care	81
8. Dietician documents description of diet instruction and assessment of patient comprehension	49
9. Nursing service documents self-care instruction and patient understanding of disease treatment	28
Posthospitalization	
1. Documentation by dietician of appropriate information for patients upon follow-up visit following hospitalization	15
2. Recording by nursing service of every Family Health Center visit, weight, blood glucose, blood pressure, and urinalysis	0
3. Review and recording by nursing service of patient's knowledge of diabetes	85

struction of a summary form by the hospital dietician to include patient's comprehension of diet and instructions during hospitalization, which would be sent to the Family Health Center dietician to facilitate a more comprehensive follow-up; and educational sessions by the Social Services Department for all hospital departments involved in direct patient care.

Various departments are planning to re-audit areas of significant variance after corrective plans have been implemented for a 12-month period. Re-audits will give a measurement of the effectivness of the actions that were initiated as a result of this audit.

This was the first time that several departments have participated jointly in assessing patient care. The opportunity of being involved in this multidisciplinary audit provided each of them with a method to objectively evaluate their department's performance. As a result of their participation, the individuals involved all expressed a new appreciation for the need of continual communication and cooperation in the providing of health care to patients with complex, chronic diseases. Also, each department gained further understanding of the roles and functions of the other departments.

REFERENCES

1. Harris AE Jr, McDowell J, Schoen RG: A longitudinal chart audit of hypertension in a family practice center. J Fam Pract 5:939, 1977
2. Dutton GB, Hoffman S, Ryan LK, et al: Ambulatory health care. NY State J Med 74:1545, 1974
3. Allen JE, Greenwald HD: An outcome-oriented audit of ambulatory care of patients with hypertension. Quality Rev Bull 3:17, 1977
4. Standard for medical audit of the accreditation council for ambulatory care. Quality Rev Bull 3:16, 1977
5. Hanson AS, Kraus ED: An outpatient medical audit. Minn Med 56 (suppl 2): 49, 1973
6. Christoffel T, Loewenthal M: Evaluating the quality of ambulatory health care: A review of emerging methods. Med Care 15:877, 1977

Psychotropic Drug Prescribing: A Self-Audit*

J. M. Wilks

In my 1971 survey of psychotropic drugs I suggested that the variety of psychotropic drugs and the use of barbiturates and minor tranquillizers ought to be reduced. Five years later these objectives had been achieved.

A comparison is made with the national prescription rate in the main categories of psychotropic drugs. The prescription rate of antidepressants was appreciably higher but that of hypnotics and tranquillizers was considerably lower. The net ingredient cost of the drugs prescribed was 33 percent of the rate for England.

Hospital referrals, suicides, and overdoses are related to the national figures.

Introduction

During 1971/2, I carried out a 12-month survey of my prescribing of psychotropic drugs (Wilks, 1975) to find out what I was actually doing with a view to possible improvement. My main conclusions were that the prescribing of a large variety of drugs, many of which were necessarily unfamiliar, was unsatisfactory and should be restricted; that the use of barbiturates should be reduced substantially; and that minor tranquillizers should be prescribed less readily.

Five years later it seemed desirable to see if these aims had been realized. In addition, I tried to compare my personal prescribing habits and consequences with those of the average general practitioner.

*Reprinted by permission from *Journal of the Royal College of General Practitioners*, 30:390–395, 1980.

Method

Since no prescriptions are given for longer than three months' treatment and I am not aware of any seasonal variation in my psychotropic prescribing, I assumed that by recording the prescribing during a three-month period and multiplying by four an approximate comparison could be made with my earlier 12-month survey.

During August, September, and October 1976 a notebook was kept with pages allocated to each letter of the alphabet. The names of all patients prescribed psychotropic drugs were entered, with the name, strength, and number of tablets of each drug prescribed. As it is a dispensing practice, all prescriptions were retained to make sure that there were no omissions. At the end of the three-month period the number of prescriptions and number of tablets were tabulated in their categories and multiplied by four.

Using the *MIMS* of September 1976 or, when appropriate, the 1976 *Drug Tariff* the cost of each drug prescribed was calculated and multiplied by four for comparison with the total net ingredient cost of prescriptions in England for 1975 (DHSS, 1976). The DHSS informed me (personal communication) that the *MIMS* prices and net ingredient cost' in the tables were identical. There were 45,560,127 people on prescribing lists in 1975 so that it was possible to calculate the number of prescriptions and net ingredient cost of each class of drugs per 1,000 patients.

The recording of hospital referrals and of cases of overdose admitted to hospital has been continued.

Table 1. *The Drugs and Number of Tablets Prescribed**

	Milligrams	March 1971–February 1972	(July–September 1976) × 4	Percentage Change
Barbiturates				
'Sodium amytal'	200	155		
	60	2,377	120	
'Seconal'	100	240	80	
	50	620		
'Nembutal'	100	335		
Phenobarbitone	60	1,398		
	30	4,300	1,920	
Phenobarbitone and theobromine		420		
'Carbrital'		590		
Total		10,435	2,120	*−80*
'Mandrax'		290		
'Mogadon'	5	1,828	2,640	*−62*
'Tricloryl'		35		
Total		2,153	2,640	*+23*
Minor tranquillizers				
'Librium'	10	3,822	600	
	5	4,273	2,900	
'Valium'	5	3,489		
	2	3,319	4,600	
'Ativan'	2.5		1,620	
Total		14,903	9,720	*−35*
Major tranquillizers				
'Fentazin'	4	1,350	120	
	2	1,362	440	
'Largactil'	50	440	1,880	
	25	2,977	2,320	
'Melleril'	50	720		
	25	82		
	10	390		
'Stelazine'	5	120		
	2	62		
'Stemetil'	25	90		
	5	1,042	2,464	
'Serenace'	0.5	740		
Total		9,375	7,224	*−23*
Antidepressants				
'Tryptizol'	25	23,252	29,160	
	10	1,459	1,984	
'Tofranil'	25	2,732	4,288	
	10	14	592	
'Lentizol'	50	30		
'Pertofran'	25	2,350		
'Triptafen'	forte	150		
	DA	100		

(*continued*)

Table 1—*Continued*

	Milligrams	March 1971–February 1972	(July–September 1976) × 4	Percentage Change
'Surmontil'	25	100	20	
'Nardil'	15	1,968		
'Parstelin'		250		
'Parnate'	10		800	
'Camcolit'	250		6,528	
Total		32,265	43,372	+34
All classes		69,131	65,076	−6

*Although nearly all the drugs are listed by their trade names, a high proportion were prescribed in non-proprietary form.

Results

Drugs Prescribed

The number of different preparations prescribed was reduced from 25 in 1971 to 15 in 1976 (Table 1).

The number of barbiturates prescribed was reduced by 80 percent but this was partially offset by an increase in the number of nitrazepam (Mogadon) tablets given. Nevertheless, there was a reduction in the total number of hypnotic tablets, both barbiturate and nonbarbiturate, of 62 percent.

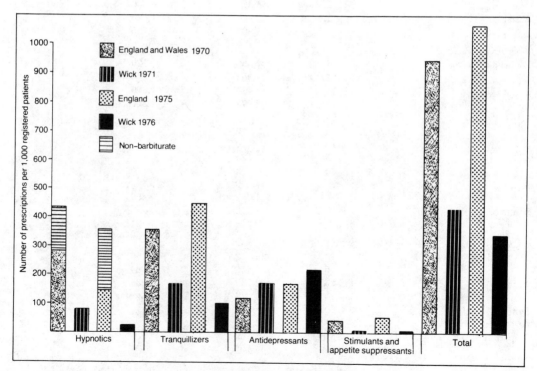

Fig. 1. Number of prescriptions per 1,000 registered patients in one year—national (1970 and 1975) and Wick (1971 and 1976) rates compared.

The number of minor tranquillizers was reduced by 35 percent and, apart from the introduction of lorazepam (Ativan) 2.5 mg, there was also a decrease in the doses used.

There was a 23 percent reduction in the number of major tranquillizers but this was due to a fortuitous change in the type of patient presenting rather than a change in prescribing policy. Again, there were no prescriptions for appetite suppressants or stimulants.

In contrast, the number of antidepressants rose by 34 percent, more than half of this rise being accounted for by lithium. In the 1971 survey the few patients on this drug were controlled by the hospital and it was therefore excluded, whereas currently they are all under my supervision which includes regular monitoring of the blood levels.

Number of Prescriptions

The changes in the number of prescriptions (Figure 1; Table 2) reflected the changes in the number of tablets prescribed, the prescription rate falling from about half the national rate to a third. The greatest disparity was in the prescribing of hypnotics which fell to seven percent of the national rate largely owing to the deaths of old regular sleeping tablet habitués and my refusal to recruit others to replace them. Again, the prescription rate of antidepressants was substantially higher than the national average; probably some patients took these drugs in lieu of hypnotics. These drugs accounted for 64 percent of my prescriptions in 1976 compared with the national proportion of 17 percent (Table 3).

Cost of the Drugs

In the classes of psychotropic drugs analysed there was a close similarity in the average net cost per prescription between my 1976 survey and that of England in 1975: £0.49 and £0.47 respectively. This is reflected in the fact that both the number of prescriptions and the net ingredient cost per thousand patients amounted to 33 percent of the national figures (Table 4). Although the prescription rate of antidepressants was higher than the national average the costs were lower, presumably because amitriptyline, imipramine and lithium, all cheap drugs, accounted for most of the prescriptions in 1976.

Hospital Referrals

During the period June 1969 to May 1979 there were 16 outpatient referrals and 11 admissions to psychiatric departments, the mean number of my patients being 2324. This is equivalent to an annual outpatient referral rate of 0.7 patients per thousand

Table 2. *Number of Prescriptions per 100 Registered Patients Compared with the National Rate (DHSS, 1976)*

	England and Wales 1970	Wick 1971	England 1975	Wick 1976
Hypnotics				
Barbiturate	276	65 *(24)*	148	10 *(7)*
Non-barbiturate	152	21 *(14)*	214	15 *(7)*
Tranquillizers	366	174 *(48)*	451	98 *(22)*
Antidepressants	114	178 *(156)*	174	222 *(128)*
Stimulants and appetite suppressants	45	0	57	0
Total	953	438 *(46)*	1,044	345 *(33)*

Figures in brackets represent the percentage of the national rate.

Table 3. *Number of Prescriptions and Percentages (in Brackets) of All Psychotropic Prescriptions per 1,000 Registered Patients by Class Compared with the National Prescribing Rate (DHSS, 1976)*

	England 1975		Wick 1976	
Hypnotics				
Barbiturate	148	*(14)*	10	*(3)*
Non-barbiturates	214	*(21)*	15	*(4)*
Tranquillizers	451	*(43)*	98	*(28)*
Antidepressants	174	*(17)*	222	*(64)*
Stimulants and	57	*(5)*	0	
appetite suppressants				
Total	1,044	*(100)*	345	*(100)*

compared with the rate of 4.1 for England and 3.5 for the South Western Region in 1975. The mean annual inpatient admission rate was 0.5 per thousand compared with 3.7 for England in 1974.

The treatment of patients in general practice is very cheap relative to the cost of treatment in hospital. In 1974/75 the cost of general medical services in Great Britain was £250 million or £5.48 per registered patient. In 1973/4 the cost per inpatient week ranged from £92 to £154 and per outpatient attendance from £4 to £6 (DHSS,

Table 4. *Net Ingredient Cost of Psychotropic Drugs per 1,000 Registered Patients Compared with the National Average (DHSS, 1976)*

	England and Wales 1970	England 1975	Wick 1976	
	£	£	£	
Hypnotics				
Barbiturate	39	35	1	*(3)*
Non-barbiturate	59	109	15	*(14)*
Tranquillizers	208	208	56	*(27)*
Antidepressants	109	200	133	*(67)*
Stimulants and appetite suppressants	45	67	0	
Total	£460	£619	£205	*(33)*

Figures in brackets represent percentages of the national rate.

1976) whereas attendance at a general practitioner's surgery cost the Exchequer on average about £1.68, apart from the cost of the prescription (calculations derived from OHE, 1979 and OPCS, 1980).

Overdoses and Suicides

In 1971 a series of measures were started in the practice to try to reduce the incidence of overdose (Wilks, 1975) and these have been maintained. Between 1966 and 1974 there were 11 overdoses by nine patients, one of them fatal, representing an annual incidence of 0.5/1000 patients (Table 5).

From 1975 to 1979 there have been three further cases of overdose requiring admission to hospital, equivalent to 0.3/1000 patients annually. A husband noting the absence of libido in his depressed wife wrongly assumed that she had a lover and took her amitriptyline (Tryptizol) tablets. Two women took simple analgesic tablets on the spur of the moment, one while she was away on holiday.

Jones (1977) noted a rise in admissions for self-poisoning to the Sheffield hospitals from under 50 in 1955 to 747 in 1970 and 1085 in 1975. He estimated that in the United Kingdom there are over 100,000 admissions yearly which is equivalent to 1.8/1000 population.

Table 5. *Summary of Outcome Compared with National Figures in Annual Rates per 1,000 Patients*

	England		Wick	
Suicide	0.328	(1975)	0.0324	(1951–1979)
Overdose	1.2–1.8		0.5	(1966–1974)
admissions			0.3	(1975–1979)
Hospital				
referrals			cost	
Outpatients	4.1	(1975)	0.7	
Inpatients	3.7	(1974)	0.5	(1969–1979)
Net cost				
ingredient	£619	(1975)	£205	(1976)

Sources: *Royal College of General Practitioners (1977).
        †Jones (1977).

There was one suicide. A retired business man had a myocardial infarction followed by a series of complications. Soon after the onset of his illness he asked my opinion as to his chances of resuming an active life and told me that he would not be prepared to live on as an invalid. Some months later, when he was obviously progressively deteriorating, he shot himself.

During the period 1968 to 1974 the national suicide rate fell by 16 percent to 3.28/100,000 population. During my 28 years in this practice there have been two suicides, giving an annual rate of 3.24/100,000 population but the figures are very small.

Discussion

Each doctor has his idiosyncratic prescribing habits which change almost unconsciously over a period of time. Some of this change is due to reading, attending lectures, or the opinions of colleagues, while the sales promotion of drug companies has proved influential enough to justify their high cost.

There is no reason why these prescribing habits should not be changed positively as a deliberate policy. For example, Wells (1973) eliminated his prescribing of barbiturates by substituting nitrazepam (Mogadon), at the same time reducing regular hypnotic takers by 41 percent. Clift (1972) reduced the long-term taking of hypnotics from 32 percent to eight percent and Lamberts (1976) showed that four partners could arrive at a common policy to prescribe tranquillizers sparingly. In each case an initial self-audit was conducted, a policy of change was decided, and a further audit showed that the objective had been achieved.

The survival of the National Health Service depends on the more effective use of limited resources. It could be postulated that the cost effectiveness of a general practitioner in his management of mental ailments is related to his practice rates of suicide, overdose, outpatient and inpatient referral and sickness, and with his psychotropic prescribing costs. I have no figures with which to measure my practice's psychiatric sickness rate but a current audit of male certification for all causes is low in relation to the national average. The low rates in the other parameters may be due to chance, the unusual mental stability of my patients, my policies, or a combination of all three (Table 5).

Conclusion

The association of the prescribing policies and outcomes described in my two papers is no evidence that they are related or would be reproducible in any other practice. Equally, there is no evidence that they are unrelated or that other doctors in other practices do not or could not reproduce them.

REFERENCES

Clift, A.D. (1972). Factors leading to dependence on hypnotic drugs. British Medical Journal, 3, 614–617

Department of Health and Social Security (1976). Health and Personal Social Services Statistics for England. Tables 5.25 and 5.26; 9.2 and 9.4. London: HMSO

Jones, D. I. R. (1977). Self-poisoning with drugs: the past 20 years in Sheffield. British Medical Journal, 1, 28–29

Lamberts, H. (1976). Pills and peer review. Update, 13, 426–427

Office of Health Economics (1979). Compendium of Health Statistics. 3rd edn. London: OHE

Office of Population Censuses and Surveys (1980). General Household Survey 1978. London: OHE

Royal College of General Practitioners (1977). Trends in General Practice. Ed. Fry, J. London: British Medical Journal

Wells, F. O. (1973). Prescribing barbiturates: drug substitution in general practice. Journal of the Royal College of General Practitioners, 23, 164–167

Wilks, J. M. (1975). The use of psychotropic drugs in general practice. Journal of the Royal College of General Practitioners, 25, 731–744

Repeat Prescribing—
A Study in One Practice*

E. John C. Parker and Victor Schrieber

A survey of the prescribing habits of a group practice of 10,500 patients was conducted during a three-month period to compare the pattern of repeat prescribing with that practised during consultations. Further analysis into therapeutic groups and categories depending on the length of treatment prescribed was performed. The results obtained were compared with annual prescribing rates and it was found that monthly figures could not be accurately extrapolated.

Introduction

Repeat prescribing accounts for a substantial proportion of a general practitioner's therapeutic activity. A short survey in the practice revealed that almost six hours of doctor time were spent on this task each week. Despite this, there has been little published research on the subject. Comparative studies are rendered more difficult because of variation in definition, classification, and research methods.

Aims

Our main objectives were to establish a profile of our prescribing habits and to reveal any differences between prescriptions issued during a consultation and those issued without the patient being seen. We also aimed to set out our rates of prescribing for the two groups, and as far as possible compare our findings with those of others. Furthermore, we wanted to compare the results given by a short (one- or three-month)

*Reprinted from *Journal of the Royal College of General Practitioners*, 30: 603–606, 1980.

analysis with those of an annual survey to see if the shorter period would give a sufficiently accurate figure.

Method

The practice is located in a Worcestershire market town with, at the time of the study, a list of 10,547 patients. There are five partners, and assistants contribute an additional six sessions per week. Requests for repeat prescriptions come via our receptionists, who pass the request to the doctor with a blank FP 10 form marked RP in the bottom righthand corner, and the patient's notes. All prescriptions issued during the months of May, June and July 1978 were subsequently obtained from the Pricing Bureau, and the marked forms were identified and separated. All the doctor's prescriptions were considered together.

After dividing the prescriptions by month of issue and into those written during a consultation (seen) and those given without direct patient contact (unseen), each item was then classified into one of 15 therapeutic sub-groups and then a further sub-division was made into three categories depending on the length of treatment prescribed.

The therapeutic sub-groups used were as follows:

Night sedation
Psychotropic
Analgesic
Other central nervous system drugs (CNS)
Cardiovascular (CVS)
Gastro-intestinal
Respiratory system (RS)
Skin
Endocrine

Musculoskeletal
Infections
Nutrition and haematinic
Eye and ENT
Allergy
Others

This is based on the classification used in *MIMS* with the following differences:

1. CNS drugs were divided into four groups, the section 'Other CNS' consisting largely of anticonvulsants.
2. Diuretics were included in the cardiovascular group.
3. All anti-infective agents, regardless of target organ, were classified together under 'infections'.
4. Drugs used for eyes and ENT were combined.
5. 'Others' includes diagnostic agents, dressings, appliances and the surgical group of *MIMS*.
6. Endocrine comprises all oral and parenteral hormonal drugs including oral contraceptives, but not topical applications.

The length of treatment categories were:

1. Long-term maintenance therapy.
2. Sporadically used drugs—'for use p.r.n.'
3. Drugs issued for a short (one-off) course of treatment.

All category 1 items issued during the study period were prescribed in a 50-day supply.

Thus, a repeat prescription request for digoxin would be classified as 'unseen', therapeutic group 'CVS', length of treatment 'Category 1—long-term maintenance therapy' and a prescription of penicillin V to a patient who attended the surgery with tonsillitis would be 'seen', 'infections', 'Category 3—one off'.

Results

During the three-month period, 9469 consultations took place (an annual rate of 3.59 per patient on the list) and a total of 9731 prescriptions were issued, bearing 16,136 items, of which 4,420 (27.4 percent) were 'unseen'. These figures give annual prescribing rates of 4.59 and 1.26 per patient for 'seen' and 'unseen' prescriptions respectively.

The numbers of prescriptions and items issued each month are shown in Table 1.

The ratio of seen to unseen prescriptions shows marked variation between the three months and thus cannot be extrapolated to give an annual rate. The annual pricing exercise (using a sample month) for our practice prescriptions, conducted by the Bureau for the years 1971 to 1978, has been plotted graphically in Figure 1. As can be seen, the annual results for unseen items derived by multiplying the sample month figure by 12 differs from the true figure of which we have records. This study is restricted to a comparison of prescribing habits during a three-month period, and any calculations of annual rates derived from this (and perhaps from the annual

Table 1. *Number of Prescriptions Issued Each Month*

	Seen			Unseen		
	FP10s	*Items*	*Items/ FP10*	*FP10s*	*Items*	*Items/ FP10*
May	2,380	4,151	1.74	869	1,312	1.52
June	2,411	4,238	1.76	1,095	1,671	1.53
July	1,985	3,327	1.68	991	1,437	1.45
Total	6,776	11,716	1.73	2,955	4,420	1.50

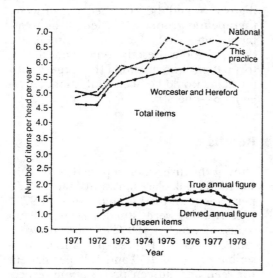

Fig. 1. Number of items prescribed per head per year compared with the national and local rates and the true and derived annual rates for unseen items.

pricing exercise) must be seen in this light.

The results of the further analyses into therapeutic and length of treatment groups are shown in Figure 2. This compares the average number of items per month (one third of the three-month totals) for seen and unseen prescriptions and shows that the overall distribution is broadly similar, with the following exceptions:

1. Some drug groups were far more likely to have been issued during a consultation. These groups were, as expected, 'infections' where the ratio of seen to unseen items was 10:1 and the 'CVS' and 'RS', both 2.5:1.

2. No group was more likely to be prescribed unseen, although 40 percent of 'night sedation' items were issued in this way.

3. The unseen items, group 3 prescriptions—the 'one-offs'—represented only a small proportion in most therapeutic subgroups. Only three subgroups, 'infections' (89 percent), 'ENT/eyes' (35 percent) and respiratory system' (23

percent) had more than one fifth of their unseen items classified into group 3. Although the figure for 'infections' seems high, it accounts for only 8.9 percent of the total (seen plus unseen). Thus few patients were given 'one-off' courses of treatment without being seen.

Discussion

The image of repeat prescribing has had a bad press, but there are few published statistics to determine its prevalence or the incidence of adverse effects. The subject is confused by variation in the use of the term; although a repeat prescription usually means one issued without a direct consultation between a doctor and a patient, Balint and colleagues (1970) use the term to describe the further issue of any drug previously prescribed to that patient, while some workers confine the usage to drugs given for long-term maintenance therapy (our group 1): (drugs in group 3— 'one-off'—are not strictly repeats).

We chose the terms 'seen' and 'unseen' which seemed to crystallize the essence of prescription without consultation, which appeared to us to be the crux of the matter. Few people mention the duration of treatment issued, and there is certainly no standardization of this.

In view of these variations, it is hardly surprising that widely differing results are obtained in calculating the proportion of prescriptions that are issued as repeats. *Update* (1977) uses the rather crude estimation of subtracting the annual consultation rate (three to four per head) from the annual prescription rate (six per head), apparently not considering those consultations that do not end in a prescription. Balint and colleagues (1970), as we have noted, used a wider definition to obtain a figure of 41 percent, while Dunnell and Cartwright (1972) arrived at a figure of 25 percent, similar to our own. Austin and Parish (1976) counted those prescriptions where the handwriting differed from the signa-

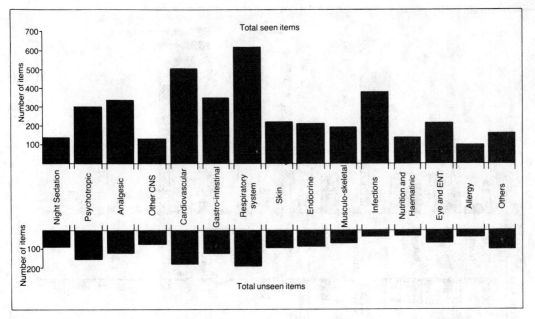

Fig. 2. Average number of items per month for seen and unseen prescriptions.

ture. Not all doctors in their study had receptionists, and many must have written unseen prescriptions themselves, perhaps accounting for their rather low figure of 10 percent. Madeley (1974), in a survey of a single practice, found a 'receptionist repeat' incidence of 22 percent.

Manasse (1974) studied repeat prescriptions issued over a four-month period in three practices serving a population of 30,600. His figures produced an annual rate of 9.65 items per patient compared with our figure of 1.86. He performed further analyses similar to ours, and his length of treatment groups (including his miscellaneous group) are compared with ours in Table 2.

Although he used different therapeutic subgroups, some comparisons may be made. In his study, 'psychiatric' and 'CNS' together account for 40.3 percent of all items, while our four subgroups 'psychotropic', 'night sedation', 'analgesic' and 'other CNS' made up 30.3 percent of our unseen prescriptions. Madeley found that 'sedatives' and 'antidepressants' represented 28.3 percent of all repeats and 'hypnotics' 18.3 percent. Our figures were 10.8 percent and 5.8 percent respectively. Freed (1976) stated that 64 percent of all drugs for 'anxiety and depression' issued during a three-month survey were receptionist repeats, a level of which he was highly critical. Our figure for this was 34.3 percent.

Table 2. *Percentage of Prescriptions by Length of Treatment Groups: Comparison with Manasse (1974)*

	1. Long Term	2. Sporadic	3. One-Off	4. Miscellaneous
Manasse (1974)	*81.9*	*10.4*	*5.5*	*2.2*
This study	62.6	24.7	12.9	—

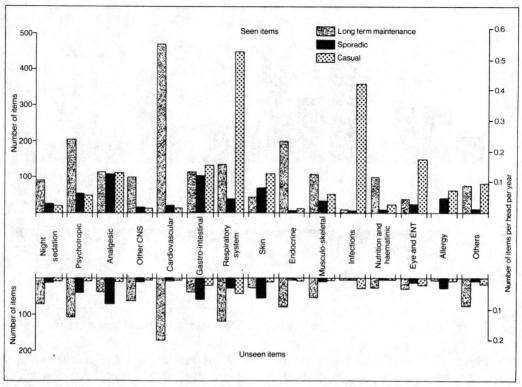

Fig. 3. Comparison of the three treatment categories for seen and unseen prescriptions.

Table 3. *Percentage of Prescriptions by Therapeutic Subgroup:*
Comparison with DHSS (1977)

	DHSS Percentage of National Total	Our Prescriptions		
		Percentage of		
		Total	*Seen*	*Unseen*
Hypnotics	4.9	4.0	5.9	3.3
Analgesics	6.5	8.5	8.5	8.5
Psychotropics	11.5	8.4	10.8	7.6
Gastro-intestinal	7.5	8.8	8.7	8.9
Cardiovascular	12.2	12.5	12.3	12.6
Respiratory	10.3	14.6	13.0	15.2
Antibiotics	13.1	7.6	2.4	10.0

As for national figures, there are statistics for overall prescriptions but none for repeats (Department of Health and Social Security, 1977). These may be used to give therapeutic subgroup rates comparable with ours as shown in Table 3.

It appears that our unseen prescribing profile bears a closer similarity to the national figures (with the exception of antibiotics) than our consultation rates. This is of uncertain significance but might reflect selection of drugs by patients rather than doctors.

One further benefit of this study has been the sight of the authors' FP10s returned from the Pricing Bureau with the cost of each item marked. This salutary experience is usually denied to non-dispensing practitioners although more useful than the histograms on relative costs issued by the DHSS. We should like to suggest that the Pricing Bureau consider returning to each doctor the month's FP10s used in the annual pricing exercise.

Acknowledgments

We should like to thank Mrs. P. M. Ball for statistical analysis and Mrs. L. Ward for typing the manuscript. Our thanks are also due to our partners, assistants and receptionists, and to Hereford and Worcester Family Practitioner Committee and the Prescription Pricing Authority for their co-operation.

REFERENCES

Austin, R. & Parish, P. (1976). Prescribing in general practice. Journal of the Royal College of General Practitioners, 26, Suppl. 1. 44-49

Balint, M., Hunt, J., Joyce, D., Marinker, M. & Woodcock, J. (1970). Treatment or Diagnosis: A Study of Repeat Prescriptions in General Practice. London: Tavistock Publications

Department of Health and Social Security (1977). Health and Personal Social Service Statistics for England 1977. London: HMSO

Dunnell, K. & Cartwright, A. (1972). Medicine Takers, Prescribers and Hoarders. London: Routledge & Kegan Paul

Freed, A. (1976). Prescribing of tranquillisers and barbiturates by general practitioners. British Medical Journal, 2, 1232-1233.

Madeley, J. (1974). Repeat prescribing via the receptionist in a group practice. Journal of the Royal College of General Practitioners, 24, 425-431.

Manasse, A. P. (1974). Repeat prescription in general practice. Journal of the Royal College of General Practitioners, 24, 203-207

Update, (1977). Repeat prescriptions, 14, 89

ABSTRACTS

Boucher F-G, Palmer WH, Page G, Barriault R, Seely J:
The evaluation of clinical competence.
Can Fam Physician 26:151–152, 1980

As governments and medical licensing bodies become more concerned with the quality of medical services and periodic re-licensing, it becomes relevant to define clinical competence in measurable terms. Medical associations in Canada and throughout the world are devoting considerable energy to this task.

During a workshop held at the Kellogg Centre for Advanced Studies in Primary Care, McGill University, the 25 participants examined methods available to evaluate clinical competence. They were all members of training programs for primary care practitioners. The workshop defined the components of clinical competence and analyzed the evaluation tools in terms of their suitability for assessing performance of selected component skills.

Clinical competence can be defined in terms of outcomes. Thus, variables such as mortality, morbidity, patient compliance and patient satisfaction can be used to evaluate competence. Unfortunately, this approach is expensive and time consuming, and it does not allow early intervention and correction. An alternative approach is to identify the skills essential for clinical competence. Each skill can then be evaluated separately and the resulting profile can be taken as a measure of clinical competence.

The workshop participants adopted the latter approach and identified 19 skills that they felt to be important components of clinical competence. These skills have been grouped according to Bloom's taxonomy; a fourth category, organizational skills or the ability to coordinate the care of multiple patients simultaneously, was included because it combines skill from each domain of the taxonomy (Fig. 1). This classification compares with, but is less elaborate than, others developed by other groups.

Using a problem-solving approach, each component skill was examined to determine the evaluation tool(s) best suited to its measurement (Fig. 1). The methods most commonly used (chart review and case presentation) were found to be very limited in the number of skills they evaluate. The large number of techniques available suggests that no single technique allows satisfactory assessment of all the component skills. The workshop participants concluded that if all the process skills are important in achieving clinical competence, then a combination of techniques is required to obtain an adequate performance profile.

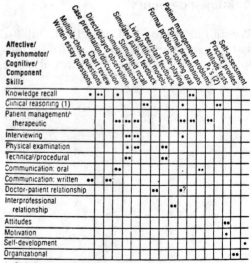

1. Clinical reasoning skills include cue perception, hypothesis generation, inquiry strategy, problem formulation and setting of priorities.
2. Portable patient problem pack[7]

•• Best technique to evaluate component skill.
• Acceptable technique to evaluate component skill.

Fig. 1. Evaluation Method

McCormick JS: Effectiveness and efficiency.
J R Coll Gen Pract 31:299-302, 1981

This paper examines some of the problems that surround measurements of effectiveness and efficiency and suggests that these terms are a proper and preferable substitute for audit and the examination of the quality of care. Physicians need to accept the technical meaning of terms used in economics such as effectiveness, efficiency, cost, input, process, cost benefit, and outcome.

The most commonly used outcomes in medicine are mortality and recovery. Mortality is useful only when it is substantial, and, conversely, recovery is useful only when it is not the rule. As perinatal mortality falls below 15 per 1,000 births, it becomes progressively more useless as an outcome measure and must be replaced by morbidity. In many instances, the outcome that is desired may be either difficult to measure or delayed and has to be replaced by a substitute or indicator: for example, dependence on tranquilizers might be used as an indicator of the effectiveness of group therapy for anxiety states or return to work as an indicator of social well-being. Outcome indicators should be acceptable only when they have been shown to be valid, that is, they truly reflect the real outcome that is desired.

Because of this relationship between costs and effectiveness, efficient use of resource demands an outcome definition that recognizes that very high degrees of effectiveness are prohibitively expensive. This is easily illustrated in the case of immunization programs, where, in the case of diphtheria, 80 percent effectiveness is probably sufficient to achieve herd immunity and to prevent the spread of the disease.

If the examination of costs and effectiveness is to produce change, it is best carried out by those whose behavior has to alter. The problem of audit is the presence in the background of an auditor. One response to this is the advocacy of self-audit or (rather more threatening) peer review. It would be better still if physicians had as an essential part of their image the thrifty use of resources. Unfortunately, since the advent of the NHS and almost universal health insurance, neither physicians nor patients profit individually to any real extent from thrift.

Improved efficiency often implies change in behavior; this can seldom be achieved by edict and usually requires conviction. One of the great strengths of self-audit is the conviction that the results carry for those who undertake the task.

Garrick CE, Cox KR, Rotem A, Whaite A:
Attitudes towards peer review.
Aus Fam Physician 8:554-558, 1979

The Australian commonwealth minister for health called on the Australian Medical Association to develop a system of peer review of medical standards in Australia. Among the initial responses was the organization of a national seminar on peer review. Participants were asked to identify questions they would like to have answered about peer review and about aspects of a peer review system that they would perceive as necessary for its acceptability.

Responses to the questions compiled by participants of the seminar are summarized according to major categories in Tables 1 and 2. Percentage responses are given for each category.

It appears from the results of the analyses that acceptance of and commitment to peer review was not widely disseminated at the time of the seminar, and in the absence of any further concrete proposals or educative efforts since, this is likely to still be the case.

Table 1. *Responses to "What Questions Would You Like to Have Answered About Peer Review?"*

Category	Approximate Percentage of Total Responses
Procedures and methods	15
Likely side effects	13
Safeguards and sanctions	13
Justifications for introduction	10
Coverage—who will be reviewed	10
Clarification of roles (profession, government)	10
Relationship to existing systems	7
Aims and purposes	6
Miscellaneous	5
Definition of terms	4
Medico-legal implications	4
Evaluation of peer review	2
Nature of criteria for review	1

Reprinted by permission from Garrick: Aus Fam Physician, 8:554–558, 1979.

If the profession is to support the concept of peer review and ensure its effective implementation, the following conditions must be met:

1. In order to influence attitudes in favor of peer review, evidence will need to be presented that indicates that present methods of medical practice and quality assurance are failing to provide optimal health care. The response of professional bodies such as the Australian Medical Association to the challenge of the government might therefore be

Table 2. *Responses to "What Is Necessary for Peer Review to Be Acceptable?"*

Category	Approximate Percentage of Total Responses
Minimal bureaucracy	12
Government finance without control	11
Improved health care as main objective	9
Locally defined criteria by true peers	9
Based on existing systems	7
Links with continuing medical education	7
Voluntary with minimal sanctions	6
Flexibility in criteria and methods	6
Coverage of whole profession	6
Adequate legal protection	5
Improved record systems	5
Provision of information about benefits of peer review	5
Adequate feedback to those reviewed	4
Need for pilot study	3
Miscellaneous	3
Acceptability to community	2

Reprinted by permission from Garrick: Aus Fam Physician, 8:554–558, 1979.

most profitably directed toward the assessment of current methods of quality assurance and the identification of their deficiencies.

2. The positive benefits to both doctors and patients of peer review should be identified and demonstrated.

3. Education of the profession in the functions and benefits of a peer review system is a high priority. This education might most effectively be accomplished in the process of designing peer review for the Australian context.

4. Methods and procedures for peer review should be developed in conjunction with all those professional groups that will be affected by it and that will work within it. The resultant shared ownership of the system would ensure acceptance of any built-in sanctions or regulatory mechanisms.

5. Open negotiation of roles for the various professional and government agencies central to the administration and decision making of peer review systems should be sought.

Berg JK, Kelly JT:
Psychosocial health care and quality assurance activities.
J Fam Pract 11(4):641–643, 1980

Quality assurance activities, although a daily practice in hospitals across the United States, center their attention on technical aspects of health care to the exclusion of psychosocial dimensions. There is no question, however, that psychosocial factors play a major role in many areas of health and illness, including etiology of disease, effectiveness of treatment, and well-being of patients and their families. This paper briefly summarizes a study that documents the extent to which one type of quality assurance activity—the medical audit—includes evaluation of psychosocial dimensions of health and disease.

In the Minneapolis/St. Paul metropolitan area, audit protocols are filed in a central criteria bank. The primary purpose of the criteria bank is to help health professionals develop audit protocols for use at their hospitals by providing, upon request, examples of audit protocols used by other institutions. This central file includes the audit protocols of 36 hospitals, comprising all acute care hospitals in the seven-county metropolitan area and including two county hospitals, a veteran's administration hospital, a university hospital, and numerous private hospitals. Each audit protocol represents a medical record audit completed by a hospital and evaluating physician performance, as required by the Joint Commission on Accreditation of Hospitals and the Professional Standards Review Organization.

At the time of this study, the central file held 448 audit protocols, representing audits completed from 1975 to 1979. Each audit protocol was examined by the authors and grouped according to topic of evaluation. A content analysis of each audit protocol was performed to identify four kinds of psychosocial criteria: (1) patient education criteria, covering areas such as use of medications, recommended activities, nutrition, and the disease process; (2) impact of illness criteria, focusing on a patient's response to his or her illness; (3) psychosocial consultation criteria, including consultation with a psychiatrist, psychologist, social worker, or other counselor; and (4) psychosocial history criteria, relating to the gathering of information from patients in the areas of family and home, work, education, finances, and personal and social life.

It was found that only a small fraction of

the 6662 audit criteria (which make up the 448 audit protocols examined) are concerned with psychosocial factors: 4 percent of criteria relate to patient education, and 3 percent relate to the other three areas combined—impact of illness, psychosocial history, and psychosocial consultation. The remaining 93 percent of audit criteria are concerned with disease-oriented aspects of diagnosis and management.

It is evident from the results of this study that medical audits, designed to assess the quality of health care, give scant attention to psychosocial health. Whereas the purpose of quality assurance activities is to guarantee that high-quality medical care is deliv-

ered, there is a failure to address psychosocial dimensions of quality, factors long recognized as important by health care consumers.

Family physicians, who have special expertise in the area of psychosocial medicine, are in a position to influence quality assurance activities in their communities. It is essential to include psychosocial evaluation when quality of health care is being measured in the following areas: health maintenance, psychiatric illness, chronic or life-threatening illness, illness that demands a change in life-style, and instances of psychological or social breakdown in patient or family.

Bull MJV: Ten years' experience in a general practice obstetric unit.
J R Coll Gen Pract 30:208-215, 1980

The aim of this survey is to record the results achieved by the Oxford Unit during a 10 year period and to examine trends apparent in this style of family physician obstetrics. The outcomes of over 8000 bookings in a general practice obstetric unit closely associated with a consultant unit were surveyed prospectively over a 10 year period.

The General Practice Maternity Unit at Oxford is a 12-bed unit. Management of the unit is supervised by a committee comprising six general practitioners (two of whom are clinical assistants in obstetrics, the remainder being nominated by the local medical committee), two consultants (including the professor of obstetrics), one pediatrician, and three nursing officers (including the divisional nursing officer, midwifery, and the nursing officer, community midwives).

Over the years, there has been a gradual increase in the proportion of patients transferred to specialist care in both pregnancy and labour (secondary and tertiary selection), with a consequent slow decline in the number of patients finally delivered in gen-

eral practice care to approximately 60 percent. To summarize, for every 100 patients originally booked, 7 will cancel (owing to change of domicile, abortion, or option for domiciliary confinement), 23 will be transferred to specialist care in pregnancy, and 8 will be transferred in labour, leaving 61 finally to be delivered in the care of the practitioner (although specialist advice or assistance may be required with two or three of these).

The perinatal death rate for each group of original bookings (excluding cancellations) is shown in Table 1. The relatively high fetal mortality rate (37.7/1000) occurring in patients referred to specialist care during pregnancy suggests that transfer was indeed justifiable, and examination of the indications reveals that toxemia, postmaturity, suspected disproportion, malpresentation, and antepartum haemorrhage are, in that order, the principal reasons and causes that would not have been apparent at primary selection. With patients transferred in labour, the perinatal loss seems reasonable (17.6/1000). This may be because most of the problems are

Table 1. *Perinatal Mortality*

	1968	1969	1970	1971	1972	1973	1974	1975	1976	1977	Total	Mortality Rate/ 1,000
Patients Transferred During Pregnancy												
Live births	144	176	179	203	218	235	214	195	162	186	1,912	
Stillbirths	10	4	5	6	6	3	5	7	6	1	53	27.0
Neonatal deaths (0 to 7 days)	2	6	2	5	2	1	1	0	1	1	21	10.7
Total number of patients	153	186	186	203	218	231	215	184	167	183	1,926	
Patients Transferred During Labour												
Live births	54	82	78	74	68	74	65	49	66	61	671	
Stillbirths	1	0	1	2	2	2	0	1	1	0	10	14.7
Neonatal deaths (0 to 7 days)	0	1	0	0	0	1	0	0	0	0	2	2.9
Total number of patients	55	82	79	76	70	76	65	50	67	61	681	
Patients Delivered in General Practice Care												
Live births	458	531	548	549	586	493	455	488	429	423	4,960	
Stillbirths	0	0	0	0	0	0	1	0	0	0	1	0.2
Neonatal deaths (0 to 7 days)	1	0	2	0	2	0	0	0	1	0	6	1.2
Total number of patients	456	530	548	548	584	493	456	488	429	423	4,955	

Discrepancy between number of patients and number of births is accounted for by multiple pregnancies.
Reprinted by permission from Bull: J R Coll Gen Pract, 30:208–215, 1980.

mechanical (failure to progress in first stage, delay in second, fetal distress, retained placenta) but is also a tribute to the technical skill of specialist colleagues and their proximity. Fetal loss in patients finally delivered in general practice care is (and should be if primary, secondary, and tertiary selection have been successful) very low indeed (1.4/ 1000).

Predictably, there was a high operative delivery rate in the first and second groups, which were selected out because of the identification of risk factors in pregnancy or of complications in labour. However, if the figures are adjusted to relate to the total number of patients booked (excluding cancellations), it was found that out of 7562 patients originally booked, 80 percent delivered spontaneously, 17 percent required forceps delivery (including breech), and the caesarean section rate was 3 percent. The operative delivery rate was thus approximately half of that which is seen in many specialist units and could equally be held to imply reasonable primary selection of cases for general practice care.

In 1968, 58.6 percent of primigravidae were delivered in general practice care, but by 1977 the rate had fallen to 43.4 percent with a commensurate increase in numbers transferred during pregnancy and labour. This trend is in all probability associated with the increasing age of women at first confinement during the last decade.

The pattern of general practice care is changing. Home confinement, in spite of sectional pressures, is now minimal, and deliveries in peripheral (NHS group A) hospitals are also shown to have declined sharply between 1970 and 1975. That *all deliveries* in general practice units fell only marginally during this quinquennium is accounted for by the significant increase in the number of patients confined in integrated general practice units of the type described. If this trend can be maintained, there may well be benefits for patients (a degree of choice with safety and continuity of care), for general practice obstetricians and community midwives (continuing experience, responsibility, and job satisfaction), and for consultant staff (reduced workload, higher-quality shared antenatal and postnatal care) alike with continuing improvement of the service that is so vital to the nation's future population.

Ryan MP, Buchan IC, Buckley EG: Medical audit–a preliminary report from general practice. J R Coll Gen Pract 29:719–722, 1979

This paper reports a study by three single-handed general practitioners, who work in the same health center, who decided to examine various ways in which clinical review can be undertaken. Clinical management of problems and preventive medicine were chosen for study. Two conditions common in general practice, minor respiratory illness and urinary tract infection, were selected as well as prescribing patterns, the influenza vaccination program, and recording patients' blood pressure.

Problem-oriented medical records were used. "Active" problems were entered in a medical information system based on feature cards. Also recorded on feature cards were data describing patients, number of contacts, drugs prescribed, and certain baseline measurements such as blood pressure. Minor self-limiting problems were not recorded routinely on the problem lists. The average number of patients registered with each doctor during the study period was as follows: Dr. A, 1530; Dr. B, 1650; Dr. C, 1390. The practices have similar age/sex structures, in general serving a young population, eight out of ten patients being under the age of 40.

The retrospective audit of 20 incidents of minor respiratory illness, randomly selected, produced some unexpected findings. The main finding was that antibiotics were prescribed in over two-thirds of the episodes and that the prescriptions covered a wide range of antibiotics. Two main conclusions resulted from this audit. First, the physicians may be prescribing antibiotics inappropriately, more often than necessary, and without any rational criteria. Second, the variation in use of "cough bottles" highlights the need for a consistent policy in the management of minor conditions in order to prevent confusion in patients about treatment. The next stage of this review will be to achieve a consensus of opinion among the physicians about the management of minor respiratory illness. The audit will then be repeated.

Sixty records of patients with suspected urinary tract infections were reviewed. In three-quarters of episodes, an initial midstream specimen was sent to the laboratory, and over half of the patients were treated with an antibiotic. Two surprising findings were the low number of positive midstream specimens (11 out of 46) and the low number of follow-up specimens (17 out of 33), although it is interesting that in several instances the request for post-treatment midstream specimen was recorded but no sample was handed in by the patient. Co-trimoxazole appeared to be the drug of first choice, with ampicillin or amoxycillin as second choice. Nitrofurantoin, nalidixic acid, and sulphadimidine were each prescribed only once. On the whole, the management of urinary tract infection was less than satisfactory, with the stated aims not always achieved.

The audit of drug prescribing revealed

Table 1. *Influenza Vaccinations*

	1975	1976	1977
Percentage acceptance in chronic heart and lung disorders	45	65	63
Percentage acceptance in over 65s	33	50	54

Reprinted by permission from Ryan et al: J R Coll Gen Pract, 29:719-722, 1979.

that antibiotics were prescribed more often than psychotropic drugs, but this may simply have been a reflection of the young practice population. The pattern of prescribing was virtually identical for all three doctors. It was noted that almost half of the patients received at least one antibiotic in a 12-month period. The most valuable outcome of the audit was a desire to examine prescribing of antibiotics and psychotropic drugs in more detail.

In 1975, it was decided to organize special clinics for influenza immunizations for those patients who were identified on the feature cards as having chronic respiratory or cardiac problems and those over the age of 65 who were considered fit enough to travel to the health centre. Table 1 shows the total acceptance rate of this effort, which was felt to justify the cost and effort of organizing the special clinics.

When the records of women using oral contraceptives were studied, it was found that the proportion who had their blood pressure noted in the preceding two years was 43 percent in Practice A, 42 percent in practice B, and 48 percent in practice C. Just over half of patients with known cardiovascular problems had had their blood pressure recorded in that period, although many may have had it noted previously. The physicians were surprised to discover their deficiencies in recording the blood pressures of the two groups known to be at risk and will use this information for improvement.

Through studying what was actually recorded, these three physicians showed that subjective views differed from objective analyses. It was found that each behaved differently in similar situations, and this has acted as an incentive to change. Clearly, local conditions always have to be taken into account, but some form of review is possible in every general practice.

Sheldon MG: Self-audit of prescribing habits and clinical care in general practice.
J R Coll Gen Pract 29:703-711, 1979

Many studies have been undertaken of the range of drugs prescribed by general practitioners and the reasons for their use, but little work has been done to examine the effect of such prescribing on the course of illnesses treated. Audit is of value only if it leads to improved clinical care.

This study was designed to discover bad prescribing habits, to formulate plans for their correction, and to monitor subsequent changes in patient management. The study was started in conjunction with the Oxford Drug Monitoring Study. The practice is rural but covers the town of Banbury and its surrounding villages. At the beginning of the study, it was a single-handed practice with 1350 patients but grew to 2090 patients in the second year and 2520 in the third year when a second partner was engaged. The age/sex and social class profile shows a marked increase in young families in social classes 2 and 3.

For the 3-year period from March 1975 to February 1978, a carbon copy was taken of each prescription issued by the practice, and the disease or problem for which each drug was given was added to the form. All doctor/patient contacts were recorded, as were prescriptions issued after telephone consultations and repeat prescriptions. For 3 months in each year, photocopies of prescriptions dispensed for random months from the Prescription Pricing Authority (PPA) were obtained without previous knowledge as to which months were selected. These were used to check the accuracy of recording methods.

For 1 month in each year, the PPA analyzed prescriptions for its annual review of prescribing costs. When all the prescriptions and encounter forms were matched during these months, less than 3 percent of forms were found not to match with a prescription, indicating that the number of prescriptions issued but not taken to the chemist for dispensing was under 3 percent of the total. During the first 12-month period, a total of 7748 prescriptions were entered on the computer file. Assuming that 5 percent of all prescriptions were not included because a carbon copy was not taken, the estimated total of prescriptions issued during the year was 8135. This did not include prescriptions for dressings and appliances, which were not included in the Oxford Drug Monitoring Study. Assuming that the average patient list was 1550 (as it rose at a constant rate from 1350 at the beginning to 1750 at the end of the first year), the prescription rate for medicines was 5.25 items per patient per year. A prescription rate of 4.79 items per patient per year was observed during the third 12-month period on the basis of the same assumptions.

The main purpose of the study was to use information obtained about prescribing habits to audit the care given in certain clinical situations. This was done for several conditions commonly encountered in general practice. Fungal skin infections were chosen, for example, because they were considered difficult to treat effectively in general practice and were often referred for consultant dermatologic advice. The following treatment protocol was developed for ringworm infection of the skin (tinea corporis):

Diagnosis

Typical clinical picture, sometimes with history of animal contacts; microscopy shows fungal hyphae present.

Treatment

1. Standard therapy: Whitfield's ointment BPC (full strength for extensor surfaces, half strength for flexor surfaces).
2. If Whitfield's ointment is too irritant use Canesten cream, 20 gm (clotrimazole).
3. If there is poor response to topical agents:
   a. consider sending scraping to laboratory for culture
   b. give griseofulvin 500 mg daily for three weeks (adult dose).
4. If the diagnosis is doubtful and no hyphae are seen on microscopy, treatment with a steroid cream is justified (assuming the condition is an eczema). In the case of false negatives, reexamina-

Table 1. *Comparison of the Number of Consultations and Items Prescribed for Fungal Skin Infections Before and After Audit*

	1975	1977
Patients treated	29	33
Illness episodes	33	33
Consultations	44	31
Repeated prescriptions	9	6
Items prescribed	60	39
Number of Prescriptions for Each Agent		
Tri-Adcortyl cream	29	0
Griseofulvin tablets	12	5
Tineafax preparations	6	4
Mycil preparations	6	5
Jadit preparations	3	0
Canesten cream (clotrimazole)	2	14
Whitfield's ointment	0	7
Others	2	4
	60	39

Reprinted by permission from Sheldon: J R Coll Gen Pract, 29:703-711, 1979.

tion at a later date may show hyphae on microscopy, as they are not affected by steroids.

During the third year of the study, the changes that occurred in prescribing habits as a result of the auditing process were monitored. Table 1 shows that in 1977 after the audit, prescribing of Tri-Adcortyl cream had been stopped, and Whitfield's ointment was being prescribed. Many fewer prescriptions for griseofulvin tablets were needed. Comparing the findings for 1975 and 1977, it was found that although exactly the same number of illness episodes were treated in both years, the total number of items prescribed fell by a third from 60 to 39, and the number of consultations required also fell from 44 to 31 following the audit of prescribing habits.

These findings suggest that the continuous use of encounter forms can accurately reveal the prescribing habits of family physicians. Self-audit can then be performed on a continuing basis with little disruption of the physician's normal routine.

Parkin DM, Kellett RJ, MacLean DW, Ryan MP, Fulton M: The management of hypertension—a study of records in general practice.
J R Coll Gen Pract 29:590–594, 1979

The beneficial effects of treating certain categories of hypertension have been established (Veterans Administration Cooperative Study Group on Antihypertensive Agents, 1967 and 1970), but little is known about its management in the community. This paper reports the results of a survey conducted between June and September 1976 into the management of hypertension in general practice, which forms part of a study of the investigation, treatment, and continuing care of hypertensive patients in hospital and general practice.

The management of a group of 322 hypertensive patients by 71 general practitioners was investigated in the Lothian Health Board Area of England by a survey of the general practitioners' records. Seventy-seven physicians, the complete complement of 16 practices, were approached, and 71 (92 percent) agreed to cooperate. This was not therefore a randomly selected group. Each physician was asked to list the first five patients whom he considered to have hypertension, regardless of whether or not they were on antihypertensive drugs, who attended the surgery for any reason after a specific date.

Only those patients who had been under the care of the practice since the diagnosis was made were included. Patients attending for a repeat prescription were eligible, but pregnant women and patients under 16 years were excluded. The level of the latest blood pressure was used as a measure of the outcome of care.

Two hundred and seventy patients (84 percent) were identified at repeat attendances, 19 (6 percent) were newly diagnosed, and 33 (10 percent) were found when attending for repeat prescriptions. There were 110 men and 212 women, with approximately twice as many women as men in each age group. The mean ages were 58.6 years for men and 58.4 years for women. The majority (75 percent) of patients had been diagnosed since 1970. The initial diagnosis of hypertension had been made by the general practitioner in 85 percent of cases; only four patients (1 percent) had been detected by screening programs.

Eighty-five percent of patients were diagnosed by the general practitioner, and 57 percent were cared for entirely by him. Hospital referral was more common in men and in patients with high initial blood pres-

Table 1. *Drug Therapy at Time of Survey (June to September 1976)*

Drug Therapy	Number of Patients	Percentage of Total Number of Patients
Diuretic only	74	27.3
Beta blocker only	55	20.3
Methyldopa only	26	9.6
Adrenergic blocker only	11	4.1
Other antihypertensive	4	1.5
Diuretic + beta blocker	32	11.8
Diuretic + adrenergic blocker	13	4.8
Diuretic + methyldopa	28 .	10.3
Other combinations of drugs	28	10.3
Total	271	100.0

Reprinted by permission from Parkin et al: J R Coll Gen Pract, 29:590–594, 1979.

sures. The amount of investigation by the general practitioner of general practitioner cases and of hospital referrals was very similar.

The initial choice of therapy was influenced by the year of diagnosis. The use of beta blockers had increased with time, whereas there were very few prescriptions of sedatives, reserpine, and ganglion blocking agents. Table 1 lists the drugs in use in the 271 patients on therapy at the time of the survey.

The means of the initial and most recent diastolic blood pressures for those receiving and not receiving treatment are shown in Table 2. Both groups show a significant fall.

Twenty-three percent of patients had a latest diastolic pressure of over 100 mm Hg and 6.5 percent of over 110 mm Hg. The result of treatment as measured by the latest diastolic blood pressure was similar for patients treated by the general practitioner and those referred to hospital, being 100 mm Hg or less in 77 percent of patients.

The main findings of this study are that the general practitioner manages the majority of patients without hospital referral and that the result of treatment as indicated by the most recent blood pressure reading is similar for both general practitioner cases and hospital referrals.

Table 2. *Means of Initial and Most Recent Diastolic Blood Pressures for Patients Receiving and Not Receiving Treatment*

	Diastolic Blood Pressure (mm Hg)		
	Initial	Latest	p value
Treated patients (271)	118.9 (SD 13.6)	96.8 (SD 11.5)	<0.001
Not currently treated (51)	108.9 (SD 10.6)	97.0 (SD 11.2)	<0.001

SD = Standard deviation.
Reprinted by permission from Parkin et al: J R Coll Gen Pract, 29:590–594, 1979.

Barley SL, Mathers N: An audit of the care of post-gastrectomy patients.
J R Coll Gen Pract 30:365-370, 1980

There are many consequences and complications of a partial gastrectomy, malabsorption of iron being the most common; a few patients also develop a vitamin B_{12} or folate deficiency anemia or calcium malabsorption presenting as osteomalacia or osteoporosis. Although a great deal of literature has been devoted to the postoperative complications of a partial gastrectomy, it is not known how many general practitioners have devised a rational and practical method of follow-up. The idea of a "birthday follow-up," that is, an annual blood test on the patient's birthday to look for evidence of malabsorption of iron, calcium, and vitamins D and B_{12} and folic acid has been recommended by some. The aim of this study was to see if the birthday follow-up scheme was a practical method of management by a general practitioner.

The birthday follow-up scheme was started in 1973; at that time, there were 2400 patients and two principals. At the time of audit 5 years later, the practice consisted of 4600 patients and three principals. Ninety-eight percent of the patients live on a council housing estate built in the 1930s, and nearly all have occupations classified by the registrar general in social classes 4 and 5. Heavy drinking and cigarette smoking are extremely common among the men.

A list of postgastrectomy patients was kept in the disease register. When a patient was found to have had a partial gastrectomy, possible ill effects that would be detected in an annual blood test were explained. Blood was obtained for a full blood count, serum iron, total iron binding capacity (TIBC), serum B_{12} and folate, red cell folate, serum calcium, serum phosphate, and alkaline phosphatase. If no abnormalities were found, the patient was asked to return on his next birthday unless this was less than nine months away. It was the responsibility of the patient to remember to come back.

There are 26 names on the disease register—19 men and 7 women. The mean age of the men was 63.4 years (range 35–84); for women, it was 68.1 years (range 57-77). The incidence of partial gastrectomy is 0.6 percent of the 1977 list. Nineteen operations were for peptic ulceration, two for carcinoma of the stomach, and one for duodenal narrowing and Crohn's disease. There was no indication for surgery in the records of four patients, although they all claimed to have had "ulcers" before operation. The mean time between operation and audit for women was 17.7 years (range 0–30 years); for men, it was 16.4 years (range 0–32 years). Apart from the two patients with cancer, all had been discharged from follow-up by the surgeons.

Of 198 possible tests (nine for each patient when seen for the first screening), only 87 (44 percent) were done; 16 (18.2 percent) were abnormal. At the 39 opportunities for annual follow-up, 71 percent of the possible tests were done; 11 of the 62 tests (17.5 percent) were abnormal. The most common abnormality was deficiency of iron (12 tests), followed by folate (four tests), serum B_{12} (two tests), and serum calcium (two tests). Appropriate action according to the review criteria was taken for 24 out of the 27 abnormalities found.

Because there were so few abnormalities found at follow-up, the plan has been modified in the following way:

One year and (arbitrarily) every 5 years after operation, all nine tests are done. Follow-up of abnormal results will be after an appropriate short interval and (arbitrarily) for two annual reviews thereafter. If all tests are normal, birthday follow-ups are confined to a full blood count and serum iron until the 5-year complete review comes round.

Jones AL: Medical audit of the care of patients with epilepsy in one group practice.
J R Coll Gen Pract 30:396–400, 1980

Epilepsy is a disease that requires adequate drug control and that has complex social and psychological implications. A past survey of epilepsy in 14 general practices found that nearly one-third of all the patients had psychological difficulties of various types; some aspects of the process and outcome of the care of epileptics are therefore difficult to quantify. A more recent study has shown that at present the follow-up of patients with seizures is not related to what patients need since some with only occasional generalized seizures still attend hospital clinics, whereas other patients with daily or weekly seizures have not been seen by a doctor for months. This suggests a need for change from patient-dictated care to care that is more under the doctor's control.

In this study, the care given in a Welsh group general practice to 47 patients with epilepsy was reviewed. This study included only patients who requested a prescription from the doctor or the receptionist for anticonvulsant drugs during a four-month period. As no more than 3 months' supply of anticonvulsants was ever given by repeat prescription, the patients were readily identified. The patients were interviewed, when possible, in the presence of a close relative. Their replies were checked against their records. They were examined for nystagmus, ataxia (by walking along a straight line of 4 m), and rombergism and observed for drowsiness, dysarthria, or hyperexcitability. Blood was taken for serum drug level estimation, full blood count, and film. In the light of the clinical, hematologic, and serum drug level findings, appropriate action was taken about management. This ranged from gradual omission of drugs for those free of seizures for over three years to changes to an alternative anticonvulsant for those with poor control of seizures and normal serum drug levels.

Forty-seven names were recorded, giving a prevalence rate of 5.5 per 1000 in a practice of 8607. There had been specialist confirmation in 41 cases. These patients had had an EEG, but this was confirmatory in only 34. Since 1960, patients have been referred for a second opinion before the diagnosis of epilepsy was applied. Twenty-nine patients had been told that they had either epilepsy or a mild form or "boundary case" of epilepsy. Seven patients could not recall being told what was wrong and did not know what the attacks were. In all, 17 had had difficulty in finding out any form of diagnosis.

Only a minority of patients had been given advice on most subjects, the exception being the availability of free prescriptions, which was known to all those who would normally have paid for their drugs. Almost

Table 1. *Numbers of Patients by Serum Drug Level and Clinical State*

Group	Serum Drug Level	Clinical State	Number
1	Low	Poor control of seizures	3
2	Low	Moderate control of seizures	3
3	Low	Good but not complete control of seizures	8
4	Low	Free of seizures for 3 years or more	3
5	Low	Children who had outgrown their dose	5
6	Normal	Good control	13
7	Normal	Poor control	4
8	High	Ataxic	4
9	High	Good control and not ataxic	1

Reprinted by permission from Jones: J R Coll Gen Pract, 30: 396–400, 1980.

a third of the relatives had been given advice on what to do if a seizure occurred, and a third of the patients had been advised on the avoidance of possible precipitating factors. Of the 23 patients eligible for driving licenses, only eight knew about the current vehicle licensing regulations in relation to epilepsy.

More than half of all patients (62 percent) had not told relatives, and 79 percent had not told friends of their epilepsy; 24 percent had not informed relatives, and 35 percent had not informed friends that they had seizures. Over half the patients considered themselves to be unacceptable to the rest of society.

Seventeen patients (38 percent) were using a single drug, 21 (48 percent) were using two drugs, and six (14 percent) were using three drugs. Thirty-two patients (71 percent) had good control, five (11 percent)

moderate control, and eight (18 percent) poor control of their seizures. Twenty-seven patients (60 percent) had drug levels outside the normal range. Five were higher, and 22 were lower than the normal ranges accepted by the local laboratory (Table 1).

Twenty-seven patients (60 percent) had not seen a doctor during the preceding year. Of the 17 patients having problems with seizure control or anticonvulsant side effects, nine were not having regular follow-up by the general practitioner or by the hospital.

Since patients with epilepsy maintain regular contact with their family physician by requests for repeat prescriptions, it should not be difficult for the physician to exercise appropriate control of the care of his patients. The more widespread use of serum drug levels should be of great value to the care of patients with epilepsy.

SECTION THREE

Continuing Education in Family Practice

COMMENTARY

COMPARED to undergraduate and graduate medical education, continuing medical education (CME) is a virtual nonsystem. Most past and current CME activities are not related to identified learning needs from the physician's practice and are more concerned with information transfer than with improving clinical competence. Several papers in this section expand on the issues and problems in providing CME that meets the individual physician's real needs and, more importantly, the needs of his patients. Inevitably, CME has to be viewed in relation to its ultimate goal, the assurance of high-quality medical care. In this respect, the papers and abstracts in this section are closely related to those in section two.

Various approaches to the identification of individual learning needs are presented in this section. In addition, several alternatives to traditional didactic CME teaching are described, including the use of simulated patients, a cardiology patient simulator, and various examination techniques.

Although the dimensions and problems of CME are starting to receive the attention they deserve among a growing number of concerned physicians and educators, much remains to be done before effective CME programs are widely available based on real learning needs. As Berg points out in his paper, there is good evidence that CME programs lead to increased physician knowledge and even behavior change. The challenge remains to tie the strategies and results of CME more directly to improved outcomes of patient care.

PAPERS

Continuing Medical Education in America*

Thomas L. Stern

Some of what may be perceived as today's failures in continuing medical education may have been caused by lack of sound educational principles in the medical education process. Others may be due to changing times and expanding knowledge. New methods need to be established which include education based on physician audit and self-assessment. Learning outcomes should be evaluated in order to assess physicians' abilities to render better patient care. The formal graduate educational program is seen as the base for the new method of delivery of continuing medical education. The residency has the ability to evaluate advances in medicine and distill them for the practicing clinician. It may also assist him with office systems which will enable him to monitor his practice and needs. Linkages with residency programs will benefit the practitioner and resident alike. In the future, other community facilities may be needed to handle problem-centered continuing medical education.

It is both timely and necessary to reassess the role, methods, and effectiveness of continuing medical education. Toward this purpose, this paper will briefly review the history of continuing medical education in

*Reprinted by permission from *The Journal of Family Practice*, 3(3):297–300, 1976. This paper is adapted from a presentation made at a conference entitled "The Challenge: Health Care, Man, the Family, the Community" in Fuengirola, Spain, November 2, 1975.

America, discuss some of its problems, and describe the operation and advantages of basing future efforts in continuing medical education in family practice residency programs.

Historical Perspective

Prior to 1910, the standards of medical education were so poor that the Carnegie Foundation for the Advancement of Education and the American Medical Association commissioned Dr. Abraham Flexner[1] to inspect thoroughly the medical colleges of the United States. The consequence of his devastating report was that almost one third of the existing schools immediately closed their doors, and, with few exceptions, those remaining either individually, or by joining forces, raised admission and teaching standards to acceptable levels. It is interesting, however, that the very report that brought about the reformation in medical education is at the root of today's problem of research oriented full-time faculty who are often unresponsive and misdirected regarding the continuing education and needs of the clinician. Flexner proposed three remedies for the problem of inadequate medical education: (1) The development of education for medicine as a university controlled discipline with the careful selection of students from those with an educational background in the liberal arts; (2) The institution of the full-time teacher/investigator; and (3) The use of the hospital as a laboratory in a way that would permit the student to gain supervised, yet responsible experience in the application of the scientific method to patient care.

From 1910 until World War II, continuing education was reparative. The postgraduate school, identified by Flexner as a necessity for American medicine, was developed in an effort to mend the machine that had broken down. Sixty-five years post-Flexner, we suffer from a new set of maladies. Most physicians have a continuing thirst for knowledge and a desire to provide better care for their patients. However, they are victims of outdated teaching and learning methodologies, medical school apathy toward clinicians' needs, research which moves ahead faster than the system is able to disseminate it, and a lack of appropriate auditing tools to inform physicians of their needs by evaluation of their current knowledge.

Shepherd[2] stated in 1960 that sponsorship for continuing medical education during the post-Flexnerian era, had gone through three stages. These are: (1) The proprietary polyclinic hospital and graduate and postgraduate school; (2) The medical society and state board of health independent of the medical school (although using medical school faculty members to a large extent); and (3) The medical school as the responsible sponsor and planner often in cooperation with a medical society. Many of the sponsorships have overlapped and, in addition, there have been sponsorships by extension of departments of universities as well as academies of medicine.

Perhaps the most important step forward in continuing medical education was the creation of the American Academy of General Practice in 1947. This marked the beginning of mandatory continuing medical education. The Academy made the first basic readjustment of assumptions underlying continuing medical education: it was proposed that the mere acquisition of education is not the ultimate end. Selection, organization, and evaluation of educational content is the means to the end, and the end is better health care for the clinician's patients.

Current Trends

Current trends in medical education are toward specific requirements for continuing medical education credits. The American Academy of Family Physicians has had these requirements for 28 years.[3] On July 1, 1975, the American Medical Association identified 13 state medical associations, five medical specialty societies, and one specialty board, the American Board of Family Practice, which have stipulated requirements for continuing medical education. Others have indicated their intention to make similar requirements.

Some educators are asking if mandatory continuing medical education is valuable as a means of improving efficacy of education. Libby[4] has recently stated categorically, "Mandatory continuing education programs as they are now administered are predictable failures." He quotes Canadian educator A. M. Thomas: "By and large, men cannot be coerced into learning." Libby also feels that academicians involved in providing continuing education for the adult practitioner are primarily skilled in child/youth education. They teach as they were taught. He then cites M. S. Knowles, who believes that for some adults, the remembrance of the classroom as the place where one is treated with disrespect is so strong that it serves as a serious barrier to involvement in adult education activities. Finally, Libby states that in his opinion, the problem-centered curriculum is the only way to achieve appropriate education for adults. He may be right.

In 1968 Hudson[5] stated that research had moved ahead of current educational methods. This is true for the family physician, and probably for all of medicine. It has moved ahead of the ability of medical education to produce organized, selected, and evaluated material appropriate for assimilation in the time the clinician has available for study.

Problems in Continuing Medical Education

Americans have always been vitally interested in the educational process. How, then, has medical education, or at least continuing medical education fallen behind? Regarding this, the following points should be made:

1. *Medical schools have been research-oriented, and unresponsive in providing educational material.* One has only to look at the federal and non-federal support for medical schools in general, and it can be seen that a great deal of this support (52 percent) comes from research-oriented funding.[6] In addition, guidelines and criteria for promotion and tenure favor only those teachers of medicine who are able to produce research material in quantity sufficient to make their way upward on the ladder of professorial stature. The following quotations from *Guidelines and Criteria for Promotion and Tenure of the University of Kansas Medical School Committee on Promotions,* approved in June 1973, illustrate this point.[7]

   Promotion to a new rank must be based principally on evidence of achievement since the last promotion. Criteria for promotion traditionally have been and continue to be teaching, research and service.... A teacher's accomplishments and contributions as a scholar bring vital recognition to the university as well as to the individual.... Promotion in professorial rank is a testimony and recognition of professional competency and productivity. The evidence of this competence is the research conducted by the teacher, the results of which are submitted for professional evaluation, review and criticism to his peers through recognized media. Publication in refereed

journals and in books is the only valid measure of scholarly productivity.

Promotion schedules that mandate research and publication as a part of scholarship are not necessarily conducive to the production of family practice teachers. Research is, however, a necessary part of family practice, particularly in the discipline's efforts to define its own core of knowledge. An equitable mix of teaching skills and health-care delivery skills must be weighed along with research as the basis for academic appointment and promotion.

2. *Family practice continuing medical education has suffered from the lack of a defined core of knowledge.* Forces in education are now making great steps toward this definition, but continuing medical education, to be most significant, must be based on the core of knowledge of the discipline. Future plans for family practice continuing medical education will gradually adopt goals and objectives centered in the definition of the discipline of family practice.

3. *There is a preponderance of the traditional content-transfer model of the educational process.* Critics of the present system see its greatest fault in being simply communicative education. But this mechanism cannot be sold short: it has performed well. Those who would measure it in terms of behavioral change have not really been able to define and measure behavior at all. We can, however, all look back on the development of the coronary care unit and find here an example of how new information was spread rapidly, safely, and usefully. We are obliged to admit that there must be something effective about a continuing medical education system that does this. Meanwhile, problem-centered education produced *en masse* is costly, logistically difficult to deliver, and not totally accepted by all of today's practitioners.

   There are other methods of communicative medical education that the physician can take part in: the blend of journals, specialty organization meetings, national postgraduate courses, and hospital staff meetings. These add up to a mixture of methods to put new information rapidly in motion. However, new methods for the delivery of continuing medical education must be designed. Perhaps this can be done best by the program director of a family practice residency who is in daily practice within his own family practice center and who is constantly aware of new events in medicine.

4. *There has been a failure to perform evaluations, both in terms of the goals and objectives of education and the results of the educational process.* The needs of the potential consumer of continuing medical education have not been measured in offices or hospitals. Instead, research-oriented medical schools have presumed to know these needs. Another method of determining the consumer's needs has been to ask him what he wishes. This is an irrational process which only reveals the subjects of greatest interest to the physician and does not take into consideration a true audit of his necessities. Measurement of learning outcomes is a necessary factor in any future continuing medical education scheme.

5. *There has been a failure to look at the motivational factors behind continuing medical education.* The American physician has exhibited a stout desire to continually upgrade himself. Yet he is irregularly motivated. The remote physician, the physician burdened with a large practice, the physician who is under financial stress or has no backup physicians to cover his practice, is under duress when it comes to obtaining continuing medical education. Systems must be devised to provide all physicians with the opportunities to partake of appropriate continuing medical education. The current system stresses man-

dated continuing medical education. This method is highly motivating, but other motivational factors should be explored. The question of punitive motivation and better educational process needs to be answered in terms of thoughtful analysis and review of the system, but without attaching "self-destruct" mechanisms to what has been an effective method of communication. The fault may lie with the process, and new processes may be needed to assist, entice, and teach the practicing physician.

General practice was criticized by its detractors as being a group of physicians without an intellectual base. Reinfrank, in his inaugural address as president of the American Society of Internal Medicine, stated,

> I suggest, therefore, that the need for competent scholarly clinicians broadly trained in disease recognition, and assessing the relationships of problems to each other in the total situation, with the ability to deal with less structured and more ambiguous problems than the subspecialties, will always remain a desirable social priority if the objective of any medical system is to obtain the best match between the physician and what he does and the patient and what he needs. Never was the old saying more appropriate. A patient says, 'I hope you treat what I got,' and the doctor says, 'I hope you got what I treat'.... I suggest that internists and other scholarly generalists will be required in the future, as they are required now, if high quality medical care is to be rationally linked to the current drive for cost containment.[8]

One would wonder if Reinfrank is referring to the family physician when he mentions "other scholarly generalists."

If our colleagues were previously able to criticize our lack of scholarly intent because of our lack of an intellectual beginning in residency, we have overcome that. But if their criticism is scrutinized, perhaps one would discover that it was the system that was at fault because the general practitioner was offered education for education's sake without regard for his needs.

The Residency Program and Continuing Medical Education

Family practice is developing its own academicians. Currently, their preoccupation is with the more glamorous undergraduate and graduate training. But the intellectualism of family practice must start here. Meaningful continuing medical education must be a part of the family practice residency and then continue in practice. The most promising place for continuing education for the graduated family physician is the family practice residency.

The three-year period of time within an organized educational environment is the ideal setting to serve as the base for continuing medical education. Each resident has the opportunity to develop and acquire lifelong habits for his continuing medical education and growth of competence. The learning process is an individual matter and each resident should be encouraged and helped to define his own style, the most effective method of learning. Within this learning process, a definite team effort needs to be made. The current American physician personality rejects any but those with an MD degree as being competent to teach physicians. Nutritionists, psychologists, and other behavioral scientists have been traditionally ignored by the physician who resents their intrusion into his intellectual sphere. This is fallacious thinking and should be overcome by introducing these professionals into the residency program. The physician who is accustomed to working with these colleagues qualified in other fields, will soon develop respect for them and accept being taught by them in future years. Evaluation, which is a part of all residency programs, may be threatening to older practicing physicians, but it is a major factor in producing appropriate education at all levels. Evaluation, begun when the individual is a student and resident and continued after he becomes a practicing physician, loses its threatening aspect.

Consideration of the residency program as the training base for continuing education is not without precedent. Hudson[5] quotes Lindsay Beaton, at an Association of American Medical Colleges teaching institute in 1962, as stating that the student graduate should never be separated from his medical school, but should be drawn periodically by ties to return to his alma mater for educational refreshment. This has not been applied to graduate training programs, and the geographical dispersion of graduates has never been addressed.

We should convert this idea to the residency program, with the development of ties to graduate training, and gradually change the method of delivery of continuing medical education. Alumni groups should have room to accept those geographically separated from their parent programs, and devices can be developed to make these educational orphans an integral part of their adopted home. This can be accomplished by the original parents "letting go" and new parents accepting without the stigma of adoption. Defining a clear-cut role for the new alumnus, such as teaching assignments and staff appointments, is imperative in this system. The function of the alumni organization will not be to rekindle the old days with meetings, but rather to serve as a support system for the residency program. No longer will content-transfer education be the graduates' only relationship to continuing education. Rather, the graduate will return periodically for refreshment and retraining as an active program participant, both as a student and a teacher. To be effective, the system must be continuous and as it grows, graduates will always be a part of the faculty. They may attend one day a week or one day a month, or daily for a week, but while present, they will spend some of their time learning certain skills, or products of new research, or reviewing a broad spectrum of care. While attending, the returning graduate must contribute to the education of his successors in the residency program. This can be done as a group leader, lecturer, or clinic supervisor, but the role is less important than the contribution of practice experience to the current crop of residents. Under this method, the practicing doctor stays fresh, enthusiastic and current professionally, and he contributes to the welfare of the residency by paying tuition as well as providing certain teaching roles. The residency director, or his designate, who is experienced in teaching and assessment of needs, assists the practicing doctor in evaluating his educational needs, while the constant infusion of practicing doctors provides patient management skills to the training program.

The logistical problems of this kind of system will grow as more and more residents are graduated and ultimately could break down under the sheer weight of numbers, but not for a long time. It is during this time that competency-based objectives for training will be established. It is also during this period that a broad core of knowledge will be established for the family physician, and that through the knowledge gained in the residency refreshment training programs, cyclical methods of retraining and review will be identified. Later, other community clinical training centers may be established specifically for continuing medical education. It is not inconceivable that in the future, as medical schools and graduate training programs decentralize and develop greater community awareness, community continuing education centers will develop around larger community hospitals. These postgraduate institutions, along with the residencies, could well provide continuing medical education for all clinicians.

This new method of education will provide the practicing physician continuing medical education through better educational methods that are appropriate to his needs. This will combat the criticism that all

continuing medical education is delivered via the content-transfer method. Content-transfer should not be totally removed, but should remain a part of association meetings. Communal learning still has a place in medical education, and until organized medicine develops new funding methods, educational association meetings need to be continued to support the work needs of the organizations. Other factors such as renewal of old friendships, contact with different perspectives, and shoulder rubbing with medical people from other areas contribute to the total learning picture in this setting.

Continuing medical education, through linkages of practicing physicians with residency programs should include practice profile methods and self-assessment as integral parts of the system. The residency program will have the responsibility of participating with the graduate in setting up systems in which educational content is geared to reality. This process will require a certain amount of time away from the individual's practice, especially in the case of doctors who are remote from the site of a residency program. Arrangements can be worked out so that senior residents spend part of their time in the office of the absent physician, under the guidance of another doctor. Current attitudes among those reviewing residency programs oppose such preceptorships, but more flexible attitudes may prevail in the future. For such a system to work, it should be meaningful to both the practicing physician who returns to the residency program and the resident who goes to the physician's office.

The role of the practicing physician has been discussed, but what about the resident who relieves him? It would seem that in order to have a positive experience, the resident would have to enter the practice while the practicing physician was still there and be introduced to the patients, the partner, or other members of the group practice in order to become familiarized with the practicing physician's methods of operation. Then, during the absence of the practicing physician, the resident would have the opportunity to apply his own attitudes and skills to the physician's practice and also receive the benefit of counseling from other members of the group practice. The resident should remain in the practice after the practicing physician returns so that fruitful discussions regarding outcomes of the resident's experience can take place and the whole process can be made into a learning experience for both the physician and the resident.

This new system of continuing medical education linked to the residency system provides the following positive features for the practicing physician:

1. Appropriate design of continuing education according to previously identified needs.
2. Immediate application of learned skills or knowledge to a patient population.
3. Opportunities for educational use of practice profiling, self-assessment, and practice audit.
4. Prospective evaluation of needs of practicing physicians and retrospective evaluation of their learning outcomes.
5. Linkages for the practicing physician to the learning centers for education and consultation.
6. Refreshment for the practicing physician both educationally and attitudinally.

The following positive points accrue to the residency program through this system:

1. Funding support through tuition charged to the returning graduates.
2. Teaching support contributed by the student-teacher returnee.
3. Constant infusion of practice attitudes in the training residents.

Author's Update

Since the publication of this article a number of changes in continuing medical education have occurred which effect the previously stated problems:

1. *Medical schools have been research-oriented, and unresponsive in providing educational material.* Since the advent of the Liaison Committee on Continuing Medical Education (LCGME), the Accreditation Council on Continuing Medical Education (ACCME), noticeable differences have occurred. The material produced by medical colleges is more relevant in terms of physicians' needs.
2. *Family practice continuing medical education has suffered from a lack of a defined core of knowledge.* This is being corrected by the Residency Assistance Program Criteria and a publication of the Society of Teachers of Family Medicine entitled *Predoctoral Education in Family Medicine.* Also, the American Academy of Family Physicians has developed a curriculum for a six-year study course.
3. *There is a preponderance of the traditional content-transfer model of the education process.* Interactive home study programs and workshops have become more popular in the years since publication of this paper.
4. *There has been a failure to perform evaluations both in terms of the goals and objectives of education and the results of the educational process.* The ACCME and the Academy's review process have helped the progress.
5. *There has been a failure to look at the motivational factors behind continuing medical education.* There still remains a problem in that the primary motivation for learning is still hazy as to whether or not the learner is motivated by mandatory CME or the desire for improvement. The author feels that physicians' desire for excellence is still the primary reason for utilization of CME.

REFERENCES

1. Flexner A: Medical Education in the United States and Canada, a Report to the Carnegie Foundation for the Advancement of Teaching. Bulletin No. 4. Boston, Updyke, 1910
2. Shepherd CR: History of continuing medical edu-

cation in the United States since 1930. J Med Educ 35:740–748, 1960

3. Continuing Medical Education Fact Sheet. Chicago, American Medical Association, July 1, 1975

4. Libby GN, Weinswig MH, Kirk KW: Help stamp out mandatory continuing education. JAMA 233:797–799, 1975

5. Hudson CL: The responsibility of the university in the continuing education of physicians. J Med Educ 43:526–531, 1968

6. Division of Operational Studies of the Association of American Medical Colleges: Medical school finances. JAMA 226:916–922, 1973

7. Guidelines and Criteria for Promotions and Tenure. University of Kansas, School of Medicine, approved by the Chancellor, June, 1973. Kansas City, Kansas

8. Reinfrank RF: The scholarly generalist known as "internist": Is there a viable future? The Internist: July–Sugust, 1975, pp 14–17

A Job Half Done*

M. P. Taylor

It is a great honour to be invited to give the William Pickles Lecture, and it is a great pleasure to give it in such delightful surroundings. I am sure that Will Pickles and Gertie would have approved for it was at Windermere that they spent their honeymoon in May 1917.

I saw Pickles on one occasion only. This was my 'short and only exposure'. It was at the opening ceremony and prize distribution at Birmingham Medical School on 3 October 1950. Pickles was giving the inaugural address and I was a very new undergraduate. I had forgotten completely until I saw a photograph of this occasion in Pemberton's (1970) fascinating biography.

I am very proud to claim at least some things in common with Pickles. He was a fellow Yorkshireman, and I too was born and bred in Leeds. We both failed finals. When I entered general practice I shared his aspirations for this College which made him its first President but rejected my first application for membership. I was rejected because I failed to demonstrate evidence of attendance at postgraduate activities.

When I was invited to give this lecture I was informed that it was "usual for it to be on an educational topic". And so, for the thirteenth William Pickles Lecture I am to speak about continuing education—not intrinsically exciting but important and topical.

I intend to review some of the developments in continuing education and to draw particularly upon my own experience as a general practitioner tutor. I will consider the relative influence of formal postgraduate education on what general practitioners actually do and draw some conclusions about what needs to be done in the future.

*Reprinted by permission from *Journal of the Royal College of General Practitioners*, 30:456–465, 1980.

Developments in Continuing Education

McKnight (1971), in the fourth Pickles Lecture, urged that continuing education should be equated with undergraduate education and vocational training. He saw formal continuing education as far less important than self-education based upon the 'need to know' and he stressed the need to inculcate the attitude of continuing education in trainees. He considered, as Byrne (1969) had two years before, that the way to improve formal continuing education lay through the activities of regional general practitioner sub-committees and departments of general practice influencing clinical tutors and devising courses. He concluded by appealing to practitioners to play their rightful part in teaching their fellows.

What, in fact, has been happening? We have a full quota of regional general practitioner sub-committees, regional advisers and associates, and an increasing number of university departments of general practice. The former have been preoccupied with vocational training and the latter with undergraduate education. Formal continuing education has come last and it probably had to. Nevertheless, there have been exciting developments and largely as a result of vocational training. Many in the audience have shared in these developments.

Vocational training has produced more than vocationally trained doctors; it has developed a body of teachers, course organizers and trainers with educational know-how and skills. It has produced in its vocationally trained doctors, practitioners with a different expectation of education, with a familiarity and preference for learning based on small-group activity, standard setting, and audit. Inevitably, continuing education has been influenced.

Some centres now have general practitioner tutors organizing continuing education in more relevant and interesting ways, providing focus and leadership.

In 1971 my experiences as course organizer for Doncaster Vocational Training Scheme encouraged me to challenge the established manner of providing postgraduate education locally. It was not that there was not considerable effort being made by a dedicated group of organizers, including clinical tutor, consultants and general practitioners, nor that there were not many enjoyable and well attended events, because all of this was true. The question was: were general practitioners changing what they were doing as a result? Was there any improvement in patient care? There was a need to decide what was to be learned first—a reversal of the tradition of inviting a 'good speaker' who would be expected to choose his own topic.

It was agreed to have small working parties to organize individual events, speakers would be briefed about objectives to be achieved, the lecture would not be seen as the only instrument of instruction, and small-group activity would be introduced where relevant. A general practitioner tutor (honorary), myself, was appointed.

Midwifery

I would like to illustrate my theme from some of my own experiences as a general practitioner tutor. In 1971 there were problems in our general practitioner maternity unit. Things were going wrong—there were delays in referring patients who developed complications in the antenatal period—toxaemia, primiparae with high heads at term—and unacceptable delays in labour, frequently requiring consultant involvement at a late stage, sometimes in unsociable hours, which were beneficial to neither doctor nor patient. The continued existence of the Unit was in danger. The main problem was the failure of general practitioners to keep up to date. The 'hands-off' expectant tradition had changed. The emphasis was now on early recognition of

abnormality in pregnancy and labour. Failure to progress in labour had criteria for active management unfamiliar to general practitioner obstetricians.

Consultants were persuaded that an educational programme would be preferable to a feud and a detailed list of the knowledge, skills, and attitudes required by general practitioner obstetricians was constructed. Important deficiencies in performance were itemized and a programme of obstetric seminars was organized. Booking policy and indications for transfer to consultant care were restated and a flow chart introduced, its most important feature being the incorporation of an action line. Failure to progress in labour past a certain point was an indication for action, usually referral. This flow chart, known as a 'partogram', had originally been devised as a job aid for use by midwives managing primigravid labour outside hospital in Rhodesia; it had been found in practice to be useful not only in the bush but also in teaching hospitals— and so why not in general practitioner maternity units?

The results of the seminars and organizational changes resolved problems in the general practitioner maternity unit and transformed general practitoner obstetrics. It would be gratifying to record that we had measured the number of deliveries by forceps and caesarean section before and those after the educational programme, but we did not. However, no-one was in any doubt that things were better afterwards.

Therapeutics

In 1975 the clinical tutor, a consultant geriatrician, proposed a study day on therapeutics relating to problems in the elderly. There were many distinct and common problems relating to side-effects, interactions and polypharmacy. Here were important educational needs, not only for local general practitioners but for others. The challenge was how to teach these complicated ideas in a way which people would understand and retain, and which would enable them to go away at the end of the day able to make some sense of their prescribing. A day of lectures would cover the ground but mainly with sleeping bodies and few residual effects. What we did was to have two lectures only. One was on 'drug treatment in the elderly', covering the more common drugs used and the more common problems, and the other was on 'drug interactions'. The other strategy for the day was to set groups of doctors to discuss a series of therapeutic problems, some of which were in the form of modified essay questions, and all illustrating differing and often multiple problems. Most of the problems used were found by the clinical tutor and myself from our own practice. Others were culled from such sources as prescribers' notes. The problems were chosen to match the lecture material. Each group had a resource leader and was allowed to use reference books. The answers to the problems were discussed further at a plenary session and a high level of discussion took place. The content was seen as relevant and was presented in a stimulating manner. Participants were able to relate their own previous knowledge and practice to the problems. The points made in the lectures were reinforced by the discussions in the groups.

What did we achieve? The response to a questionnaire seeking subjective opinion about the value of the day, its organization, and reaction to the teaching methods used was encouraging. As to a change in general practitioner behaviour, we had an unexpected indication that we might have achieved something unusual when pharmaceutical representatives asked what we had been up to—there was surprise at the level of questioning from general practitioners who had attended. Other than that we do not know.

Group Work

Sheffield Medical School has a tradition of week-long refresher courses for general practitioners. In the past these have consisted of a week of lectures and demonstrations, but in recent years we have introduced group activity aimed at setting criteria for the management of common conditions in practice. Groups have been provided with literature and specialist resources to assist them. It has been encouraging to see in members of such groups the acceptance of new ideas, particularly relating to continuing care and surveillance. This has been borne out by requests after courses for advice and material, such as simple morbidity indexes.

Last year we had a contrary experience: for several reasons the group activity was curtailed and on the final session of the course the reaction of members to concepts of continuing care and surveillance of such conditions as asthma and epilepsy were negative. There were responses such as: "We can't be specialists in everything!" "Not paid to do it." This may have been a characteristic of course members, but my belief is that with carefully organized courses, attitudes can be shifted and enthusiasm generated.

Epilepsy

In my final example I propose to go into more detail. If we consider epilepsy, a condition in which it is now possible to provide greatly improved care, at a topic for continuing education, we find that in order to identify standards of practice to aim for we need to know what is possible. In order to plan a programme which is relevant we need information about current performance and especially about deficiencies.

Recent literature gives us information about both possibilities and deficiencies. The British Epilepsy Association (S. McGovern personal communication) has described problems encountered by patients with their general practitioners. Table 1 summarizes some of the main points. Jeavons (1975), reviewing 470 patients attending two epilepsy clinics in Birmingham, identified 20 percent as not having epilepsy. Parsonage reports similar experience (per-

Table 1. *Management of Epilepsy*

Performance Deficiencies	New Knowledge/Skills
Wrongly diagnosed	Drug level monitoring
Polypharmacy	Single drug effective
Failure to explain	Daily or twice daily
Ignorance about blood	dosage
level monitoring	
Poor records	
Poor supervision	

sonal communication). The most important reasons were found to be inadequate history taking and ignorance of the nature of epilepsy.

Amongst the many problems described by the British Epilepsy Association were: polypharmacy in response to repeat seizures, failure to explain about the disease or the purpose of medication, and ignorance about blood level monitoring.

That, in general, records are inadequate cannot in honesty be denied: it is a feature of British general practice and none of us can afford to be complacent. Long-term supervision depends upon good record keeping.

Drug level measurement has led to greater understanding of the pharmokinetics of anticonvulsants, especially phenytoin. It has been demonstrated (Cocks *et al.*, 1975) that this drug works effectively in a once-daily dosage and other anticonvulsants work in the majority of patients in a twice-daily dosage.

In hospital series it has been shown that 76 to 88 percent of new patients may be controlled with a single drug (Shorvon *et al.*, 1978). It has also been shown (Shorvon and Reynolds, 1979) that polypharmacy may be reduced in chronic epilepsy with reduction to a single drug in 72 percent of patients, with improvement in seizure control in 55 percent, plus a striking improvement in mental function in 55 percent. (It must be noted that a small number may become worse.)

Phenytoin dose adjustment is known to be particularly critical (Mawer *et al.*, 1974); above a certain serum level small increases

in dose, as small as 25 to 50 mg, are needed to avoid toxicity. Conversely, to forget only the occasional dose brings the level below the therapeutic range. On the standard 300 mg per day dosage the majority of patients are likely to be under- or over-treated.

Improvement in care, however, will not result from the general practitoner improving his knowledge alone. Laboratory services must also be available, and available, I would like to stress, means specimen collection services—there is evidence that such a service can be cost-effective (G. E. Leyshon, personal communication).

Here then are educational needs to indicate learning objectives. What sort of learning situation is necessary to translate these into improved patient care? A lecture could be a start, but really the problem cries out for a standard-setting exercise carried out by groups of doctors with the emphasis on activity at practice level. The basic steps are familiar to many of you: first of all, preliminary meetings to set standards aided by discussion with experts and a search of the literature; secondly, identification of the patients and of deficiencies either by a review of the records, if adequate, or of the patients, or both; thirdly, action to remedy deficiencies; and finally, a further review to check the effectiveness of the exercise.

Audit of Epilepsy

I am aware that it is not wise to organize other people's standard-setting exercises and do nothing personally, and so, two weeks ago, I carried out an audit on the records of patients with epilepsy in my practice. This was neither research nor a model standard-setting exercise, rather a look at the state of affairs after several years in which we have gradually changed the management of epilepsy, but with increased activity in the past 6 to 12 months. Certain implicit criteria had been adopted, a requirement for:

1. As precise a diagnosis as possible, based on a description of any seizure; where

a description was missing, one was sought.

2. A regular review, at least yearly.
3. Adequate records, especially of the incidence of seizures, side-effects of drugs and the problems patients were facing.
4. A policy of improving seizure control with a decreasing number of drugs, in simpler dosage, enquiring for and avoiding side-effects.

The results are shown in Tables 2 and 3. Thirty-seven patients were identified in a practice population of 6498, giving a prevalence of 5.7 per 1000. This number included only three children under the age of 16. There was a description of seizures in 78 percent and from this doubts about the certainty of the diagnosis in three, one of whom was an ex-barbiturate addict who had had seizures which appeared to be related to barbiturate withdrawal and who, in any case, was no longer on anticonvulsants. Three patients had not been reviewed in the past year and one of these had escaped for 18 months. Out of the five handicapped, improvement in control has made it possible for one to return to work and another to contemplate it. Another with previously

Table 2. *Audit of epilepsy (from records). Practice population = 6,498, N = 37 (19 male, 18 female), (5.7 per 1000)*

	Total	Percentage
Description of seizure	29	78
EEG	26	70
Seen in year	34	92
Seizure record	32	86.5
Seizure-free	21	57
Drug side-effects	4	11
Handicapped	5	13.5
Number of drugs		
3	2	
2	14	
1	17	46
0	4	
Reduction from 3+ in two years	9	24
Blood levels	13	35
(Of value)	8	21

Table 3. *Audit of epilepsy–results.*

Seizure control over two years	Improved in	10 (6 male,
	Worse in	4 female)
Drug levels	Critical in	1 male
	improving	7 (mainly phenytoin)
General move to twice daily or daily dosage		

apparently intractable epilepsy was noted to have very variable and often low serum levels of anticonvulsants and improved magically on the simplicity of a daily dose of phenytoin. Polypharmacy has been reduced in 24 percent, and 46 percent of patients are now on one drug.

Seizure control appears to be improved in 27 percent. Improvement in general well-being in some patients has been dramatic.

These few examples demonstrate a range of educational activity. They are not unique—others in other places have done similar or better. I have presented them in order to show the need for thoughtful planning and skill; that there is a structure to the process of education which, if understood, can be of enormous assistance. I have to say something about this process.

Educational Theory

Unfortunately, educational theory is often seen as a burden (Figure 1) rather than something to ease progress. It is shown in a variety of forms fundamentally the same. The educational paradigm in its triangular form is familiar to you all (Pereira Gray, 1979). I personally prefer to think of it as a cybernetic cycle as described by Miller (1967), also known as Miller's carousel.

The pathway is common. We start with objectives through appropriate learning experiences to evaluation. Objectives indicate what we intend the learner to do as a result of the process.

What is the overall objective for continuing education? Byrne (1969) suggested that it should seek to initiate and promote

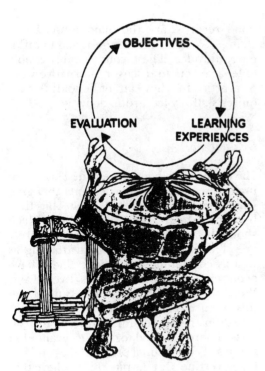

Fig. 1. The educational paradigm.

change; I suggest that such change be towards improved patient care, and that it is necessary to work towards a model and that the model is fundamental. What models do we have?

The job description of our terms and conditions of service is as follows: "A doctor shall render to his patients all necessary and appropriate personal medical services of the type usually provided by general practitioners" (NHS Reg., 1974). A comprehensive description of the work of the general practitioner which has travelled from Manchester to Europe in various forms and has been the model for vocational training is equally appropriate for continuing education: "The general practitioner is a licensed medical graduate who gives care to individuals irrespective of age, sex, and illness. He will attend his patients in his consulting room and in their homes and sometimes in a clinic or a hospital. His aim is to make early diagnoses. He will include and integrate physical, psychological, and social factors in his considerations about health and illness. He will make an initial decision about every problem which is presented to him as a doctor. He will undertake the continuing management of his patients with chronic, recurrent, or terminal illnesses. Prolonged contact means that he can use repeated opportunities to gather information at a pace appropriate to each patient and build up a relationship of trust which he can use professionally. He will practise in co-operation with other colleagues, medical and non-medical. He will know how and when to intervene through treatment, prevention, and education to promote the health of his patients and their families. He will recognize that he also has a professional responsibility to the community" (Leeuwenhorst Working Party, 1977).

The lowest level to which general practitioners retreat is to provide an on-demand service which responds to wants. A fuller job description is: "Comprehensive continuing care which responds to needs." The latter does not yet in any true or complete sense exist in British primary care. Objectives for continuing education programmes should have this model in mind.

Objectives

Objectives need to be derived from training needs and I suggest that training needs may be identified by looking for deficiencies in performance and those arising out of new medical knowledge and skills (Table 4). Care must be taken in reviewing performance since shortcomings may not be due to lack of knowledge or skill so much as failure in execution; this may be due to heavy workload, high morbidity, the certification burden, or common-or-garden laziness. Lack of resources, for example lack of access to contrast radiology or absence of specimen collection services and laboratory facilities, would negate increases in knowledge or skill gained from an educational programme.

Table 4. *Selecting Learning Objectives*

Performance Deficiencies	
Knowledge/skill	
Execution	

From Practice	From Outside
Ask	Use of hospital services
Audit	Referrals
	Diagnostic services
	Prescribing data

New Medical Knowledge and Skills
Postgraduate organization

From outside we can look at the use of hospital services; we can ask patient groups; we can look at prescribing data. The possibilities from new medical knowledge and skills should be forthcoming from the postgraduate organization, universities, and specialists (the latter in a general sense), and this College.

Learning Experiences

Learning experiences should be both appropriate to the objectives and optimal for older learners. As Miller (1967) has pointed out, there is no one superior method and individuals learn in different ways. However, different methods suit different objectives. Acquisition of knowledge comes by reading or listening; skills are acquired by demonstration, practice, and correction; attitudes are more readily influenced by peer interaction. In general, methods which actively involve learners are more effective and adult learners are no exception. Their main problem is difficulty in accepting new ideas, especially when this means discarding the security of established practice. Since attitudes about role, for example, concepts about continuing care, preventive health, health education, and the need for good records, are the major obstacles to change, we need courses designed to influence attitudes. These courses must enable older learners to discover alternative ways of practice for they cannot be told; this requires skilfully led group activity.

Evaluation

Have objectives been achieved? Has learning taken place? Are participants changing what they do? Have any new objectives been identified? These are questions which should be asked of every activity, but rarely are. This is true of vocational training as well as continuing education. There have been very few validated studies (Evered and Williams, 1980). We generally assume from unstructured comment or uncontrolled observation the success or failure of our efforts. There is a need to conduct evaluation studies of educational programmes and it is long overdue. But despite this I believe that we can accept that well designed and executed activities can lead to changes in what doctors do.

Let me now pull the threads together:

What can we say about formal continuing education?

1. It is possible to provide more effective learning leading to improved patient care.
2. It is complicated and to do it properly requires skill.
3. It is most effective if it leads to self-learning.
4. However, it reaches only a small number.

What is the case for formal continuing education?

1. It gives direction and indicates standards.
2. It gives structure and support.
3. It reduces the effect of professional isolation.

Skill and leadership are required and my experience and that of others confirms my belief that this should be provided primarily by a general practitioner tutor at district postgraduate centre level—not to replace the clinical tutor, since his work is different and complementary. He should be paid and have secretarial support. Both he and the clinical tutor should have local budgets.

Secondly, at regional level, an improved postgraduate organization is needed which is able to provide resources—to link general practitioner tutors and provide more ambitious, long courses.

Pemberton (1970, pp 98–99) described and McKnight (1971) reminded us how Pickles, at the age of 40, comfortably settled in practice, was inspired by reading Mackenzie's (1916) classic *Principles of Diagnosis and Treatment in Heart Affections*. Soon afterwards in 1927 he undertook a correspondence course to bring himself up to date and, finding this inadequate, in 1929 he took a month's refresher course in hospital and continued to do so each year until 1939. Pickles, an exceptional man, took exceptional steps to keep himself up to date and he did this in early middle age onwards. So perhaps there is hope for many of us yet.

What about the young doctors entering general practice at present? Let us consider our young ex-trainee entering general practice. Has the desire to continue his education been inculcated in him? Are his attitudes 'tuned'? He will have many responsibilities including a wife and family. What if he settles in a busy underresourced practice with high demand? Will he cope and maintain his standards? Will he experience difficulty in keeping up to date like 55 percent of the practitioners responding to a recent survey on continuing education in Nottinghamshire (A. J. Pickup, personal communication)? Will it become harder as he becomes older? Will he, like the majority of Nottinghamshire general practitioners, find the job enjoyable or satisfactory despite over-demand and heavy workload? Will he be able to lead a balanced life essen-

tial to health and good practice, sharing in activities enjoyed by the rest of society, all very proper pursuits, or will it all prove too much and will his standards fall despite the early promise?

Will he sink into professional obsolescence? Will he and colleagues, as Carr (1979) asks, face the challenge of our inner cities or opt out and leave it to the hospitals? Will they seek out vulnerable patients or leave it to community medical officers and community nurses? Will he become our ideal general practitioner providing comprehensive continuing care?

The Relative Influence of Continuing Education

Apart from pressures of work, leisure, and the family, what external forces will be influencing the young doctor in the way he practises? Figure 2 shows the major influences and these are seen to be largely organizational or educational. Our colleague has, of course, views about where he is going: he has aspirations and attitudes. Changes in payment since the Charter have had a profound impact on general practice, in particular in providing improved premises and ancillary staff. Item-of-service payments influence a range of activity; the burden of certification will restrict it. Attached community nurses, open access services and specimen collection services expand what it is possible for him to do.

Of educational influences, the major contenders are the pharmaceutical industry and activities financed under Section 63. The former will reach the doctor whether he likes it or not and the latter only if he wishes. Over 40 free magazines will reach him, all financed by advertising. Numerous representatives will call and there will be the opportunity to attend sponsored meetings. Much of the information provided in this way is found helpful and informative, but many doctors complain about the sheer volume and variable quality of the material,

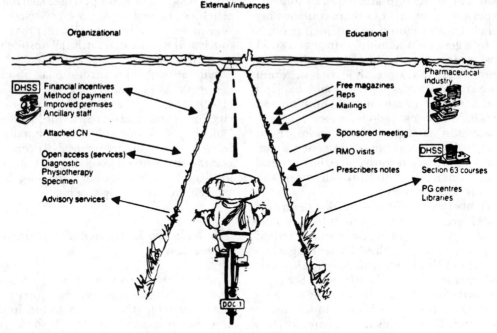

Fig. 2. External influences on a young doctor.

described as 'overkill' (A. J. Pickup, personal communication). The pharmaceutical industry spends 10 percent of its home sales on promotion, according to recent information from APBI, that is £80 million a year. About 80 percent of prescriptions are written by general practitioners so, at a rough estimate if these sums are correct, something like £64 million is spent in influencing the prescriber. In contrast, the Department of Health and Social Security relies upon Regional Medical Officer visits, prescribers' notes, and funds postgraduate centres, postgraduate deans, clinical tutors, and regional advisers. The annual allocation for Section 63 courses, to cover both vocational training and continuing education, is £660,000. This is controlled at regional level and local centres have to request funds for specified activities from postgraduate deans well in advance. There are in addition, as you know, funds for travelling and subsistence which account for another £500,000.

Who and What Are We Trying To Change?

Taylor (1954) described general practice as consisting of a quarter which is of a high standard, a half sound and reliable, if unexciting, and a quarter unsatisfactory. Within that quarter was one-twentieth of the whole which was inexcusable. He considered that Collings (1950), in his damning description, was looking at the unsatisfactory quarter. He asked (p. 468): "Is it right for a doctor in a northern industrial town to have to do three times as much work for each of his patients as a doctor in a healthy London suburb, while receiving the same amount of remuneration?" He observed (p. 470): "The lowest standards of practice were seen more frequently in the large list industrial areas than elsewhere and appeared to result in part from excessive pressure of work on too few doctors." "Distribution of doctors should follow morbidity."

What is the situation in 1980? I offer an

image of general practice as a piece of elastic nailed down at one end and being pulled out at the other (Figure 3), the best getting better and better, the worst changing little if at all; the unsatisfactory portion limits the whole, its failure causing others to seek to fill the gap in primary care: hospitals, deputizing services, and a more recent and worrying arrival in London.

What is the nature of this nail? It is not just the weight of apathy. Good men as well as bad are pinned down by it. It is high morbidity, high workload, established patterns of practice. Taylor's (1954) statement is still applicable today. Vocational training and continuing education alone cannot change general practice, and the part of general practice pinned down is the most important part of general practice today: removing that nail is the most important single thing to be done. How this should be done is not for me to say, but suggestions such as those of the Greater Glasgow Local Medical Committee advocating special payments linked with accepted indices of social deprivation, which are themselves linked with high morbidity, deserve serious consideration. Remove that nail and away he goes.

Perhaps William Pickles' (1951) optimism in his inaugural address at that opening ceremony 30 years ago will be justified. "I have faith that even in general practice we have the makings of a first-class Health Service, if only some means can be devised to make it unnecessary for doctors to have enormous numbers of potential patients on their medical lists. The impossibility of giving adequate attention to patients is a source of great unhappiness to many of us, but I believe this can be remedied and we shall continue to have, as we always have had, the finest medical service in the world."

I have outlined what I believe needs to be done in continuing education. Although the practitioner of the future is likely to be greatly assisted by the microchip and improved information systems and self-assessment packages, the immediate problems relate to setting standards and shifting attitudes: this requires leadership, group activity, and general practitioner tutors.

General practitioners are busy people. It is nonsense to consign continuing education to lunchtimes, evenings, and Sundays and although surveys still find these times to be convenient (Reedy et al., 1979), I submit that they are not truly desired. Rest, recreation, and family life are important and

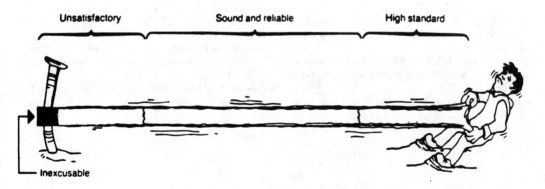

Fig. 3. Model of a general practitioner.

make for a better doctor. Time is the main obstacle and I believe that paid study leave is necessary and will provide the opportunities to lead to more satisfactory and effective continuing education.

I have an egg-cup. It is made of old English oak, five or six hundred years old. I turned it myself and I am rather pleased with it. I am pleased with it not just because of its appearance and feel, but because it is the first egg-cup that I have turned which will actually hold an egg. It does what it was intended to do.

So it is with this lecture in honour of William Pickles. It matters that it should lead to our doing something as a result of it.

REFERENCES

Byrne, P. S. (1969). Postgraduate education for general practitoners in the Manchester region. British Journal of Medical Education, 3, 50–57

Carr, T. E. A. (1979). Whither general medical practice? Health Trends, 11, 83–88

Cocks, D. A., Critchley, E. M. R. & Hayward, W. H. (1975). Control of epilepsy with the single daily dose of phenytoin sodium. British Journal of Clinical Pharmacology, 2, 449–453

Collings, J. S. (1950). General practice in England today. Lancet, 1, 555–585

Evered, D. C. & Williams, H. D. (1980). Postgraduate education and the doctor. British Medical Journal, 280, 626–628

Fulton, W. & Riddell, A. (1980). Getting doctors into the inner cities. General Practitioner, 28 March, 18–19

Gray, D. J. Pereira (1979). A System of Training for General Practice. Occasional Paper 4. 2nd ed. London: Journal of the Royal College of General Practitoners

Jeavons, P. M. (1975). The practical management of epilepsy. Update, 10, 269–280

Leeuwenhorst Working Party (1977). The General Practitioner in Europe. Statement of a Working Party appointed to the Second European Conference on the Teaching of General Practice (1974). Journal of the Royal College of General Practitioners, 27, 117

Mackenzie, J. (1916). Principles of Diagnosis and Treatment in Heart Affections. London: Henry Frowde & Hodder & Stoughton

McKnight, J. E. (1971). The art so long to learn. Journal of the Royal College of General Practitioners, 21, 315–324

Mawer, G. E., Mullen, P. W. & Rodgers, M. (1974). Phenytoin dose adjustment in epileptic patients. British Journal of Clinical Pharmacology, 1, 163–168

Miller, G. E. (1967). Educational science and education for medicine. British Journal of Medical Education, 1, 156–159

Pemberton, J. (1970). Will Pickles of Wensleydale. London: Geoffrey Bles

Pickles, W. N. (1951). And this is my path. Queens Medical Magazine, 44, 13–15

Reedy, B. L. E. C., Gregson, B. A. & Williams, M. (1979). General Practitoners and Postgraduate Education in the Northern Region. Occasional Paper 9. London: Journal of the Royal College of General Practitioners

Shorvon, S. D., Chadwick, D., Galbraith, A. W. & Reynolds, E. H. (1978). One drug for epilepsy. British Medical Journal, 1, 474–476

Shorvon, S. D. & Reynolds, E. H. (1979). Reduction in polypharmacy for epilepsy. British Medical Journal, 2, 1023–1025

Taylor, S. (1954). Good General Practice. London: Oxford University Press

Continuing Education and General Practitioners*

Leeuwenhorst European Working Party

Introduction

This statement is written for all general practitioners, for all those responsible for organizing continuing education and those who create the conditions in which it can flourish.

We have already published reports on the contribution of the general practitioner to the basic education of all doctors and on the objectives for the special training of those who choose this career, based on an agreed definition of this role in medicine. These objectives include one which states that the established practitioner will continue to improve and refine his skills during his professional lifetime; he will need to add to his knowledge as new medical discoveries are made, and to adapt his attitudes in response to changes within society itself.

Medical education forms one developing process, of which continuing education is the longest part. Like the others, it needs to be planned. There are problems common to all our countries.

A New Balance

One intention dominates this document—to help to establish a new balance between the contribution of general practitioners to their own continuing education and the contribution of others—medical specialists, biological and social scientists, and workers in professions related to medicine.

We believe that general practitioners should have the basic responsibility at this stage for seeking their own education; for

*Reprinted by permission from *Journal of the Royal College of General Practitioners*, 570–574, September 1980.

identifying their own deficiencies; for helping to plan, organize and contribute to the training of their fellows. General practice is developing as a research and teaching discipline, with its distinctive features of accessibility, breadth, synthesis, continuity and the use of the simplest appropriate methods in the care of patients. The increasing self-consciousness and self-criticism which result make it now capable of developing in certain ways its own continuing education.

But all clinicians have a responsibility for helping each other to discover what they see as needs in other clinicians' knowledge and practise in their own subject. In this way each can act as a resource for the others. We all need help in acquiring new knowledge and revising the old.

The planning and production of continuing education is a joint activity, in which the general practitioner's participation is crucial. This statement sets out the broad aims and discusses motivation, content, methods and organization. Evaluation will be considered separately.

The Aims of Continuing Education

Continuing education is concerned with the maintenance, development and improvement of the care which a doctor provides for people throughout his professional life. It starts for the general practitioner in most of our countries when he or she assumes professional responsibility.

This aim can only be promoted by continuing education if it is based on people's needs for care and on appropriate application of the biological, social and clinical sciences; and if it is related to the particular situation, personality and interests of the general practitioner. Success depends on the mutual understanding and respect of those who work in different parts of the health care system, since all have something to learn and something to teach.

Its purposes should be:

1. To review knowledge, skills, and attitudes already acquired in undergraduate and vocational training, eliminating those which are obsolete, while retaining those which are still valuable.
2. To help the doctor to discover his deficiencies and to deal with the difficulties which he already recognizes in his own work, by sharing experiences with his colleagues, both medical and non-medical.
3. To help the doctor to recognize and apply new evidence and ideas, using the experience of general practice as a basis for their evaluation and application. By giving as well as receiving training in this way, he will be enabled to develop new competences and learn new roles effectively.
4. To help the doctor's capacity to think creatively and to appraise his own work critically, by means of education and research activities.

Motivation

If general practitioners are to assume such varied responsibilities for their own re-education, their motivation becomes a dominant issue. It will depend first on their basic education. If curiosity and self-criticism are to become habits of mind, they must be developed long before the doctor starts to practise. Basic university education should accustom students to regard knowledge as transient and replaceable, preparing them for a life-time of changing problems, changing solutions, and even changes

which they themselves will initiate. In most countries it is no longer the intention to provide students at this stage with all the knowledge and skills which are thought to be essential for making them into safe general practitioners. A less crowded programme can result.

It is the period of specific training which has to ensure the competence of the general practitioner. But this period also has to foster the desire to continue learning. Not all countries yet provide specific training; its absence causes some doctors to search for it during the period of continuing education. Although this may be temporarily unavoidable, it is a wrong use of time intended for a different purpose. Continuing education cannot be a substitute for specific initial training.

Strong motivation can also stem from current experience. There is great satisfaction to be had by sharing in a science and art which is growing and offering increasing benefits to mankind. New challenges are stimulating. Without a constant stream of new problems for solution medicine would lose some of its fascination for the doctor. Difficult clinical problems, difficult patients—even failures—are challenges which immediately face him with the need to continue learning. But he does not always recognize the difficulty in a problem, for example, that it may be mainly in his relationship with a person; he may not see himself as others see him or be prepared to acknowledge his own failures. It is hard to become both self-critical and self-confident as a clinician; yet this is what is needed.

When general practitioners themselves contribute to continuing education, they come to recognize and discuss their successes and failures, so that they and others can learn from them. If some do this, it is easier for others to do the same, and easier still if they have acquired the habit as students. Discussion and interaction with peers tend in themselves to motivate.

The absence of a doctor from all organized forms of continuing education is no proof that motivation is lacking; there are hidden activities—from reading to research work.

Clearly, the best motivation lies in the satisfaction of daily work in a professional field which is developing; in the spirit of enquiry and self-criticism; and even in that sense of personal inadequacy which spurs to greater efforts. But these qualities can and must be supported by practical arrangements which will allow the doctor to participate. These are discussed later under the heading 'Organization'.

Some advocate that the doctor should be *compelled* to educate himself throughout his professional life. If this is understood literally, we believe that compulsion can diminish motivation to learn. If it is understood to mean, for example, the pressure of opinion of colleagues or patients, it is an acceptable incentive.

The Content and Methods of Continuing Education

We said above that continuing education can improve the quality of health care only if it is based both on people's need for care and upon the appropriate application of the biological, social and clinical sciences. The general practitioner's role is also at the centre of the problem of selection and must act as a continuous focus for every contribution. In our first document we stated this as follows:

> The general practitioner is a licensed medical graduate who gives personal, primary and continuing care to individuals, families and a practice population, irrespective of age, sex and illness. It is the synthesis of these functions which is unique. He will attend his patients in his consulting room and in their homes and sometimes in a clinic or a hospital. His aim is to make early diagnosis. He will include and integrate physical, psychological and social factors in his considerations about health and illness. This will be expressed in

the care of his patients. He will make an initial decision about every problem which is presented to him as a doctor. He will undertake the continuing management of his patients with chronic, recurrent or terminal illnesses. Prolonged contact means that he can use repeated opportunities to gather information at a pace appropriate to each patient and build up a relationship of trust which he can use professionally. He will practise in co-operation with other colleagues, medical and non-medical. He will know how and when to intervene through treatment, prevention and education to promote the health of his patients and their families. He will recognize that he also has a professional responsibility to the community.

The educational aims which follow this statement in our first document apply as much to continuing education as to specific training.

Content

The content must relate to the setting in which the general practitioner works, the range of problems he faces, the knowledge, skills and attitudes which he brings to their solution, and what he does and is as a person.

The field is vast—the actual content will vary from country to country and from year to year. We make no attempt even to outline it here, but only to indicate how we think it might best be selected if the aims described above are to be achieved.

1. "Reviewing what was already acquired in the periods of undergraduate and specific training."

   This will happen naturally in the process of discussing new knowledge.

2. "Helping the doctor to discover his needs and deficiencies and to deal with the difficulties which he already recognizes in his work."

   The main responsibility lies on the

doctor himself, but the extent to which each doctor discharges it will vary greatly. Daily experience in practice—particularly the requirements and reactions of patients—are unavoidable lessons. They alone give rise to a range of content far too extensive for description here.

The contact with colleagues and the mutually constructive criticism which play such an important part in raising the standards of medicine in hospital demand from the practitioner more initiative in making contact, particularly if he practises single-handed. A group practice offers one learning situation, but only if the members of the group meet regularly and talk freely. If it contains related disciplines, it is all the more stimulating. The daily working contact of a group practice provides an intimate and continuous setting in which successes and failures can be discussed, but it must not become an exclusive setting.

There are other ways of identifying needs and deficiencies. One example is the self-administered questionnaire. Another is created when a small group of doctors come together to define and agree their methods for managing a particular type of clinical problem, so that they can observe afterwards the degree to which their own performance differs from their standards.

Some doctors identify their own deficiencies by reading specialist reports on their cases, by reading books and papers, or by attending lectures in which specialists point them out.

Educational needs cannot necessarily be inferred either from the views of educators or from those of practitioners about what ought to be taught. The essential is to emphasize the systematic identification of personal and corporate needs, and the selection of priorities, and to respond by careful design of educational programmes.

The general practitioner's main concern is with the people for whom he cares. What he can extract in knowledge and skills from others must be constantly sifted and adjusted to his needs. It is this process which can ensure the practitioner's interest in his own education and the selection of content which is relevant.

3. "Helping the doctor to recognize new evidence and ideas."

This has hitherto been regarded as the sole responsibility of the specialist, who teaches while the general practitioner listens. We believe this to be wrong. It is the particular intention of this report to emphasize the integrated experience of general practice as an important source of continuing education. It is developing as a research and teaching discipline, already established within universities in many of our countries. Its distinctive features should be accessibility, breadth, synthesis, continuity, and the use of the simplest appropriate methods. It can link prevention with care and cure, concern for the individual with concern for the community, the physical with the psychological and social; it is the putting together of these elements which we mean by 'synthesis'.

But it would be a serious mistake to suggest that we want to manage on our own. There must be a balance. We still need new information from outside our discipline. Help from others is as necessary as ever to bring new knowledge, to revise and modify old knowledge and to help us to discover valuable ideas of which we could be unaware.

Specialists are increasingly trying to ensure that their contributions are relevant to doctors who deal with a different range of problems, work in a different setting, and have responsibilities and resources which are not precisely the same as their own.

4. "Helping the doctor to think critically about his own work."

This can be achieved if the previous aims are pursued. It is achieved more rigorously when a practitioner undertakes formal research which will be subject to the scrutiny of colleagues. Both research and teaching are excellent methods of continuing to learn.

Methods

The choice of methods should depend as much as possible on the content, but geography or lack of resource may in fact have an important influence; it should certainly not depend merely on the preference or habits of teachers.

Traditionally, continuing education has been associated with lectures by experts to large groups. We believe that this method should be used rarely, because it places adult learners, who have much to give, in the passive role of receivers. Active methods of learning are known to be the most effective. Moreover, listening to a sequence of experts, general practitioners have been led to feel that expertise lies in every branch of medicine except their own. Continuing education is meant to increase, not to decrease, the confidence of the doctor in his role and his skills.

Like others, doctors see, hear and build upon mainly what they know already and can already do; what they bring to a learning situation, therefore, will largely determine what they take from it. Because of this and because they are likely to retain only what they can use, it is crucial that continuing education should be as relevant as possible to their work; teaching has to help them to widen, enrich and sometimes change knowledge, skills and attitudes which are already within them. Totally new concepts or knowledge will be introduced most successfuly if the doctor can see that it relates to those which he already possesses.

We see the small group as the most appropriate method for most of the established practitioner's learning needs. It is an active method which allows a responsible experienced adult to give as well as to receive. It provides a way for discovering deficiencies and dealing with recognized difficulties. It is one way in which continuing education can answer the individual needs of a particular doctor. It can help him to think creatively and to examine his own work critically, notably by sharing opinions about the clinical or organizational methods most likely to achieve improvement in health ('peer-review'). It has a profound influence on the development of attitudes, social and interpersonal skills and self-understanding. It can deal with the overconfident doctor or help one who lacks confidence and fears to expose himself, since within the group ignorance can be admitted without penalty or humiliation.

Small group learning lends itself as well to topic teaching as to the discussion of particular patients. It can start from a short presentation, or from questions, as often as possible by members of the group. It should end with 'feedback', in two senses—was it a good session? What will each member take from it that he can use? How useful the session proved for practice can be checked later if the group meets regularly.

In the small group a specialist has a most important part to play, but this depends on his capacity to imagine himself in the general practitioner's situation and to apply his own expertise to the general practitioner's problems. He is there as a resource, not as a leader. For most people this role is more demanding than that of lecturer.

Planning and Organization

The general practitioner should have the basic responsibility for seeking his own continuing education, for identifying his deficiencies, and for helping to plan, organize, and contribute to the education of his fellows. Trust in a doctor and the assurance that he will do his best for his patients are traditional. The responsibility of individual doctors to demonstrate their own continuing competence is therefore heavy. It is nevertheless prudent for patients, whether through local, regional, or national arrangements, to make sure that the doctor is able to fulfil this responsibility. Clearly the community has an interest in supporting this means both to the improvement of health status and to the containment of costs.

Whoever undertakes it—doctors or others—some degree of planning and organization is essential if continuing education is to be undertaken by all general practitioners, as the development of society and medicine in our countries so clearly demands.

As examples, there is a need for central and local sources of literature review; for encouragement to general practitioners to contribute material from their own work and for support in their own more active involvement in teaching. The range of content needed is now so large that systematic review of the material for inclusion needs to be organized. Group 'leaders' need to be trained. Meetings of many sorts need to be arranged and co-ordinated.

The extent to which responsibility for these tasks is shared by the general practitioner, as consumer, with the other providers varies greatly even among our countries. So does the extent to which professional bodies, social security organizations or the state intervene by paying expenses, compensating for loss of earnings, organizing replacements or exerting pressure towards regular, or even compulsory, attendance at courses in relation to the right to practise.

Unquestionably in all our countries continuing education must be recognized as essential and given its proper priority for time otherwise devoted to patient care, by whatever means this can be achieved.

For the selection of content, teachers and teaching methods, general practitioners should have the dominant, but not the only, voice. Universities have both educational expertise and administrative machinery, without which planning, organization and evaluation would be far less effective than it can be through co-operative effort. Where universities include a department of general practice, this is an obvious focal point at which co-operative planning and organization can occur, but it will need to relate to other more widely distributed centres, whether in hospitals or group practices, where the actual work of education takes place continuously.

Addendum

Members of the working party are as follows: N. Bentzen (Denmark), R. B. Boelaert (Belgium), P. S. Byrne (United Kingdom), S. Häussler (Federal Republic of Germany), G. Heller (Austria), J. P. Horder (United Kingdom), S. Hummerfelt (Norway), Z. Jaksic (Yugoslavia), J. D. E. Knox (United Kingdom), B. S. Polak (Netherlands), A. M. Reynolds (France), M. Simunic (Yugoslavia), M. Szatmari (Hungary) and J. C. van Es (Netherlands). I. Hügel (German Democratic Republic) remains a member, but was unable to contribute to this part of the work. K. M. Parry (United Kingdom) has helped in the drafting of all our reports.

The terms used in each country represented in the working party, equivalent to the English term 'general practitioner' are as follows: Austria, *Praktischer Arzt;* Belgium, *Médecin de Famille/Huisarts;* Denmark, *Alment Praktiserende Laege;* France, *Médecin Généraliste;* Federal Republic of Germany, *Arzt für Allgemeinmedizin;* German Democratic Republic, *Facharzt für Allgemeinmedizin;* Hungary, *Altalános Orvos;* Netherlands, *Huisarts;* Norway, *Almenpraktiker;* Yugoslavia, *Liječnik Opće Medicine.*

A New Look at Continuing Education in Family Practice*

John P. Geyman

The rapid increase of medical knowledge in recent years, together with continuously changing methods and patterns of practice, have made continuing medical education today a critical and challenging problem. It is now recognized that the large majority of a physician's medical knowledge over a practice career is derived from post-graduate learning after his initial formal undergraduate and graduate medical education. Despite the present importance of continuing medical education, we still have a relatively ineffective system which is not easily accessible to the practicing physician and which often fails to meet his individual learning needs. This paper critiques our past efforts in this area, describes some principles of learning, and suggests some new approaches to make continuing education in family practice more accessible and effective.

Continuing medical education today is a complex problem. In recent years we have witnessed an information explosion, and we have all been deluged with an informational overload. For example, there are approximately 20,000 journal articles published each month. The half-life of biomedical knowledge is now on the order of five years.[1] It is further estimated that some 75 percent of a physician's medical knowledge in the course of his practice career falls into the area of continuing medical education.[2] We can, therefore, no longer depend on our initial formal education to sustain our professional competence over time. This

*Reprinted by permission from *The Journal of Family Practice* 2(2):119-122, 1975. Adapted from an address presented at the Panel on Education, Sixth World Congress on General Practice/Family Medicine, Mexico City, November 4, 1974.

applies to all fields, but the breadth of family practice poses a particular challenge especially as the role of the family physician expands to include preventive medicine, counseling, rehabilitation, and related areas.

The purpose of this paper is to give an overview of continuing medical education as it applies to family practice, to briefly critique our past efforts in this area, and to describe some principles of learning and new approaches to continuing medical education. Some useful directions for departments of family practice will be proposed and specific recommendations will be offered to the family physician concerned with his own continuing medical education.

Traditional Approaches to Continuing Medical Education

Dr. Clement Brown, who has done a great deal in recent years to advance the art of audit in community hospitals, recently pointed out the inadequacies of our standard approaches to continuing medical education:

The concept of continuing medical education conjures up a roomful of preoccupied but hopeful attending physicians at a community hospital, anticipating a learned presentation by the medical school faculty either in person or by way of educational television, two-way radio or other media. The members of the audience are caught between the demands of their practices and the hope that such an educational program will somehow be useful in the care of the patients. But such a teacher or planner-oriented approach is both limited and limiting since it may only incidentally or accidentally meet the needs of the learner and possibly less often the patient. Diagnosis of patient care needs seldom precedes educational therapy. Also, most current learning experiences in continuing medical education are designed to achieve only information transfer, implying that most patient care deficits derive from lack of physician-learner knowledge. This implication is seldom tested, just as many other assumptions concerning continuing medical education are not tested, and so there is no real measure of knowledge deficits, skill deficits, whether intellectual or psychomotor, or the need for attitudinal change. Furthermore, the current standard approach is not based on sound principles of adult learning.[3]

The few studies which have looked into the effectiveness of continuing medical education in improving the quality of patient care have failed to show a positive correlation. Dr. George Miller has asked two major questions: "What is continuing medical education for?" and "What care needs improvement?"[4] Dr. Miller replies to the first question by saying that continuing medical education aims at improving the quality of patient care. The second question, however, is not an easy one to answer. We have seen an incomplete though enthusiastic response among medical educators to develop many approaches to the transmission of information. Unfortunately, this has been a shotgun approach and has contributed to the ineffectiveness of continuing medical education. Miller points out that our past emphasis has been on small areas of knowledge benefiting relatively few patients. He has suggested that continuing medical education should stress more areas which relate to larger numbers of patients.

A recent report by an expert committee of the World Health Organization on continuing medical education made this comment:

Although some countries have made significant progress in organizing a system of con-

tinuing education for physicians and all countries have acknowledged the importance of doing so, the present efforts in this field are often unsystematic, poorly supported, little influenced by contemporary educational science, episodic, focused more on transmitting new information than on improving competence, and are only incidentally related to health needs and national health priorities.[5]

We have, therefore, in contrast to undergraduate and graduate education, a nonsystem for continuing education with these problems: content is not based on individual learner need; learning is episodic, passive and often not related to patient care; educational aids are frequently inaccessible to the physician; and the process is often measured by the wrong standards (eg, hours of attendance at courses).

Some Principles of Learning

Dr. Miller suggests that,

it would seem that the time has come to try a different educational model—one built on solid evidence about the way adults learn rather than on the time honored method of teaching them. There is ample evidence to support the view that adult learning is not most efficiently achieved through systematic subject instruction. It is accomplished by involving learners in identifying problems and seeking ways to solve them. It does not come in categorical bundles but in a growing need to know. It may initially seem wanting in content that pleases experts, but it ultimately incorporates knowledge in a context that has meaning. It is in short a process model of education.[6]

He goes on to say that,

men learn what they want to learn. The first step in this long process is not to tell them what they need to know, it is to help them to want what they require. It means involving participants in identifying their own educational needs, in selecting the learning experiences most likely to help them to meet these needs, and assessing whether they have learned what was intended, not merely determining whether they took part in the learning experience, or even whether they liked it.[7]

Beyond these points, we now know that there is a forgetting curve—information which is not related to one's continuing practice is easily forgotten. In addition, each of us has our own individual style of learning. Some will learn best by reading, others by small group patient-oriented discussions, and still others by self-instructional media. We now know that effective continuing medical education requires: (1) a need to know (preferable related to patient care itself), (2) an active process, (3) a continuous relevance to everyday practice, and (4) a format which fits our individual learning style.

Newer Approaches to Continuing Medical Education

There are a number of new directions in continuing medical education which it would be useful to summarize briefly here.

1. *Increased emphasis on small group interactive teaching and self-instruction rather than the lecture method.* Many of our postgraduate courses now involve small group discussions on specific subjects. These are both popular and effective, and they facilitate learning based on clinical problems from the practices of participating physicians. We are also seeing an increased use of multimedia learning methods, including video tape, tape-slide programs and programmed learning units.

2. *Profiling of one's practice.* There is an increasing awareness that it is important and useful to gain insight into the content of the physician's practice. The May, 1971, issue of *Patient Care* magazine was devoted entirely to continuing education. It is an excellent reference describing several methods of gaining a profile of one's prac-

tice.[8] More recently, the Illinois Council on Continuing Medical Education has developed a handbook for physicians which suggests another method for profiling and also for developing a personal learning plan based on individual needs.[9]

3. *Increasing use of the problem-oriented record.* We continue to see gaining emphasis on the problem-oriented medical record which was developed by Dr. Lawrence Weed. This approach to recordkeeping not only allows for better organization of medical care and communication among peers and consultants, but it also facilitates examination of the quality of care through audit.

4. *Increasing use of medical audit.* Audit of medical records both in the office and in the hospital is increasingly emphasized. It is becoming clear that this should be a valuable way of identifying our own specific needs for continuing medical education. We are all aware of the basic approach of the audit process which includes identifying a major problem area for audit, setting of criteria (by our peers on a local basis), conduct of the audit (principally by paramedical personnel), development of an educational response to deficits noted, and finally, reaudit of the problem at a later date to see if improvements in medical care have actually occurred.

5. *Self-assessment.* The audit, both in the hospital and in the office, is certainly an important method of self-assessment. A second major approach is through self-assessment examinations which allow an individual physician to discover his own areas of weakness and help him plan more specifically for his continuing education.

6. *Learning through teaching.* With the development of more training programs in family medicine in medical schools and community hospitals, there is a greater opportunity for practicing family physicians to become involved with teaching in various ways. Some serve as preceptors for medical students in their own practices, some are active in resident teaching in model family practice units, others participate in collaborative research projects involving their

practices and nearby teaching programs, and still others associate themselves in other ways with undergraduate or graduate education in family medicine. The teaching process exposes us to younger, more recently trained students and physicians, and the interchange is inevitably a learning process for all involved.

Roles for Departments of Family Practice

Departments of family practice in medical schools have new responsibilities and opportunities to improve continuing medical education for large numbers of practicing family physicians. The following approaches are suggested as being of particular value in this regard.

1. *Develop educational programs in family practice as a continuum involving undergraduate, graduate, and postgraduate phases.* Medical schools for years have placed most emphasis on undergraduate medical education. Although they are now assuming increased responsibility for graduate education, the area of continuing medical education continues to receive too low a priority. As competency-based curricula and more effective teaching methods for family practice residency training are developed and refined, there should be more overlap between graduate and postgraduate education in family practice. Departments of family practice should respond to the need for continuing education of family physicians within their region. Family practice refresher courses should be more than didactic sessions; they should provide opportunities for self-assessment, self-instruction and learning of self-audit technique.

2. *Decentralize educational programs on a regional basis.* Of particular value here is the development of a regional network of affiliated family practice residency programs. Such a network allows new relationships to be established with practicing physicians over a wide area. It affords closer com-

munication with the medical school and visiting faculty, opportunities to teach in community hospital settings, and access to the newer techniques of patient care utilized in model family practice units.

3. *Establish improved linkages between primary, secondary, and tertiary care.* Departments of family practice are in an ideal position to facilitate improved linkages between primary, secondary, and tertiary care within their regions. They can interface actively with other faculty and resources of the medical school, with community hospitals of various sizes in outlying communities, and with practicing family physicians over a wide area. Efforts should be directed toward improving consultation services on a regional basis. Telemetry for electrocardiographic and electroencephalographic interpretation are examples of two methods of demonstrated value. Interactive radio or television linkages with outlying affiliated hospitals could make consultation more readily available and better utilize specialty resources of the medical school.

4. *Involve practicing family physicians in part-time teaching.* Practicing family physicians have much to offer in both undergraduate and graduate teaching. Students and residents require "real world" role models and the teaching input from those engaged in active practice in varied settings. Departments of family practice have a particular responsibility to help family physicians learn problem-oriented record and audit techniques, and improve their teaching skills.

5. *Develop specific educational support methods.* There are several approaches to serving family physicians on a regional basis. A teaching bank can be established for multimedia self-instructional materials. These can be made available to affiliated hospitals and physicians in outlying communities. Self-assessment examinations can be developed which allow for individual profiles of test results and specific identification of educational needs. Methods for

profiling one's practice can likewise be made available to practicing family physicians. Locum tenens exhcanges can be established between third-year family practice residents and individual family physicians. Such exchanges allow residents to gain a better perspective of anticipated practice settings while providing family physicians with someone to cover their practices while they pursue further training at the university.

6. *Engage in collaborative research with practicing family physicians.* Research in family practice is a wide open field with many areas requiring study. Such efforts are now being facilitated by the establishment of departments of family practice in medical schools, the development of improved audit and record retrieval systems, and by refinements in disease coding for common clinical problems. Participation in collaborative research projects should be of real educational value to all physicians involved.

Recommendations for the Family Physician

Although this paper has pointed out some of the difficulties involved with continuing medical education, I would propose the following specific recommendations to the individual family physician:

1. *Assess your own attitudes.* It is useful to look at ourselves in terms of our need and desire to learn, our priorities for continuing medical education, our sense of guilt in committing time to this and taking it from our practice, our willingness to expose ourselves to our peers or others concerning our areas of educational need, and how each of us feels we learn best.

2. *Identify your needs.* Several approaches have been suggested for this process, including profiling of one's practice, taking self-assessment examinations, the use of the problem-oriented medical record and audit technique.

3. *Explore available educational resources.*

This involves looking in one's community for potential help from colleagues and consultants, and looking at resources within the region and nearby teaching programs including medical libraries, journals, courses offered, and self-instructional media.

4. *Individualize your approach to specific needs.* Each physician's approach should be adapted to his own needs and learning style. A number of options are available. Selected courses and locum tenens exchanges have been mentioned. To this could be added study through self-instructional media, reading and teaching.

5. *Utilize consultation as a teaching process.* Consultation affords an important and often neglected avenue for continuing medical education. If we choose our consultants not only for their competence in dealing with a difficult problem, but also for their willingness and interest in teaching, we can make each consultation a valuable learning experience.

6. *Set a habit for continuing medical education.* This involves organizing our practice so we can allocate time for continuing medical education. Our own personal priorities may have to be reorganized to make this happen.

7. *Further information in various areas can be obtained.* Several specific sources are recommended. Bjorn and Cross' book on the problem-oriented private practice of medicine is a good reference on the problem-oriented record and audit in a small group practice.[10] The recent work by Easton on the problem-oriented medical record is useful to the same area.[11] Several recent articles describe newer methods of audit as one type of continuing education.[12-14] The AHME Journal is recommended for other articles of this nature.* Beyond these references, it should be pos-

*The AHME Journal is published by the Association for Hospital Medical Education, 1911 Jefferson Davis Highway, Suite 1003, Arlington, Virginia 22202.

sible to identify physicians within your hospital and community who are interested and informed about newer techniques in continuing education.

Discussion

An expert committee on continuing education of the World Health Organization recently stated that "the primary purpose of continued medical education is to assist in the maintenance and improvement of competence of delivering preventive and curative health care, not merely to impart knowledge and to spread information."[15] Continuing medical education is continuing self-education. It is an active approach which should be based on specific needs. Help is increasingly available within our communities and from adjacent medical schools to aid us with this process. The American Board of Family Practice has pointed the way to a new emphasis on continuing medical education. Recertification (every 6 years) is now a reality and goes beyond the written examination to include audit of family physicians' office and hospital records. Our challenge now is to make continued learning more accessible, more specific, and more meaningful to each individual physician.

Many years ago Sir William Osler said, "In what may be called the natural method of teaching, the student begins with a patient, continues with a patient, and ends his studies with the patient, using books and lectures as tools, as means to an end."[16] Today we may add other methods to books and lectures, but the essence of this statement is unchanged and the responsibility for continued education remains ours.

REFERENCES

1. Meeting the challenge of family practice. Report of the Ad Hoc Committee on Education for Family Practice of the Council on Medical Education. Chicago, AMA, 1966, p. 28
2. Farber SM: In, Relevance today and tommorrow in medical education. Calif Med 112(5):69, 1970
3. Brown CR, Uhl HSM: Mandatory continuing education—Sense or nonsense? JAMA 213:1660-1668, 1970
4. Miller GE: Continuing education for what? J Med Educ 42:320-326, 1967
5. Continuing Education for Physicians. Report of a WHO Expert Committee. Geneva, World Health Organization, 1973, pp 28-29
6. Miller GE: op. cit. p 322
7. Miller GE: op. cit. pp 322-323
8. What about your continuing education? Patient Care 5(9):7-61, 1971
9. Stein LS: Your Personal Learning Plan, A Handbook for Physicians. Chicago, Illinois Council on Continuing Medical Education, 1973
10. Bjorn JC, Cross HD: The Problem-Oriented Private Practice of Medicine. Chicago, Modern Hospital Press, 1970
11. Easton RE: Problem-Oriented Medical Record Concepts. New York, Appleton-Century-Crofts, 1974
12. Phillips TJ, Bratrude AP, Wood FC: Peer review of a small group practice. J Fam Prac 1(1):28-33, 1974
13. Campbell HJ: Do physicians satisfy their own diagnostic and treatment criteria in the care of patients with urinary infections? J Fam Prac 1(2):19-23, 1974
14. Smith SR: Application of the tracer technique in studying quality of care. J Fam Prac 1(3/4):38-42, 1974
15. Continuing Education for Physicians. Report of a WHO Expert Committee. Geneva, World Health Organization, 1973, p 30
16. Osler W: Aequanimatis, with other Addresses to Medical Students, Nurses and Practitioners of Medicine, ed 2. Philadelphia, Blakiston's Son & Co. 1932, p 315

Does Continuing Medical Education Improve the Quality of Medical Care? A Look at the Evidence*

Alfred O. Berg

Although continuing education has a long tradition within the medical profession, mandated continuing medical education is of very recent origin. The conceptual framework used to justify continuing medical education is that it exposes physicians to new knowledge, changes physician behavior, and favorably alters patient outcomes. Considerable evidence exists that physician knowledge can be increased, and that behavior can be changed, but there is very little to show an effect on patient outcomes. The effectiveness of continuing medical education is further clouded by such issues as consumerism, licensure politics, and professional standards review organization legislation. Family physicians should have a role in determining the outcome of the continuing medical education debate, as participants, as policy-setters, and as informed critics.

The education of physicians has long been acknowledged to be a lifetime process. Observe:

> John Shaw Billings: The education of the doctor which goes on after he has his degree is, after all, the most important part of his education.[1] (1894)
> Sir William Osler: Post graduation study has always been a characteristic feature of our profession.[2] (1900)
> Karl Marx: The education of most people ends upon graduation; that of the physician means a lifetime of incessant study.[3] (1865)

The advent of mandatory continuing medical education (CME) in the last decades, however, has been dramatically abrupt: 35

*Reprinted by permission from *The Journal of Family Practice*, 8(6):1171–1174, 1979.

states have legislated required continuing medical education as a prerequisite to relicensure, and at least 22 medical specialty boards are moving toward recertification procedures, all with CME requirements. The impact of required continuing medical education has been substantial if measured in terms of dollars and time spent by physicians in CME activities (to say nothing of dollars accruing to CME-sponsoring institutions).[4,5] The impact of continuing medical education on the quality of medical care in the United States is, however, substantially unknown.

The traditional conceptual framework justifying continuing medical education is that it exposes physicians to new medical information, increases physician knowledge, changes physician behavior, and favorably alters patient outcomes.[6] It has further been assumed that completion of the first step guarantees the last three.

This paper will briefly review the effects of continuing medical education on physician knowledge, on change in physician behavior, and on patient outcome, listed, unfortunately, in descending order of the quality of information available. In the end, the data will allow very limited conclusions regarding the efficacy of continuing medical education, but will permit a broader discussion regarding the relationship of CME to other quality assessment and assurance mechanisms.

Continuing Medical Education and Physician Knowledge

The idea that systematic exposure of physicians to new medical information will lead to increased physician knowledge does not require a very large leap of faith. Yet this first, basic step of documenting increased knowledge must be taken in order to allow interpretation of studies focusing exclusively on later results. Failure to demonstrate increases in knowledge would allow suspicion of results showing large changes in subsequent behavior or patient outcome, or may partially explain results showing no changes at all in behavior and outcome.

On the face of it, the demonstration of increased knowledge following continuing medical education should be a straightforward affair: do a pretest and post-test and measure any significant difference between the two. A much more rigorous approach, however, is necessary if generalization to other programs and situations is desired.

Typical of studies demonstrating increased knowledge is that of Neu and Howrey, who showed significant increases in post-test scores in a large sample of physicians exposed to a nationally distributed televised program dealing with antibiotic use. Since the post-test was part of the presentation, however, the retention of the knowledge gained is open to question.[7] A more indirect approach to demonstrating the efficacy of continuing medical education in increasing physician knowledge is that by Chang's group, which showed in a community survey that those who scored higher on a test dealing with child abuse and neglect were likely to have reported continuing medical education as their source of information on the subject.[8] A similar study by Hunter and Portis showed that those physicians scoring higher on a mailed survey dealing with placebos, heart disease, and new drugs were likely to have viewed televised CME programs on those subjects three to six months earlier.[9] Both of these studies indicated that CME knowledge is retained beyond the few days or weeks immediately following the presentation.

Several investigators have gone further by comparing different methods of continuing medical education on increasing physician knowledge given similar subject material. Hogben demonstrated similar increases in knowledge following two CME courses in cardiology, differing only in length. The study is subject to criticism because of poor documentation of comparability between groups, and the lack of adequate controls.[10] Donnelly's study of weekend seminars for physicians learning about new drugs addresses issues regarding methods, but his findings were inconclusive.[11]

Other examples are available, of varying methodological quality. Research in the area has been less than enthusiastic, presumably because few have seriously questioned that continuing medical education increases physician knowledge; nearly all studies published have shown increases in knowledge, independent of methodological rigor. The notion has some face validity, and is indirectly supported by a large volume of research in educational psychology and teaching methods. Knowledge assessment has, for better or worse, become entrenched as the only necessary and sufficient evaluation technique in many CME programs.[12]

Continuing Medical Education and Behavior Change

Evaluation of CME's impact on the behavior of physicians presents obvious methodological difficulties. In the arena of perhaps the greatest interest, that of the practicing physician's private office, the literature is practically silent. A single study, by Mock's group, failed to demonstrate an impact of a medical television network on physician behavior, largely because medical records reviewed were inadequate for the analysis.[13] Caplan showed high physician compliance 6 to 12 months after a CME course on tonometry, but the numbers were very small, and not all those taking the course were evaluated.[14]

The issue is less difficult and the endpoints easier to measure in hospital based studies of physician behavior. Setting aside the (literally) hundreds of testimonial reports from hospitals to the effect that an audit/continuing education program has "changed behavior," there are a few studies which have attempted to look at the question in more depth. Reed has shown that audit generated continuing medical education was effective in changing a variety of physician behaviors in the coronary care unit setting, although the definition of continuing medical education (eg, suspension of hospital privileges) and the small numbers of physicians involved, limit generalizability.[15] Dramatic changes in behavior were documented by Rubenstein following continuing medical education directed at the use of blood products and the work-up of pulmonary embolism in a large hospital setting.[16] A similar study was reported recently showing reduction in blood products ordered for elective surgery.[17]

Within the framework of a large well-designed study on the quality of care in Hawaii, Payne and co-workers demonstrated significant improvements in appropriateness of hospitalization, length of stay, and staff assessment of quality of care following seminars dealing with identified problems in six hospitals. The study was hampered by a follow-up of only five months and by inadequate measurement of some relevant outcomes, but offers convincing evidence of changes in physician behavior in defined areas.[18]

What is certainly clear from these and other studies is that physician behavior can be changed. However, the active agent is not always clear. Few studies have randomized physicians to exposed and nonexposed groups in experimental fashion, nor have selective, historical, situational, and maturational effects generally been taken into account. Further, the intervention itself has frequently been a confusing mixture of continuing education coupled with administrative fiat (as in reducing availability of certain tests or drugs).

Given the enormous number of testimonial reports and anecdotal comments from hospitals and practitioners that behavior does change in response to continuing edu-cation, the complacency of the medical profession in not demanding more rigorous "proof" is not difficult to understand. There is certainly even less evidence that continuing medical education *negatively* affects behavior. Perhaps that is proof enough.

Continuing Medical Education and Patient Outcome

The fog of imperfect evidence that surrounds the effect of continuing medical education on physician knowledge and behavior becomes no less dense when considering patient outcome. Good outcome measures are difficult to come by in any event, and attempting to causally relate them to antecedent CME appears virtually impossible.

Lewis and Hassanin attempted to relate short courses in obstetrics and pediatrics to measurable outcomes, such as perinatal mortality and maternal complications, without showing a positive effect. The report has been widely criticized, however, because the endpoints chosen were sensitive to many other uncontrolled factors.[19] Improved patient knowledge and compliance, and better control of blood pressure were demonstrated among patients in a general medical clinic cared for by resident physicians receiving a single teaching session on hypertension. The study included a comparison group of physicians not exposed to the teaching session, but ability to generalize is weakened by follow-up of less than one year.[20]

Unfortunately, the most valid evidence for the most part ends here. The few other reports of the effect of continuing medical education on patient outcome are very small anecdotal studies with negligible external validity. Not surprisingly, all such studies have shown dramatic effects of continuing medical education on measured outcomes. Perhaps the consistency of the findings is in itself useful.

Discussion and Conclusions

The evaluation, at any level, of continuing medical education has been meager. Of the nearly 200 listings on CME in the 1977 *Index Medicus*, over three quarters are editorial comments, and nearly all the rest are reports of "how we do it at our place"—documentation of a given CME program. Only a handful, fewer than ten, are attempts at evaluation, and few of those are worth examining beyond the abstract.

The evidence that continuing medical education assures quality care is weak, but the association between continuing medical education and quality assessment is certainly stronger. Suggestions that continuing education be linked to perceived deficiencies in physician knowledge (examination or self-assessment), physician behavior (process measures, medical audits), or patient outcome (audits of outcome) have been exhaustively pursued in the literature, mostly in editorial comment.[21] Particularly popular has been the notion that data collected as part of mandated peer review (through the professional standards review organizations—PSRO) be integrally linked to the design of continuing education programs.[22-24] This conceptual framework certainly has intuitive appeal, and neatly fits the current input-output-feedback mentality. In this respect, there is little doubt that deficiencies in medical care identified by process or outcome evaluations can be corrected in many cases, but the precise role of CME in the process remains to be defined.

If a new evaluation were to be initiated, demonstration of efficacy and effectiveness of continuing medical education with respect to patient care and physician knowledge, behavior, and satisfaction should be the first steps. These may yet be examined, more rigorously than has been done, but the examination is increasingly difficult with the overlay of other issues, such as licensure, certification, politics, CME as big business, professional standards review organizations, and the consumer movement. On the other hand, surely the high costs implied by these other issues argue even more urgently for thoughtful analyses of benefits and overall effectiveness.

The precise role of family physicians in this controversial area is not clear. Certainly as "consumers" of continuing medical education, the profession has a great deal at stake in arguing for high quality programs of demonstrated effectiveness. Further, as the first specialty to require both CME and an examination for recertification, family practice is in a unique position to evaluate the effects of CME over time. Many family physicians are in positions of leadership in local, state, and national medical organizations where issues related to CME requirements frequently surface. Overall, I would argue for a more critical approach, with emphasis placed upon problem-directed continuing medical education meeting known needs of the participants, followed by rigorous evaluations of effectiveness. A healthy skepticism should remain: continuing medical education will not in itself solve all the problems of assuring quality medical care. The problem is far too complex for that.

Author's Update

Interest in CME remains high, but may be waning in some areas—at least one specialty board has dropped CME requirements: several states with CME requirements for licensure have chosen not to enforce them; and the number of state medical societies requiring CME for membership has declined. Dollars expended for CME have increased, however, even after adjustment for inflation.

The quality of research in CME has, unfortunately, not changed. Published evaluations are few, and virtually none comment on resulting improvements in medical care. Thus the questions raised in my article of 1979 remain unanswered.

REFERENCES

1. Billings JS: Educating the physician. Boston Med Surg J 131:140, 1894
2. Osler Sir W: The importance of post-graduate study. Lancet 2:73, 1900
3. Marx K, quoted by Garrison FH: The evil spoken of physicians. Bull NY Acad Med 5:145, 1929
4. Continuing medical education. In Medical Education in the United States, 1970–1971. JAMA 218:1258, 1971
5. Storey PB: Mandatory continuing medical education: One step forward—two steps back. N Engl J Med 298:1416, 1978
6. Scott AJ: Continuing education: More or better? N Engl J Med 295:444, 1976
7. Neu HC, Howrey SP: Testing the physician's knowledge of antibiotic use. N Engl J Med 293:1291, 1975
8. Chang A, Oglesby AC, Wallace HM, et al: Child abuse and neglect: Physician knowledge, attitudes, and experience. Am J Public Health 66:1199, 1976
9. Hunter AT, Portis B: Medical education television survey. J Med Educ 47:57, 1972
10. Hogben MD, Schorow M, Caine T: Shorter training in cardiology for practicing physicians. J Med Educ 47:806, 1972
11. Donnelly FA, Ware JE, Wolkon GH, et al: Evaluation of weekend seminars for physicians. J Med Educ 47:184, 1972
12. Turiel SM, Kummer TG (eds): Goals and Techniques in Continuing Education. Arlington, Association of Hospital Medical Education, 1970
13. Mock RL, McLoard BF, Prestwood R: Northern California postgraduate medical television: An evaluation. J Med Educ 45:40, 1970
14. Caplan RM: Measuring the effectiveness of continuing medical education. J Med Educ 48:1150, 1973
15. Reed DE, Lapenas C, Rogers KD: Continuing education based on records audits in a community hospital. J Med Educ 48:1152, 1973
16. Rubenstein E: Continuing medical education at Stanford. J Med Educ 48:911, 1973
17. Mintz PD, Lanenstein K, Hume J, et al: Expected hemotherapy in elective surgery. JAMA 239:623, 1978
18. Payne BC, Lyons TF, Dwarchius L, et al: The quality of medical care: Evaluation and improvement. Chicago, Hospital Research and Educational Trust, 1976
19. Lewis C, Hassanin R: Continuing medical education: An epidemiologic evaluation. N Engl J Med 287:254, 1970
20. Inui TS, Yourtree EC, Williamson JM: Improved outcomes in hypertension following physician tutorials. Ann Intern Med 84:646, 1976
21. Hutchison D: The process of planning continuing education programming; AND Fleisher D: Priorities and data bases: Their relationship to continuing education. In Health Resources Administration, Bureau of Health Resource Development (Rockville, Md): Fostering the Growing Need to Learn. DHEW publication No. (HRA) 74-3112. Government Printing Office, 1973
22. Nelson AR: Orphan data and the unclosed loop: A dilemma in PSRO and the medical audit. N Engl J Med 295:617, 1976
23. Inui TS: Continuing medical education and the professional standards review organizations. Johns Hopkins Med J 139:37, 1976
24. Geyman JP: Toward performance-based continuing medical education. J Fam Pract 5:333, 1977

ABSTRACTS

Brandt EN: Preferences of family physicians for subject matter in continuing education programs. J Med Educ 50:395–398, 1975

Continuing education for the family physician presents a particularly difficult challenge since few curriculum guidelines have been established. In recent years, there has been much discussion of a core curriculum for family physicians, although the responsibility they bear for continuing comprehensive care of families suggests that each physician will have individual needs for knowledge and skills that depend on his practice. Therefore, continuing education programs for family physicians must have breadth of subject matter if they are to be of value.

Since 1966, the Scientific Program Committee of the Texas Academy of Family Physicians has conducted periodic surveys of the attendees of its annual meeting and has used other methods to select topics for the annual meeting. This paper reports

Table 1. *Questionnaire Results on Meeting Topics Selected by Physicians Attending Three Annual Meetings of the Texas Academy of Family Physicians (TAFP)**

	Year					
	1966		*1967*		*1970*	
Topic	*No.*	*Percent†*	*No.*	*Percent†*	*No.*	*Percent†*
Dermatology	67	16.9	102	23.8	83	23.3
Gynecology	115	29.0	128	29.8	94	26.4
Internal medicine	197	49.6	252	58.7	203	57.0
Neurology	22	5.5	40	10.2	43	12.1
Obstetrics	72	18.1	81	18.9	66	18.5
Ophthalmology	16	4.0	56	13.0	33	9.3
Otolaryngology	40	10.1	53	13.5	65	18.3
Pathology	4	1.0	28	7.1	17	4.8
Pediatrics	57	14.4	98	25.0	84	23.6
Psychiatry	51	12.9	98	25.0	64	18.0
Surgery, general	107	27.0	120	28.0	90	25.3
Surgery, subspecialties‡	147	37.0	255	59.4	172	48.3
Athletic medicine	—	—	50	12.8	50	14.1
Industrial medicine	16	4.0	22	5.6	29	8.1
Other§	55	13.9	72	18.4	53	14.9
Total votes cast	966		1,455		1,146	
Total number voting	397		430		356	

*The response rate each year exceeded 80 percent of those attending. Multiple responses were accepted.
†This figure is the percentage of persons selecting this topic.
‡Includes orthopedics, urology, pediatric surgery, and others.
§Includes medical-law and medical-economics.
Reprinted by permission from Brandt: J Med Educ, 50:395–398, 1975.

the results of these findings, which represent the perceived needs of one group of family physicians who are concerned about continuing education.

In the preference surveys conducted at the 1966, 1967, and 1970 meetings, the respondents were asked to check those disciplines that should be included in future annual meetings, and on the average approximately three topics were selected by each respondent (Table 1). The response patterns for the three years are consistent. Internal medicine, general surgery, surgical subspecialties (such as orthopedics and urology), and gynecology were the areas of greater preference, although pediatrics, psychiatry, and obstetrics were also frequently selected.

The goal of continuing education for physicians is to effect and maintain high-quality patient care. Thus, the ultimate evaluation of its effectiveness must rest on measurement of the quality of patient care delivered by those who participate in continuing education programs. No such evaluation was attempted here. One approach to defining continuing education requirements, however, is to assess the physician's preceptions of his own needs, based upon the principle of adult learning that a person must become aware of his own deficiencies before he will undertake to correct them through further learning.

Metcalfe DHH, Chir B, Mancini JC: Critical event outcome studies used as a teaching tool. J Med Educ 47:869–872, 1972

One of the stated goals of the Family Medicine Program at the University of Rochester School of Medicine and Dentistry is to teach residents a "system of practice." This means that they are taught to keep patient records and cross-index them in such a way that their practice generates data as a basis for self- and peer-review, continuing education, operational planning, and outreach. Accordingly, the teaching methods used in the program utilize these techniques as a demonstration of their potential. Residents are taught to learn by analyzing "cohorts" of patients—those having certain characteristics in common such as age or socioeconomic status or disease entity—to determine the quality of care given to that cohort; and where any patient has received care falling short of the optimal, the physician responsible is notified. Thus, the learning process is shown to depend on a research technique and is immediately reinforced by clinical utilization.

The 15 residents of the Family Medicine Program are divided into four teams, each led by a member of the faculty. Each month

one team has the responsibility for presenting a topic at family medicine rounds. Some members of the team carry out a literature review and evolve from their reading a "profile" of the well-managed patient with the disease in question. Other members of the team then carry out a chart review, utilizing one of the cross-indexing systems in use in the Family Medicine Group Practice and measuring care against the "profile." The presentation consists of a verbal summary of the literature review, reinforced by a "handout" bibliography, the results of the chart audit with appropriate graphics, and discussion of the problem in depth; afterward, each physician whose care was found to fall short of the ideal is notified of the particular patients involved. Where possible, the analyses are in the form of "critical event outcome studies." In these, the physician's response to a clearly defined and well-documented clinical situation can be assessed. Since the starting point is easy to establish and the possible responses are limited, an algorithm for the outcome can be drawn. This provides the framework for the chart review, and the physician's performance is assessed by counting how many patients followed the correct pathways in the algorithm and how many followed the incorrect pathways. Obviously, not all clinical situations are amenable to this form of study. The example to be used in this paper is the study of the management of patients with infected urine.

The team then turned its attention to the patients in the Family Medicine Group Practice who had had urinary findings consistent with, or significant of, infection. Sixty-two names were found in the laboratory log as having "positive findings" in October 1970 (during which time there had been 1435 patient visits). The results of the chart review are shown in Fig. 1. It should be noted that of the 17 abnormal urines "missed" at the first level (recognition and action), several were of doubtful significance. Nevertheless, the correct response by the physician should have been to arrange for further urinalysis. At the second level (action and follow-up plan), of the eight who were not followed up after treatment, one had been admitted to a subspecialist renal unit for a congenital ab-

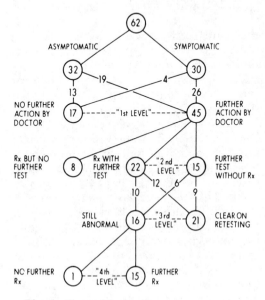

Fig. 1. First critical event outcome study.

Reprinted by permission from Metcalfe et al: J Med Educ, 47:869–872, 1972.

normalities work-up; follow-up had been arranged for four who did not return for further urinalysis and who were not contacted further; no follow-up had been arranged for three. Thus, not only were the physician's control of patient management shown to be lacking, but also the administrative arrangements for communicating with these patients who did not keep appointments were not operating properly. As an immediate result of this teaching session, the procedure for collecting "clean-catch" specimens was improved, and so was the procedure for contacting patients who did not keep follow-up appointments.

Two months later, a further chart audit was carried out on the 26 patients whose management had been inadequate. Of the 17 at the first level, 7 had been retested and found to have clear urine and 10 had been retested and found to have infected urine and had been treated; of the latter, one was still under treatment and the rest had been found to have clear urine after treatment. Of the eight at the second level, all had been retested after treatment (except the patient admitted for work-up) and found to have clear urine. The one patient at the fourth level had been retested and found to have clear urine. Thus, 10 patients with urinary tract infections who would not have gotten any treatment if the chart review had not been carried out had been successfully treated, and the rest of the 26 patients were found to need no further treatment.

Six months after the original presentation, a further 62 consecutive abnormal urines were culled from the laboratory log, and the chart review was repeated. At each point of recognition and mangement, improvement was noted between the first and second critical event outcome study:

	First	Second
Recognition in symptomatic cases	26 of 30 (87%)	34 of 35 (97%)
Recognition in asymptomatic cases	19 of 32 (59%)	20 of 27 (74%)
Treatment with adequate follow-up	37 of 45 (82%)	45 of 54 (83%)

In the chart review described in this paper, the comparable figures of recognition of infected urine from patients without symptoms suggestive of urinary tract infection were 19 out of 32 (59.3 percent) before the teaching session and 20 out of 27 (74.1 percent) six months later. It is disappointing that even in a teaching unit like the Rochester Family Medicine Program, where teaching, service, and research are closely integrated, the improvement was not greater. It shows that teaching must be backed up by continuous chart review, nonverbal reinforcement (such as modification of report forms to have more impact), and repetition of learning experiences.

Rakel RE: Indexing in office practice: a system for monitoring high-risk patients and filing medical literature. Cont Educ Fam Phys 9(1):30–35, 1978

Medical records are playing an increasing role in the practice of medicine, especially family practice. Concomitant with modernization of the office medical record have come assessment techniques used to analyze these records for recertification and relicensure purposes. Recertification requires that selected patient records be re-

Table 1. *Advantages of Problem Indexing*

1. Identify patients with similar problems or medications.
2. Simplify recall when updating of treatment is necessary.
3. Identify patients for whom medications must be changed to avoid newly recognized hazards.
4. Simplify recall for periodic evaluation of chronic problems.
5. Assist with self audit by:
   a. assessment of diagnostic accuracy
   b. identification of areas to be stressed in continuing education
   c. identification of conditions rarely encountered (or missed)
6. Analysis of practice content for design of teaching objectives.
7. Simplify collection of data for clinical research.
8. Identify new syndromes or unique associations between problems.
9. Retrieve cases for recertification.

Reprinted by permission from Rakel: Cont Educ Fam Phys, 9(1):30–35, 1978.

trieved and analyzed. This can be a time-consuming and difficult process because the physician must recall names of patients who received treatment for problems in the required categories.

This article describes an indexing system for the easy retrieval of the medical records of patients with selected problems and a method for filing and retrieving interesting articles gleaned from the family physician's ongoing review of the medical literature. Both of these systems use the PriCare classification as the common basis for indexing. Two new card files are suggested—a problem index that lists patients who have problems that the physician wishes to index in order to be able to analyze the practice or to keep track of high-risk conditions and an article file that utilizes the same classification scheme to code the file articles from the medical literature.

Problem indexing systems can be unduly complex. The best filing and indexing system is one that is simple, flexible, and practical (Table 1).

The problem index is a separate, 4- by 6-inch or 5- by 7-inch card file that lists the names of patients who have any specific problem indexed. For example, a physician may list only those patients who have diabetes mellitus and are on oral hypoglycemic agents, those who have had a coronary

Table 2. *Categories Utilized for Office Record Review By the American Board of Family Practice*

Abnormal vaginal bleeding	X:6260/6262/6263/6264/6269
Acute cystitis	X:595–
Acute duodenal ulcer	IX:532–
Appendicitis	IX:540–
Chronic bronchial asthma	VIII:493–
Chronic obstructive pulmonary disease	VIII:492–
Colitis	IX:564–
Congestive heart failure	VII:4270
Coronary artery disease	VII:415–
Depression	V:296–/3004
Diabetes mellitus	III:250–
Hypertension	VII:400–/401–/4012
Lumbar disc disease	XIII:725–
Normal pregnancy through delivery	XI:650–/XVIII:Y60–/Y61–
Obesity	III:277–
Otitis media	VI:3810/3811
Pediatric patient	XVIII:Y00–/Y62–
Postoperative carcinoma of the breast	II:174–/XVII:Y17–
Rheumatoid arthritis	XIII:712–
Vaginitis	X:6221

Reprinted by permission from Rakel: Cont Educ Fam Phys, 9(1):30–35, 1978.

bypass procedure, and those with carcinoma of the breast or other common problems requiring unique attention. Most physicians will, as a minimum, wish to list patients who have problems that fall within the 20 categories identified by the American Board of Family Practice since patient records in these areas will need to be retrieved and audited during the recertification process (Table 2). The problem index card can also include whatever procedures the physician is most interested in following. In addition to patient name, age, and telephone number (and perhaps chart number), it can include medication, other diagnoses, or complications. This system promotes an investigative approach to problems and enables the physician to analyze the effectiveness of his diagnostic and therapeutic skills.

The article filing system need be no more complicated than a series of manila folders placed in a traditional filing cabinet or expanding cardboard file. Each of the 18 PriCare categories serves as a major divider, with secondary dividers identified by the 100-plus specific subcategories previously described. Once a category has over ten or so articles, subcategories should be established to maintain efficiency of retrieval and avoid cluttering. Most articles will have more than one subject, concept, or topic as a significant feature. Since an original article can be filed under only one of these various categories, a cross-index is therefore necessary to permit its retrieval when the review of one of the other subject areas is desired. The cross-index can be based either on the PriCare classification, or it can consist of a key word file. In this system, key words are chosen that most appropriately represent the alternate subjects covered in each article.

Sivertson SE, Meyer TC, Hansen R, Schoenenberger A:
Individual physician profile: Continuing education related
to medical practice.
J Med Educ 48:1006-1012, 1973

A major problem for a physician is to relate his continuing medical education accurately to the knowledge and skills necessary to meet the needs of his patients and community. The faculty of the University of Wisconsin Department of Postgraduate Medical Education identified the following factors as being significant in dealing with this dilemma: problems patients bring to their physician, organization of the practice, community setting, and the physician's personal likes and dislikes relating to his practice and his apparent interest in continuing medical education. All are determinants of the type of practice he builds and the quality of care he delivers. It was out of the need to describe these variables for any physician that the Individual Physician Profile (IPP) was created.

The Individual Physician Profile is a three step process: *practice profile, examination,* and *educational consultation and design of a continuing medical education program.* The practice profile is obtained by issuing the physician a small tape recorder on which he records, one different day each week for four weeks, the age and sex of every patient encountered in the office, in a hospital, on the telephone, and at home, presenting symptoms, significant findings, major diagnosis (patient problem), contributing diagnoses (other patient problems), tests ordered, and disposition. The tape is then transcribed and the diagnoses codified in the categories of the International Classification of Diseases, Adapted (ICDA). The numbers of diagnoses in the categories form a practice profile, that is, a histogram such as that shown in Fig. 1, which is a "typical" profile of a family practitioner in Wisconsin. That practice profiles vary is shown in Fig. 2, which reflects on atypical family practice.

The physician is tested with 125 ques-

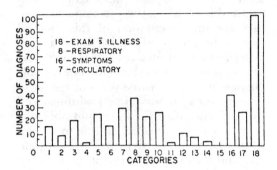

Fig. 1. Profile of a typical family practitioner.

Reprinted by permission from Sivertson et al: J Med Educ, 48:1006-1012, 1973.

tions obtained from a large pool of questions stored in the computer; these questions have been cross-indexed in the ICDA. For example, if he sees a large number of diabetic problems, he will receive a greater number of questions on diabetes; the complexity of the questions also increases with the number of questions. The test takes approximately two hours to complete.

In order to design an appropriate educa-

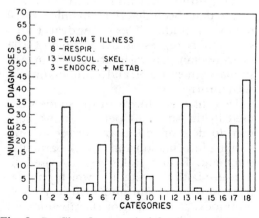

Fig. 2. Profile of an atypical family practitioner.

Reprinted by permission from Sivertson et al: J Med Educ, 48:1006-1012, 1973.

tional program, an educational consultant who is a member of the medical school faculty meets with the physician, and together they study the practice profile and the test results and other information elicited by asking the participant questions of a general and personal nature. Resources necessary for implementation of this method were a computerized test bank and a computerized educational resource index. The testing procedure underwent considerable change during the three years of research. The examination was initially administered in the physician's office over a portable teletype that was connected on-line to a computer in Madison. This proved to be expensive and technically incompatible with the many telephone companies in Wisconsin. The test is now printed out and mailed to the physician, who returns the answer sheet for scoring.

A subjective analysis of educational recommendations for 58 physicians who had completed the procedure by July 1, 1971,

was made. The assumption was that an educational diagnosis based on the three steps of IPP, that is, practice profile, testing, and the subjective information obtained during consultation, was effective. When all three steps contributed to the end result, the project staff assumed IPP to be highly effective in relating recommendations to a practice. When two factors pointed to an educational need, IPP was considered to be effective. (This occurred, for example, when the practice profile indicated a high volume of patients in a specific area of medicine and the consultation indicated a need for study but the test results were inconclusive.) Where only one step supported an educational diagnosis, IPP was considered to be ineffective. It was concluded that 35 (62 percent) of the 58 physicians involved received a highly effectual educational diagnosis, 18 (31 percent) received effective program planning, and the results for 5 (7 percent) were ineffective.

Gambrill J, Bridges-Webb C: Use of sources of therapeutic and prescribing information by general practitioners. Aus Fam Physician 9:482–484, 1980

The use of sources of therapeutic and prescribing information available to physicians has, to date, been described in only a small number of studies. This paper deals with a survey of a representative sample of 104 metropolitan general practitioners in Australia on their use of, and attitudes toward, such information.

Two different forms of questions were used in the survey. Open questions were used to determine the overall use of prescribing information and to seek particular comment. Rating scales were devised to measure both the extent to which publications were read and also their perceived usefulness as a source of therapeutic and prescribing information.

Table 1 summarizes the responses for the five most frequently mentioned sources.

Table 1. *Sources of Information About Therapeutics and Prescribing*

Source	Percentage of Respondents		
	Most Recent Source	*Regular Sources*	*Most Useful Source*
Journals	46	91	50
Drug company representatives	22	56	17
Consultants and colleagues	9	33	13
Drug company literature	10	20	0
Clinical meetings	8	25	9

Reprinted with permission from Gambrill, Bridges-Webb: Aus Fam Physician, 9:482–484, 1980.

Journals rank highest for all three criteria of measurement, and the descending order for the other four sources is also consistent, with one major exception. Drug company literature, while ranking high in regard to being the most recent and a regular information source, was not ranked as the most useful by any of the practitioners.

The results suggest that general practitioners read journals quite widely. How-ever, there is always a temptation for groups under survey to overstage usage, particularly in a face-to-face interview situation. The study has shown less variation in usage of different journals than would have been expected. Only 19 practitioners offered suggestions for new forms of information. There were a few suggestions for a standard summary form of publication related to therapeutics and prescribing.

Law R: The ages of man.
J R Coll Gen Pract 30:21–27, 1980

This paper describes a new approach to continuing education for the experienced general practitioner. It makes use of small group work, provides a longitudinal framework for planning over several years, and by its flexibility permits the participants to shape the content to their needs.

This series was divided as follows:

1. The infant—0–4 years
2. Toward maturity—5–18 years
3. The years of struggle—19–35 years
4. Middle age—36–59 years
5. The elderly—60 onward

Objectives were established for each phase. For example, the following content areas were outlined for the first phase (The infant—0–4 years):

Objective 1. Normal Development and Behavior

1. Fetal development and factors affecting this
2. Measurement and the place of regular assessment
3. Factors affecting development and behavior
4. Place of intervention in early departures from normal
5. The National Child Development Study

Objective 2. Health and Disease

1. Margins of normality—bruits, hernias, orthopedics
2. Congenital disease
3. Neonatal problems
4. Emotional disorders
5. Diagnosis—rashes, the feverish child, convulsions
6. Long-term illness and its management at home—asthma/eczema, urinary abnormalities, mental subnormality
7. Therapeutics

Objective 3. Ways parents Relate to the Child

1. The new family—its tasks, problems, and fears
2. Social problems—broken home, battered baby, immigrants and their problems

Objective 4. Practice Organization

1. Age/sex registers
2. Baby clinics
3. Research projects
4. The team and referral agencies
5. Parental education and counseling

The Ages of Man Series has Four Main Ingredients:

1. It is centered on a longitudinal time view of the patient rather than on diseases, in accordance with the job definition of the general practitioner as "a doctor who provides personal, primary, and continuing care to individuals and families...."
2. An emphasis is placed on the individual in society and on the need for health education and preventive medicine.
3. The series takes place over several years, and by feedback it is possible for a core of attenders to shape it to their needs rather than to the preconceptions of a course organizer.
4. It is based on small-group work, especially with the subsequent presentation of questions to specialists. This was one of the most successful innovations of the series. Small-group work enabled the physician to compare himself with his peers.

Gordon MS, Ewy GA, Felner JM, Forker AD, Gessner IH, Juul D, Mayer JW, Sajid A, Waugh RA: A cardiology patient simulator for continuing education of family physicians. J Fam Pract 13(3):353–356, 1981.

"Harvey," the cardiology patient simulator (CPS), is the result of a new type of simulation technology that allows for repetitive practice of bedside skills and provides feedback to the learner. The CPS realistically represents an essentially unlimited number of both common and rare cardiac diseases. It is currently programmed to faithfully simulate the blood pressure, bilateral jugular venous and arterial pulsations, and various precordial movements and ausculatory events of a core curriculum of 20 commonly encountered cardiovascular conditions (Table 1).

This report describes the use of the CPS in continuing medical education programs conducted for members of the American Academy of Family Physicians.

A postgraduate medical education symposium entitled "Practical Diagnosis of the Cardiac Patient" was conducted at both the 1979 and 1980 annual scientific sessions of the American Academy of Family Physicians. The major emphasis of the program was on the bedside diagnostic skills used in evaluating patients with suspected cardiovascular disease. Eight sessions of approximately four hours' duration were held with an average attendance of over 200 physicians. Over the two meetings, a total of

Table 1. *Core Curriculum of CPS Diseases*

Normal
Innocent murmur
Hypertension
Angina pectoris
Mitral valve prolapse
Mitral stenosis
Mitral regurgitation, chronic
Aortic stenosis
Aortic regurgitation
Cardiomyopathy
Idiopathic hypertrophic subaortic stenosis
Atrial septal defect
Ventricular septal defect
Patent ductus arteriosus
Primary pulmonary hypertension
Mitral regurgitation, acute
Ventricular aneurysm
Mitral stenosis and regurgitation
Pulmonary stenosis
Coarctation of the aorta

more than 1500 physicians participated. Although the audiences were large, the use of individual stethophones for cardiac auscultation and closed-circuit television monitors for visualization of the CPS's pulses allowed each physician to participate in the evaluation of most of the nonauscultatory as well as all the auscultatory physical findings. A panel of clinical cardiologists experienced in teaching with the CPS discussed the significance of each physical finding as well as the pathophysiology, natural history, and management of each disease. In each four-hour session, many of the cardiovascular problems encountered by the family physician were reviewed, including the innocent murmur, coronary artery disease, hypertension, mitral valve prolapse, chronic rheumatic mitral regurgitation, mitral stenosis, aortic stenosis, and aortic regurgitation.

Well over 90 percent of the participants felt that the technical quality of the CPS was excellent and that it was very useful as a teaching tool. In addition, 88 percent of the physicians in 1979 and 97 percent in 1980 would like to be taught with the device in the future. Many also expressed the desire to work with the CPS in an individual, "hands-on" mode of learning. The very positive acceptance of the CPS was also confirmed independently by a survey carried out by the American Academy of Family Physicians. They found that among all those presented at the scientific sessions, the CPS training programs were ranked highest by their membership. Based on these findings, the CPS has a great potential for providing an innovative, well-received, interactive type of postgraduate medical education.

Lamont CT, Hennen BKE: The use of simulated patients in a certification examination in family medicine. J Med Educ 47:789-795, 1972

The performance of physicians as they relate directly with patients is perhaps the most important aspect of their professional behavior. Family physicians especially depend on their skills in interviewing to elicit information and establish rapport. The quality of the relationship between the physician and patient affects continuity of care, a major diagnostic and therapeutic tool of the family physician. Also, most of his time is spent in office management of the ambulatory patient. Evaluating office patient-side physician skills is therefore a necessary part of assessing the competency of family physicians. This paper describes how the "simulated office" portion of the 1970 Certification Examination of the College of Family Physicians of Canada (C.F.P.C.) assessed the performance of candidates.

The total examination included a written component followed by an oral component.

The written examination consisted of a 180 multiple-choice question paper, a series of three film strips with accompanying questions that tested the candidate's powers of observation and interpretation, and three patient-management problems of the erasure type to test ability at problem solving. The oral portion consisted of a one-hour formal oral, a half-hour role-playing patient-management problem in which the examining physician played the role of the patient, and a simulated office oral.

Every candidate was allowed up to 12 minutes to interview three simulated patients. Each had been "programmed" to portray an individual with a problem that is commonly encountered in family practice. For example, the protocol for one of the simulated patients contained such information and instructions as: "You are a 41-year-old, happily married housewife and mother of four healthy children. You are apprehensive, having been called in to discuss the results of a Pap test taken one week ago. The candidate will tell you that your test is positive. If he is sympathetic, clear in his explanation, and reassuring, indicate less acute anxiety. If he is insensitive, break down completely. If the candidate does not tell you, ask: "Is this cancer, doctor?" All three patients had problems that required the candidate to exhibit desirable attitudinal skills, to elicit pertinent information quickly, to show skill in problem solving, and to allay the patient's anxiety. One patient, in addition to the interview, required a partial physical examination.

A simulated office oral has several advantages. It introduces realistic variables into the medical problem-solving model that are identical to those that operate in a family physician's office. The simulated patient can be interviewed and examined repeatedly. Clinical problems can be preplanned, and examiners can control content to provide attitudinal changes and to elicit the clinical and behavioral science knowledge and skills they wish to evaluate. The simulated patient can report his impressions of the candidate's performance.

There are also disadvantages to the simulated office oral. The use of human models establishes considerable individual differences of the interpersonal reactions between the physician and the patient. Two actors playing the same role cannot be programmed to give precisely the same performance. Two physicians cannot be expected to behave the same way with the same patient.

Assessment of the simulated office oral revealed the following:

1. That it was a valid simulation of the context in which family physicians interact with patients.
2. That the simulated patients accurately represent the kinds of patients that present to family physicians in their office.
3. That simulation performance scores correlated positively with the formal oral and role-playing oral portions of the 1970 Certification Examination of the C.F.P.C. and with the assessments made by the simulated patients of the candidates' performance.
4. That simulation performance scores did not correlate well with parts of the examination intended to measure recall or problem-solving ability or with the part intended to measure observational skills. This may also relate to the assessment methods; only in this case they would appear to differ.
5. That it is an effective method of assessing physicians' ability to utilize their personal skills in interacting with patients.

Van Wart AD: A problem-solving oral examination for family medicine. J Med Educ 49:673–680, 1974

Problem solving is a daily task for a family physician. The variety and scope of the primary care field require the development of skills in data collection, problem recognition, and organized thinking as well as the ability to make a decision and relate to patients.

The College of Family Physicians of Canada has used in its certification examination a new type of structured problem-solving examination called the Formal Oral. Over a thousand candidates have been tested with this tool in the past 5 years. The problem-solving oral simulates what happens in daily practice. The candidate is told that during the oral he is in charge and that the examiner is his information source. The candidate then, during the interview, must find his own way through the patients' problems based on the data he collects and the decisions he makes.

Unlike the traditional medical oral examination, this oral has a tight structure from which the examiner is not allowed to deviate. The clinical content and the protocols on how to conduct the examination are determined in advance. The examiner does not on his own quiz the candidate; instead, he must provide information to the candidate on the preselected case. He then scores the candidate on what the candidate says and does. The pathway through the case is determined by the positive findings. For example, in a case of carcinoma of the cecum in a patient presenting with fatigue, the route through the case would be from fatigue to anemia, to positive occult blood, to a positive barium enema; then there would be preparation for surgery, and follow-up management.

A good candidate, after collecting pertinent data, will make acceptable patient-management decisions. If the examiner needs to assist the candidate, the latter loses marks. A series of preselected problem areas such as the complaint, relevant data base, investigation, and treatment are scored by two independent examiners under the headings Suspicion, System and Diligence, and Judgment. The candidate's ability to relate to patients and his overall coordination of clinical skills are also scored.

An oral examination of this type has certain advantages over a written or a computer-terminal test.

1. It more closely simulates the true practice situation.
2. This oral does not offer a choice of a certain number of fixed alternatives. It need not even identify the problem. It can, therefore, test suspicion, problem sensing, and identification of important issues.
3. In this oral examination, the candidate must gather data, a process that can be easily observed and scored. Scores are tabulated under the headings of system and diligence.
4. An oral examination that simulates the data base and personal contact pressure of real practice offers an opportunity to test judgment in a clinical setting.
5. Because an oral examination is a dialogue between two people and because the candidate must describe his method of interrogation and management of the patient, observations can be made on the candidate's affective skills and his ability to relate to others.
6. The final advantage of the oral examination technique is that it allows the examiner to judge the candidate's coordination of clinical skills.

A vehicle for observing and measuring problem solving in a simulated practice setting has been perfected to a degree that the members of the examination committee are pleased with its validity and reliability. However, it is an expensive tool. Many hours of preparation are required to produce the written script and protocols. Good examination facilities with one-way mirrors are used to improve the quality of the oral. Videotapes are made and scored in advance. To examine 300 candidates, 36 examiners, 3 validators, and 3 coordinators, all of whom are practicing family physicians, must give up over 3 full days of their time. The real total cost of oral examinations is so high that skills are now being developed in the use of other methods of peer-group evaluation, such as ongoing evaluations of clinical training programs, auditing of clinical records, and a measurement known as a tracer study, which demonstrates how specific health problems are actually dealt with in an active clinical practice.

Dickie GL, Bass MJ, Spitzer WO, Roberts R:
Multiple choice questions for continuing
education in family medicine.
J Fam Pract 13(7):1031–1035, 1981

Many types of continuing medical education have been instituted to help the family physician, and these have enjoyed a greater or lesser success as measured by the subjective impressions of participants. One such mode that enjoys considerable popularity is the self-assessment exercise using multiple choice questions. These have been developed and distributed by academies and colleges of family medicine. This study examines the content of one such program to determine the characteristics of those questions that seem to be most relevant to family physicians.

The questions examined in this study were prepared by the Connecticut and Ohio Academies of Family Physicians and constitute part of their Core Content Review Programme for 1974–1975. A panel of 48 certificated family physicians, 24 from academic practice and 24 from private practice in the same communities, assessed the Core Content Review. Three of the six exercises offered in 1974 and 1975 were examined. One exercise was randomly allocated to one-third of each group so that each of 308 questions was assessed by eight academic and eight community family physicians. In addition to answering the questions, the physicians answered probes concerning the subject matter of each question. These dealt with the frequency of occurrence of the problem, its ability to discriminate between family physicians providing high- and low-quality care, the usefulness of the question as a learning experience, and its usefulness in the management of patients. A question was considered relevant if 12 or more of the 16 physicians answering it indicated that it discriminates between the family physician providing good-quality care and the physician providing less than adequate care, *or* the question deals with a problem reported to be seen at

least once a year, and it is useful either for physician education or in patient management.

Of the 72 percent of questions that were considered educationally useful, those relating to adult medicine were significantly more useful, while those relating to psychosocial aspects were significantly less educationally useful. Of the 44 percent of questions considered to be discriminators of high- or low-quality clinical practice, ques-

Table 1. *The Relevance of Question Content Areas*

Content	Number	Percent Relevant
Specialty Orientation		
Adult medicine	168	53
Pediatrics	59	53
Psychosocial (includes family dynamics)	33	52
Obstetrics	22	73
Surgery (includes gynecology)	27	78*
Strategies of Practice		
Prevention (includes health maintenance)	1	100
Office organization	11	9†
Clinical Activity		
Related to given diagnosis	67	39†
Complaint or symptom	36	72*
Clinical investigation	48	60
Basic science	54	46
Management/therapy	97	68†
Severity of Illness		
Conditions with minor degrees of severity	154	60*

*P < 0.05.
†P < 0.01.

tions on surgery and patient management were significantly more frequent. Only 23 percent of questions were considered useful in patient management, with no particular content area being specifically identified.

Fifty-four percent of the 308 questions achieved the agreed composite criterion of relevance. Table 1 shows the number of questions with given content areas and the percentage of relevant questions in each group. These data indicate that questions involving management and therapy have high relevancy rates, while questions on office management and specific diagnoses are of little relevance. In addition, items involving surgery or symptoms may have higher relevancy rates, but the strength of the evidence is somewhat weaker.

Nearly half of the questions required only simple recall of isolated information to answer them. Questions considered most relevant, however, require recognition of meaning, total situation evaluation, or problem solving of a familiar type (Table 2).

The apparently low overall relevance figure of 54 percent may seem surprising in a program such as this designed specifically for family physicians, but the criterion of relevance used was stringent and probably resulted in a conservative estimate. In formulating the criterion, the authors recognized that many questions might be educationally useful, but unless they dealt with problems reportedly seen at least once a year, they could not be regarded as relevant to the continuing medical education of family physicians.

Self-administered multiple choice questions constitute part of the Maintenance of

Table 2. *Intellectual Process and Relevance*

Process	Number	Percent Relevant
Recall of isolated information	143	51
Recognition of meaning or implication	44	59
Relevant generalization to explain phenomenon	17	29
Simple interpretation	10	60
Application of simple principles in a familiar situation	76	59
Application of combination of principles in new situation	7	14
Evaluation of total situation	11	82
	308	

Reprinted with permission by Dickie et al: J Fam Pract, 13(7):1031-1035, 1981.

Certification process recently introduced by the College of Family Physicians of Canada and play an important part in the continuing medical education of many family physicians. The characteristics of the best questions for this purpose must be defined so that the physicians involved will obtain the maximum benefit from participation. It would seem that questions that are thought to discriminate between high- and low-quality clinical care are most important for this purpose, but there is a need to demonstrate a correlation between answering such questions and providing good-quality care in practice. Confirmation of the external validity of our findings would be of great assistance to those who design multiple choice questions for continuing medical education.

Index